OXFORD MEDICAL PUBLICATIONS

Men's Health

Men's Health

Oxford General Practice Series • 41

Edited by

Tom O'Dowd

Professor of General Practice, University of Dublin,
Trinity College, Dublin, Ireland

and

David Jewell

Consultant Senior Lecturer in Primary Health Care,
University of Bristol, Bristol, UK

Oxford : New York : Tokyo

OXFORD UNIVERSITY PRESS

1998

Oxford University Press, Great Clarendon Street, Oxford OX2 6DP

Oxford New York

Athens Auckland Bangkok Bogota Bombay Buenos Aires
Calcutta Cape Town Dar es Salaam Delhi Florence Hong Kong
Istanbul Karachi Kuala Lumpur Madras Madrid Melbourne
Mexico City Nairobi Paris Singapore Taipei Tokyo Toronto Warsaw

and associated companies in
Berlin Ibadan

Oxford is a trade mark of Oxford University Press

Published in the United States
by Oxford University Press Inc., New York

© Tom O'Dowd, David Jewell & contributors listed on p. ix, 1998

A catalogue record for this book is available from the British Library

Library of Congress Cataloging in Publication Data
Men's health / edited by Tom O'Dowd and David Jewell.
(Oxford medical publications) (Oxford general practice series; 41)
Includes bibliographical references and index.
1. Men—Health and hygiene. 2. Men—Diseases. 3. Andrology.
I. O'Dowd, Tom. II. Jewell, David, Dr. III. Series.
IV. Series: Oxford general practice series; no. 41.
[DNLM: 1. Men. 2. Health. W1 OX55 no. 41 1988 / WA 300 M5478 1998]
RC 48.5.M46 1998   613'.04234–dc21   97-22778
ISBN 0 19 262581 0 (Pbk)

Typeset by Jayvee, Trivandrum, India
Printed in Great Britain by
Biddles Ltd., Guildford & King's Lynn

PREFACE

Men tighten the knot of confusion
Into perfect misunderstanding,
Reflecting a pocket-torch of observation
Upon each other's opacity
Neglecting all the admonitions
From the world around the corner
                    T. S. Eliot, *The family reunion*

The health profiles of men and women show clear differences. More males than females are conceived but fetal mortality is higher in males at all stages of fetal development (Shaw 1989). Infant mortality is about 20% higher for boys than for girls and higher death rates occur in males for each age group throughout life thereafter. While life expectancy has increased for both sexes this century, it is still lower in men than in women. There are international differences also with men in Japan living 6.1 years longer than men in Portugal.

However, mortality is only one index of health and morbidity is likely to be more informative for those of us in clinical practice. A range of conditions causes more morbidity in men than in women, a few are gender specific, and others occur more commonly in men than in women. Men are more prone to accidents, violence, and cancer than women (McCormick *et al.* 1995). The epidemic of cardiovascular disease targets men in the most productive time of their lives. Factors such as stress, smoking, poor diet, and alcohol misuse are commoner in men, but general practitioners' efforts to communicate this information and influence patients' behaviour have not been notably successful. Prostatic disease is gender specific and common with one man in four in the 40–79 age group having benign prostatic hypertrophy (Garraway *et al.* 1991). All too often such men present to the doctor with acute retention, and, in 1990, in Britain, 16% of transurethral resections and 35% of retropubic prostatectomies were performed as emergency operations (Donovan *et al.* 1992). Prostatic carcinoma is on the increase with occult cancer being found in up to 30% of men over 50 years of age. It is likely that pharmacological advances in this area of medicine will be reaching such men in the next decade, with the general practitioner playing an important role.

However, gender differences are not fixed and many of the chapters in this book

Preface

point to the shift in areas such as smoking and alcohol-related diseases, sexually transmitted diseases, and unemployment, which may lead to a convergence of morbidity patterns.

Despite the greater morbidity among men, doctors see them less often than women. The Fourth National Morbidity Study (1995) covered over half a million patients on the lists of 60 British general practices. Between the ages of 15 and 64 years the overall consulting rates for men were less than those for women. Men consult less often for a variety of conditions such as genito-urinary conditions, mental disorders, haematology, and ill-defined conditions. This is not a new finding. John Graunt, the founder of demography, observed in 1662 that physicians had two female patients for every one male. However, examination of the burial statistics led him to conclude that women were cured by their physicians and died of the infirmities of their sex while men died of their vices without recourse to a doctor (Glass 1963).

The tendency of men not to consult their doctors, despite their greater risk of ill health, is reflected in the organization and structure of health care services. Because women consult more frequently than men, both for themselves and for their children, general practitioners have responded by providing the necessary services. General practitioners of both sexes are equipped to provide sound family planning advice, good maternity care, screening for cervical cancer, and advice on breast self-examination and mammography. Practice nurses too spend much of their time dealing with women's health and problems. There are gender-specific services provided in the form of clinics in general practice (although some 'well man clinics' exist, they are much less common than well woman clinics), family planning clinics, which in reality provide more of a service to women than men, and, despite recent threats to their existence, some hospitals catering exclusively for women. There have been many books written about women's health but hardly anything about men's health.

Recently, there has been more interest in men. The 1992 annual report of the Chief Medical Officer of the Department of Health devoted an entire chapter to men's health. It includes an eloquent exposé of the state of men's health and concludes that 'the scope for men to improve their health and to prolong active, healthy life is considerable' (Calman 1993). Several magazines for men have been launched, including one entitled Men's health, although such magazines contain much information on sexual performance and advice on how to have even more sex.

With increased interest, and in the absence of firm evidence, commentators have been free to ascribe men's health problems to whatever cause most suited their ideas. As will be seen, the possible candidates include biological, lifestyle, and behavioural explanations. Men's reactions to illness, unemployment, and retirement are poorly understood and not often discussed, an example where men's unwillingness or inability to express their emotional selves is matched by a failure of researchers to explore them. Any theory that attempts to explain the evidence will need to look beyond purely biological concepts of gender to social ones of masculinity. Until very recently, masculinity was invisible, with maleness being seen as the norm and femaleness defined in contrast to it. However, if we wish to tackle the burden of male illness we shall need to understand why men take more risks than women, why they are more reluctant to see their doctor, and to what extent such behaviours are bound up with core ideas of masculinity. We can be sure, however, that there will be enormous diversity of masculine models. Traditional masculine models are under threat with changing patterns of work and domestic responsibility as well as rapidly changing female roles. The pressure to adapt causes movement in all directions: many men cling to traditional roles, some (although the evidence is that they are few in number) become 'new men', keen to share domestic and parenting responsibilities with women, others look for links with more primitive models as 'wild men'. The feeling of crisis has recently reached down to the schools with the evidence that schoolgirls are now achieving their full intellectual potential and outstripping schoolboys. Given that women are expected to be able to combine better interpersonal skills with better intellectual skills, there are fears for the future employability of men and worries about their feelings of self-worth.

Despite signs of recent changes in patterns of provision and use of health care, the paradox remains, and has been the central and abiding motivation in the planning and writing of this book. Men are less likely to see the doctor than women and are generally less likely to be thought to need medical services, yet by any objective criteria they experience worse health. In what way is their health worse, and is it possible to explain the paradox?

When we first planned this book it was not obvious whether there was enough material to justify discussing the issues at such length. Very quickly we became aware of a lack of experts in the area of men's health. In clinical areas, where men are the main users of services, it was with dismay that we discovered how little thinking doctors had done about treating their patients as men rather than as genderless, biological machines. This was in contrast to the amount of knowledge the doctors had about the diseases concerned. In an attempt to address the central paradox we have taken a broad view, borrowing from many disciplines that we feel could make a valuable contribution to the debate, such as epidemiology, sociology, and psychology, as well as the more traditional clinical disciplines. We have encouraged general practitioners to apply their specialized experiences to an exploration of men's health in areas such as sexuality, violence, alcoholism, unemployment, and phases in the male life cycle. We have also sought a specialized perspective when necessary and general practitioner readers will find the chapters on infertility, and AIDS both demanding and informative. Each chapter starts with an editorial summary. The intention is to tell readers why we chose the topic and to highlight any aspect of the content that we think needs emphasizing or being challenged.

The first chapter is a general overview of disease patterns among men. There is then a series of chapters devoted to phases in the life cycle, exploring the processes of change and adaptation. Next there are chapters dealing with aspects of male behaviour and their interaction with health. These include work, recreation, alcohol, and sexuality. While alcohol is intertwined with violence, we felt each merited a chapter on its own. It is likely that attitudes to alcohol will continue to change over the next decade. Patterns of alcohol consumption will also change as the behavioural consequences of heavy drinking become more socially unacceptable. General practitioners are still reluctant to take alcohol histories even though there is evidence that asking about it makes a difference to patients' consumption. In nearly all violence, the protagonist is male whether the context is international warfare or the home with spouse and children. Successful self-poisonings are much commoner in men as are road traffic accidents. Indeed, many stressed males will admit to barely controllable feelings of aggression at the wheel of the car. Several chapters then cover those clinical problems which predominantly affect men.

Finally, since men are slow to come forward to get help, we have devoted a chapter specifically to this area. Services for well men are becoming more available in both private and state sectors of health care. Barriers exist both within men themselves and in the services provided for them. Men are less likely to interpret their symptoms as arising from physical symptoms, which may be a form of denial. They are poor at remembering and disclosing health information and this may have something to do with the way men use language. Women are socialized into the health culture from an early age and develop the terminology for the consulting room and the confidence to use it (Verbrugge 1985).

Inevitably, focusing on men's health makes compartmentalization of health care more explicit. However, this book is emphatically not an attempt to take attention away from the women's health agenda or to deprecate the attention that women rightly receive in the health arena. Almost all the people, men and women, lay and professional, with whom we have discussed this project have welcomed it warmly as an overdue step to identify a male health agenda. Over the years that it has been taking shape such an agenda has begun to emerge, and we hope that ultimately what has been created here is more than the sum of its parts. What we have learnt is that, in the end, there is not a single unifying answer to the paradox. There are many disparate forces at work that influence men's health, and if the overall agenda is to be addressed, it will require input from people coming from many different disciplines, working together to achieve a shared objective.

Dublin   *Tom O'Dowd*
Bristol   *David Jewell*
December 1997

References

Calman, K. (1993). *On the state of the public health*. The annual report of the Chief Medical Officer of the Department of Health for the year 1992. HMSO, London.

Donovan, J., Frankel, S., Nanchahal, K., Coast, J., and Williams, M. (1992). *Prostatectomy for benign prostatic hyperplasia*. Department of Health, London.

Garraway, W. M., Collins, G. N., and Lee, R. J. (1991). High prevalence of benign prostatic hypertrophy in the community. *Lancet*, **338**, 469–71.

Glass, D. V. (1963). John Graunt and his *Natural and political observations*. In *A discussion on demography* (ed. P. B. Medawar and D. V. Glass). *Proceedings of the Royal Society B*, **159**, 1–37.

McCormick, A., Fleming, D., and Charlton, J. (1995). *Morbidity statistics from general practice. Fourth national study 1991–1992*. HMSO, London.

Shaw, C. (1989). The sex ratio at birth in England and Wales. *Population Trends*, **57**, 26–9.

Verbrugge, L. (1985). Gender and health: an update on hypothesis and evidence. *Journal of Health and Social Behaviour*, **26**, 156–82.

CONTENTS

Contents

CONTRIBUTORS

Ken Addley
Director of the Northern Ireland Civil Service Occupational Health Service, Belfast

Richard Anderson
Lecturer, Department of Obstetrics and Gynaecology, University of Edinburgh, Edinburgh

Peter Barrett
General Practitioner, Nottingham; Member, Institute of Psychosexual Medicine; Specialist in Psychosexual Medicine, City Hospital, Nottingham

Norman Beale
General Practitioner, Calne

Hugh Bethell
General Practitioner, Alton

Fiona Bradley
General Practitioner, Dublin; Lecturer in Community Health and General Practice, Trinity College, Dublin, Ireland

Gerard Bury
Department of General Practice, University College Dublin, Dublin, Ireland

Brian Cox
Senior Research Fellow, Department of Preventive and Social Medicine, University of Otago Medical School, Dunedin, New Zealand

Charles Freer
Medical Director, Health-Sure, Glasgow

David Gillatt
Consultant Urologist and Honorary Senior Lecturer, Department of Surgery, Southmead Hospital, Bristol

David Jewell
Consultant Senior Lecturer in Primary Health Care, University of Bristol, Bristol

George Kinghorn
Directorate of Communicable Diseases, Royal Hallamshire Hospital, Sheffield

Aidan Macfarlane
Consultant Community Paediatrician, Oxford

Ann McPherson
General Practitioner, Oxford

David Mant
Regional R & D Director, South and West Region, NHS Executive

Stephen Rollnick
Principal Clinical Psychologist, South Glamorgan Health Authority

Christopher Silagy
Professor of Evidence Based Medicine and General Practice, Flinders University, Adelaide, Australia

Delia Skan
Senior Employment Medical Advisor, Employment Medical Advisory Service, Belfast, N. Ireland

Richard Slack
Consultant in Communicable Diseases, Nottingham Health Authority, Nottingham

Simon Smail
Sub-Dean and Director of Postgraduate Education for General Practice, University of Wales College of Medicine

Andrew Wilson
Senior Lecturer in General Practice, Leicester General Hospital, Leicester

CHAPTER ONE

The epidemiology of men's health

David Mant and Christopher Silagy

It is easy, as so many commentators have done, to make off the cuff explanations of why men die younger than women. This chapter sets out the context in which the rest of the book is set. It takes a broad view in order to identify all conditions which are more common in men and discusses possible explanations.

Excess male mortality

The average man in England and Wales can expect to live to age 73 – five and a half years less than the average woman. The female mortality advantage continues throughout life but peaks in late adolescence and early adult life (Fig. 1.1). Each year in England and Wales 5.3 million years of male life are lost because of premature death before age 65.

The four most important causes of premature death in men are diseases of the circulation, cancer, accidents, and suicide (Fig. 1.2). Ischaemic heart disease accounts for the bulk (about 70%) of circulatory disease deaths. The most important cancer is lung cancer, which accounts for 25% of premature deaths from neoplasms. Over 60% of accidental deaths occur in motor vehicle traffic accidents.

Drones syndrome

Nature caters for this premature mortality in men by arranging for more boys to be born than girls – about 5% more in the UK. Until the 1950s the high mortality rate among young males, particularly in times of war, meant that the excess of men had been eliminated by age 20. However, since 1951 the reduction in child mortality rates and a period of relative peace have led to an increase in the age at which the crossover between an excess of males and an excess of females occurs. By 1981 this had risen to 50–54 years and it is continuing to edge upwards. By the turn of the century it is likely that for every 10 women

Fig. 1.1 *Death rates per 1000 population by age and sex, and sex ratio, 1990 (OPCS 1990)*

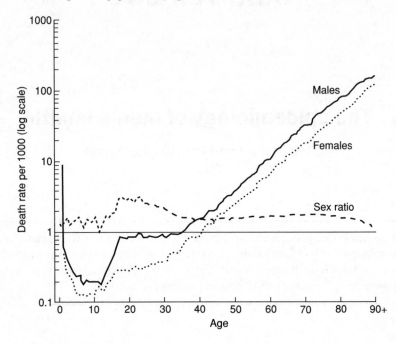

Fig. 1.2 *Main causes of premature death (under age 65) – males* (OPCS 1990)*

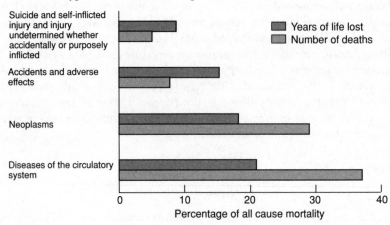

* Deaths aged under 28 days excluded from table

aged 20–34 there will be 10.4 men. This phenomenon has been referred to as the Drones syndrome, on the grounds that men who remain single for longer than they might wish are likely to adopt the behaviour pattern of the drone bee which consists of the

Table 1.1 *Comparison of morbidity in males and females: patients consulting/1000 persons at risk/year by ICD chapter (McCormick et al. 1995)*

	All			Serious		
	M	**F**	**M/F**	**M**	**F**	**M/F**
Infection and parasitic diseases (1–139)	114	165	0.69	1	1	1.00
Neoplasms (140–239)	19	29	0.66	8	10	0.80
Endocrine, nutritional, and metabolic diseases & immunity disorders (240–279)	30	45	0.67	14	23	0.61
Diseases of blood & blood-forming organs (280–289)	5	14	0.36	1	1	1.00
Mental disorders (290–319)	50	94	0.53	8	14	0.57
Diseases of the nervous system & sense organs (320–389)	154	192	0.80	17	23	0.74
Diseases of the circulatory system (390–459)	84	102	0.82	38	35	1.09
Diseases of the respiratory system (460–519)	272	340	0.80	59	57	1.04
Diseases of the digestive system (520–579)	76	97	0.78	24	22	1.09
Diseases of the genitourinary system (580–629)	36	188	0.19	26	35	0.74
Diseases of the skin & subcutaneous tissue (680–709)	127	163	0.78	0	0	
Diseases of the musculoskeletal system & connective tissue (710–739)	129	174	0.74	42	65	0.65
Congenital anomalies (740–759)	5	5	1.00	3	3	1.00
Injury & poisoning (800–999)	136	142	0.96	6	6	1.00

NB: Episode rates given to nearest integer, ratios to two decimal places

continuing production of a loud and irritating noise, interrupted by intermittent, and almost invariably unsuccessful, attempts to mate (Lancet 1987). After the crossover point in middle age, a striking excess of females develops rapidly. Little more than one-third of the population aged 75–84 are men; at 85 and over this proportion has fallen to less than a quarter.

Excess male morbidity

There are three readily available sources of information on morbidity: cancer registration, general practice morbidity data, and hospital discharge data.

Gender differentials across all disease groups are shown in Table 1.1, which gives male and female disease episode rates according to ICD chapter from the 1991–92 National General Practice Morbidity Survey. Overall episode rates are lower in men for all chapters except congenital abnormalities (740–759). However, when account is taken only of episodes of illness classified as 'serious', diseases of the circulatory, respiratory, and digestive system are more common in men, more closely reflecting mortality differentials. In contrast, the excess of musculoskeletal disease in women is accentuated rather than attenuated if account is taken only of 'serious' episodes.

Table 1.2 shows common illnesses with a twofold gender difference in episode rates, according to the individual ICD codes used in the 1991–92 National Morbidity Survey. (Common is arbitrarily defined as an episode rate > 0.2% per annum.) There are more than five times as many 'female excess' as 'male excess' illnesses. Some have an obvious physiological explanation: candidiasis, iron-deficiency anaemia, varicose veins, phlebitis, and renal tract infection. The reasons for the female excess of thyroid disease, obesity, affective psychosis, migraine, and rheumatoid arthritis are less obvious. The reasons for the male excess of gout, peptic ulcer, and hernias as well as ischaemic heart disease, chronic bronchitis, ankylosing spondylitis, and Reiter's syndrome are discussed later in the chapter.

One of the issues in comparing male and female morbidity is the different age structure of the male and female populations. Diseases which are prevalent mainly in the elderly will tend to show a female excess simply because there are more elderly females than males. Table 1.2 therefore also shows age-specific episode ratios: in the majority of cases the gender difference is greater in younger than in older age groups.

Table 1.3 presents RCGP diagnostic codes from the 1991–92 National Morbidity Survey, where the ratio of male to female episode rates is two or more, irrespective of frequency of occurrence. The fourfold male excess of episodes of gout is discussed in more detail in the context of joint disease. The male excess of duodenal ulcer and chronic lung disease has already been noted. The ratios for angina, acute myocardial infarction, and other forms of chronic ischaemic heart disease are shown to demonstrate that they do not reveal a twofold male excess. This was not the case in the previous (1981–82) National Morbidity Survey, where acute myocardial infarction showed a M/F ratio of 2.5; also in the 1991–92 study there is a twofold excess in all age groups below the age of 75. Within the group of injury and poisoning the codes for foreign body in the eye, fractured tibia and fibula, and open wound of hand show a twofold male excess, and these are not shown in the table. The specific injuries reflect work, sport and home maintenance activities. The issue of alcohol abuse is taken up in Chapter 8.

Table 1.2 *Comparison of morbidity in males and females: common conditions showing a twofold gender difference in rates of patients consulting/1000 persons at risk/year by ICD chapter (McCormick et al. 1995)*

	Rate per 1000	Ratio M/F	Age-specific M/F ratios in adults				
			25–44	45–64	65–74	75–84	85+
Illnesses more common in females							
Herpes simplex (54)	8	0.45	0.33	0.36	0.80	0.68	1.80
Candidiasis (112)	31	0.19	0.09	0.19	0.50	0.77	0.71
Hypothyroidism (244)	5	0.14	0.13	0.12	0.17	0.24	0.46
Obesity (278)	8	0.30	0.25	0.34	0.46	0.41	
Iron-deficiency anaemia (28)	5	0.23	0.04	0.20	0.69	0.57	0.69
Affective psychosis (296)	6	0.44	0.39	0.49	0.38	0.63	0.79
Neurotic and other non-psychotic mental disorders (300–316)	65	0.53	0.46	0.55	0.54	0.55	0.83
Migraine (346)	11	0.34	0.26	0.28	0.48	0.57	0.38
Mononeuritis (354)	2	0.37	0.29	0.39	0.88	0.79	1.13
Disorders of lacrimal system (375)	3	0.40	0.31	0.33	0.50	0.61	0.69
Varicose veins (454)	9	0.49	0.32	0.52	0.75	0.76	0.95
Acute sinusitis (461)	25	0.47	0.42	0.41	0.59	0.67	0.61
Diverticula of intestine (562)	2	0.42	0.75	0.42	0.59	0.54	0.64
Functional digestive disorders (564)	21	0.45	0.28	0.42	0.73	0.98	1.11
Cystitis (595)	11	0.07	0.04	0.09	0.14	0.17	0.36
Other disorders of the urethra and urinary tract (599)	28	0.29	0.15	0.34	0.64	0.84	0.80
Rheumatoid arthritis and other inflammatory polyarthropathies (714)	4	0.42	0.41	0.50	0.49	0.40	0.20
Illnesses more common in males							
Gout (274)	4	4.00	10.75	5.95	3.72	2.65	2.44
Duodenal ulcer (532)	3	2.19	2.72	2.02	2.29	1.82	1.27
Inguinal hernia (550)	3	9.50	8.33	11.86	15.60	14.56	7.63

NB: Episode rates given to nearest integer, ratios to two decimal places. Common is arbitrarily defined here as any condition with an episode rate of two or more per 1000 persons at risk per year. The group Neurotic disorders contains four related conditions, all of which show a twofold excess in women.

Table 1.3 *All illnesses showing a twofold excess in men, in rates of patients consulting/1000 persons at risk/year by ICD chapter. Rates are shown for ischaemic heart disease where the excess is less than twofold, for comparison (McCormick et al. 1995)*

	M	F	Ratio (M/F)
Other venereal disease (99)	0.8	0.3	2.67
Malignant neoplasm of bladder (188)	0.6	0.2	3.00
Gout (274)	6.4	1.6	4.00
Sexual deviations and disorders (302)	2.3	0.8	2.88
Alcohol dependence syndrome (303)	2	0.6	3.33
Acute myocardial infarction (410)	*3.8*	*2*	*1.90*
Old myocardial infarction (412)	0.9	0.3	3.00
Angina pectoris (413)	*13*	*9.8*	*1.33*
Other forms of chronic ischaemic heart disease (414)	*6.2*	*3.3*	*1.88*
Aortic aneurysm (441)	0.5	0.1	5.00
Deflected nasal septum (470)	0.8	0.3	2.67
Nasal polyps (471)	1.1	0.5	2.20
Emphysema (492)	1.1	0.5	2.20
Duodenal ulcer (532)	4.6	2.1	2.19
Inguinal hernia (550)	5.7	0.6	9.50
Abscess of anal and rectal regions (566)	1	0.4	2.50
Congenital anomalies of genital organs (752)	1.3	0.1	13.00

NB: Episode rates given to nearest integer, ratios to two decimal places

Table 1.4 reports hospital discharge diagnoses from the 1985 Hospital In-patient Enquiry where the male discharge rate is at least 50% higher than the female rate. As in the mortality data, hospitalization for ischaemic heart disease, malignant neoplasm of the bladder and lung, congenital abnormalities, and trauma are all more common in men. The excess hospitalization rate for peptic ulcer and hernia reflect the increased episode rate seen in the general practice data. The excess male trauma rates reflect occupational and road-traffic hazards as well as the sports and home maintenance injuries evident from general practice data.

Table 1.4 *Excess male morbidity: discharge diagnoses from the 1985 Hospital In-patient Enquiry where male discharge rate exceeds female rate by 50% or more (DHSS/OPCS 1987)*

	Discharge rate/1000 population		
	Males	**Females**	**Ratio**
Hernias of the abdominal cavity (D 343)	32.7	9.4	3.5
Fractures of the skull or face (D 470)	7.4	2.3	3.2
Malignant neoplasms of bladder (D 126)	15.6	5.1	3.1
Open wounds and injuries to blood vessels (D 50)	12.8	4.8	2.7
Malignant neoplasms of lung, bronchus, or trachea (D 101)	17.2	6.5	2.6
Intracranial and internal injuries (D 49)	30.1	15.0	2.0
Burns (D 52)	3.0	1.6	1.9
Ischaemic heart disease (D 27)	52.5	27.6	1.9
Congenital abnormalities (D 44)	18.9	11.1	1.7
Birth asphyxia and other respiratory conditions (D 454)	3.8	2.4	1.6
Peptic ulcer (D 341)	8.2	5.3	1.5

Male and female health service use

Data on general practice consulting patterns are available from the General Practice National Morbidity Survey 1981–82 and from the OPCS General Household Survey 1992; the latter also records hospital admissions (Table 1.5). Overall, males make less use of health services than females from age 15–64, but at the extremes of life hospital in-patient stays are more common in males. Similarly, adult men aged 15–64 visit their general practitioners (GPs) much less often than women, but consultation rates in the young and elderly are similar in both sexes.

Epidemiology and risk

The rest of this chapter is about the epidemiology of excess male morbidity and mortality for specific diseases, but a brief reminder of the terms used may be helpful. Epidemiologists try to identify the causes of disease by comparing the characteristics of ill and healthy people. The characteristics which are more common in the ill than in the healthy are termed 'risk factors'. A 'relative risk' of 10 for smoking means that people who smoke are 10 times more likely to become ill than those who do not.

Table 1.5 *Health service use by males and females: age-specific GP consultations, in-patient stays, and long-standing illness reported in the General Household Survey 1992 and GP consultation rates from the General Practice National Morbidity Survey 1981–82 (RCGP/OPCS/DHSS 1986; Thomas et al. 1994)*

Age		0–4	5–14	15–44	45–64	65–74	75+
In-patient	M	17	7	7	11	24	26
stays/1000 persons/	F	12	5	16	12	15	24
12 months	M/F	1.4	1.4	0.4	0.9	1.6	1.1
GP consultations	M	22	10	9	13	20*	–
by adult	F	22	11	18	18	21	–
in previous	M/F	1.0	0.9	0.5	0.7	1.0	–
14 days							
GP consultations	M	99	66	58	63	72	78
in previous year	F	98	67	79	72	75	80
(% of population	M/F	1.0	1.0	0.7	0.9	1.0	1.0
consulting)							

* *data for 65+*

Much of what follows is expressed in terms of risk factors and relative risk and it is important to understand three things about these terms. Firstly, risk factors are predictors of disease but they may predict only by association with the true cause. Eliminating the risk factor does not necessarily eliminate the cause of disease. Secondly, the importance of a risk factor depends not only on the relative risk it imparts but also on its frequency of occurrence. Familial hyperlipidaemia is associated with a relative risk of early death from ischaemic heart disease of up to 100, but because the condition is rare it contributes little to total mortality from this cause. The relative risk associated with smoking is much less, but smoking contributes a great deal more to total mortality from ischaemic heart disease because so many people smoke. Thirdly, high relative risks are unimportant if the baseline risk to which they are relative is negligible. A twofold relative risk of myocardial infarction in a woman aged 20–24 years is trivial because the baseline risk is about one in 2 million per year; a twofold relative risk in a man aged 65–69 is important because the baseline risk is about one in 100 per year.

Ischaemic heart disease

Men below 50 years of age have a sixfold higher risk than women (Fig. 1.3), and there is some evidence that hormone replacement therapy may extend this relative disadvantage beyond the female menopause. Box 1.1 shows those risk factors for ischaemic heart disease which are thought to be important and where the risk could possibly be reduced by preventive activity in general practice.

The most ignored risk factor for death from ischaemic heart disease is established vascular disease as evidenced by angina, diabetes, hypertension, or previous infarction.

Box 1.1 *Modifiable risk factors for death from ischaemic heart disease*

- Smoking
- High saturated fat diet
- High blood pressure
- Obesity
- Evidence of existing circulatory disease (e.g. angina, previous MI, diabetes)
- Lack of physical fitness

The latter imparts a four- to eightfold increased risk of further infarction and the value of risk modification by lifestyle and therapeutic intervention is well-established (Weinblatt *et al.* 1968).

The most important lifestyle factor is smoking, which accounts for about 25% of coronary heart disease deaths. (Male smoking habits are considered further in the section on lung cancer.) Dietary fat intake, and particularly saturated fat intake, is higher in men

Fig. 1.3 *Death rates from ischaemic heart disease, England and Wales 1991 (OPCS 1993)*

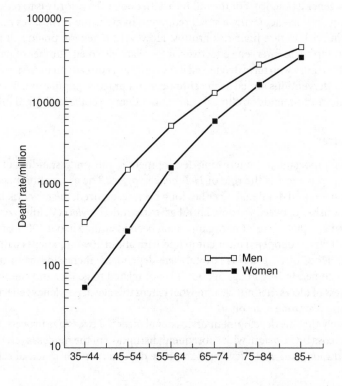

than in women and is strongly associated with heart disease: a 1% increase in total cholesterol is associated with about a 2% increase in risk. Exercise is also important – it is now clear that much of the early uncertainty about the benefit of exercise was due to inadequate epidemiological measurement of physical fitness. Formal meta-analysis and review of 37 studies published between 1953 and 1987 gives a summary risk of death from coronary heart disease of 1.9 (95% CI 1.6–2.2) for men in sedentary occupations over those in active occupations. It also indicated that the methodologically stronger studies show greater benefit (Berlin and Colditz 1990). Lack of physical fitness is now endemic among middle-aged men in the UK (Allied Dunbar National Fitness Survey 1992). Generally, however, males exercise more than females and any protective effect against ischaemic heart disease will tend to work in men's favour.

Some established risk factors are not included in Box 1.1 since they are not modifiable. For instance, mild to moderate vertex baldness is related to a 40% increase in myocardial infarction and severe baldness with a 340% increase (Lesko *et al.* 1993).

All the risk factors cited in Fig. 1.4 are cumulative: although the interaction is less than multiplicative, it is certainly more than additive (Silberberg 1990). This implies that men at only moderate risk from a number of individual factors can accumulate high overall risk. It does not imply that one should encourage patients to try to modify more than one risk factor at a time.

The continuing debate about the value of preventive activity in general practice does not reflect epidemiological uncertainty about risk factors. The uncertainty stems from inadequate evidence for the effectiveness of much of the preventive activity currently promoted in general practice. For the public health doctor the priority is to reduce risk in the entire population – achieving a small reduction in everyone's risk saves more lives than eliminating risk in rare high-risk groups. However, in general practice it may be more productive to try to intervene effectively on a relatively small number of patients at high risk, such as those who have diagnosed ischaemic heart disease, than to spend time on less effective interventions aimed at the entire general practice population. The final answer to this question depends on clinical trials rather than on epidemiological inference.

Peptic ulcer

The most important and interesting development in our understanding of the epidemiology of peptic ulcer is the role of *Helicobacter pylori*. The association between chronic antral gastritis and duodenal ulcer has long been recognized; the new link in the chain is the relationship between chronic antral gastritis and *H. pylori* (Veldhuyzen van Zanten and Sherman 1994). The latter organism has been identified in over 90% of patients with active gastritis or duodenal ulcer compared with about 10% of patients without gastritis. The prevalence of *H. pylori* is strongly age dependent, increasing from under 10% in teenagers to nearly 50% at age 50, but it is not related to gender and cannot explain the male excess of ulcers. It is not clear to what extent this age dependency reflects cumulative acquisition over time or a cohort effect.

It is likely that the development of duodenal ulcer is a two-stage process. Colonization of the mucosa by *H. pylori*, with subsequent disruption of the mucus layer, inflammatory cell infiltration, and ulcer development, may depend on prior mucosal cell metaplasia.

Metaplasia is associated with the traditional, so-called 'male' risk factors for peptic ulcer such as smoking, excess alcohol consumption, and 'stress', which induce production of gastric acid.

The association of *H. pylori* with gastric ulcers and gastric cancer is also important but may reflect a more complicated pathogenesis. Forman *et al.* (1994) have argued that the process is similar but with severe gastritis *H. pylori* colonization ceases and immunoglobulin G (IgG) levels return to normal, thus leading to an underestimate of the causative role of the bacteria. This view is supported by data showing that the estimated risk of gastric cancer associated with *H. pylori* seropositivity is strongly related to the interval between serum testing and cancer diagnosis (Webb *et al.* 1994). The mode of acquisition of *H. pylori* is still uncertain although clustering in families and high prevalence in institutions suggest environmental transmission. Housing conditions in childhood seem to be important (Forman *et al.* 1994). The value of antibiotic agents in the management of gastritis and peptic ulcer is now well-established, and reinfection after proven eradication is uncommon. There are issues about the prevention of gastric cancer by population screening and antibiotic treatment which have yet to be resolved.

Chronic obstructive airways disease

There is scientific unanimity that cigarette smoking is the major cause of chronic obstructive airways disease (COAD), and that the present excess of COAD in men is a reflection of smoking habits earlier this century. Industrial exposure to dust is also responsible for excess pulmonary disease in men and is the most important factor in some sectors of the population, but even in an industrial disease such as asbestosis there is a clear synergistic effect in pathogenesis between asbestos and cigarette smoking. Nevertheless, epidemiologists are still taxed by the problem of why some smokers develop significant COAD while many do not (Sparrow 1988).

The classic explanation of the pathogenesis of COAD in smokers has been the excess secretion of mucus and local inflammation in the pulmonary airways. This is thought to encourage recurrent infection and consequent structural damage, leading to the clinical syndrome of chronic bronchitis. However, the evidence for this pathological sequence of events has been questioned and there is no clear evidence that development of COAD can be predicted by the initial degree of mucus hypersecretion. An alternative theory which has gained some support is that progression to COAD reflects the degree of airway responsiveness and atopy in the individual. In support of this theory is evidence that smoking increases immunoglobulin E (IgE) secretion and blood eosinophil counts, but it is not possible to be sure whether this means that smoking induces atopy or simply influences the markers of atopy.

Congenital malformations

In 1991 in the UK there were 4195 notified congenital malformations in males compared with 2802 in females (Office of Population and Census Studies 1994). Three sites of malformations accounted for the bulk of the male excess: external genitalia (849 in males, 37 in females), limbs (1347, 999), and cleft lip (347, 167). Malformations of the heart and circulatory system, alimentary tract and ear, face and neck are also more common in males;

congenital dislocation of the hip is more common in females (64, 205). Apart from the obvious anatomical association between male sex and hypospadias, the gender difference in congenital malformation remains largely unexplained. Interestingly, Table 1.1 indicates that the differences between males and females in the incidence of congenital malformation is not reflected in the rates of general practice consultations.

X-linked genetic disorders

Most X chromosome-linked genetic disorders are recessive and only men can be expected to display the full syndrome (as women have two X chromosomes); females are affected only if an affected male fathers a child of a female carrier. There is no male to male transmission (as men pass on only the Y chromosomes) but all female children of affected males are carriers. Sisters have a 50% chance of being carriers and in many cases the carrier state can be identified and appropriate genetic counselling given. The most frequent forms of X-linked recessive disorder are shown in Box 1.2: all of these disorders are extremely rare. It is important to remember that affected males with a number of these disorders, such as Duchenne muscular dystrophy, do not reproduce. The majority of such cases will therefore result from new mutations in the patient or mother and no affected uncle will be identifiable.

Dominant X-linked disorders (such as Vitamin D-resistant rickets) are rare. Females transmit to half their children (sons and daughters); males transmit to all daughters and no sons. Females are therefore affected twice as often as males but the syndrome is more variable, and usually less severe, in females than in males.

Box 1.2 *X-linked recessive disorders*

- Haemophilia A
- Nephrogenic diabetes insipidus
- Lesch–Nyhan syndrome
- Duchenne muscular dystrophy
- G6PD deficiency
- Testicular feminization
- Fabry's disease

Joint disease

This is a fascinating area of epidemiology with differences in incidence between males and females that are still not well-understood; a readable and authoritative account of the aetiology of joint disease and its management in general practice is given by Curry and Hull (1987). Table 1.2 shows that rheumatoid arthritis (RA) is more common in women than in men; osteoarthritis (OA) is also more common in women at all ages although the excess is less than twofold. Gout, anklylosing spondylitis, and Reiter's disease are more common in men than in women, although only in gout is the excess twofold.

The definition of OA is based on pathological features – focal cartilage loss and sub-chondral bone reaction – which bear an inconstant relationship with radiological and clinical findings. Radiographic surveys suggest that OA is present in the knees of about two in three adults aged over 65, with only a slight excess in women, but the prevalence of symptomatic disease is almost twice as high in women than in men. Traditionally, the causes of OA have been divided into 'primary' and 'secondary', the latter being explicable in terms of identifiable pre-existing joint disease (e.g. gout), metabolic predisposition (e.g. chondrocalcinosis), or mechanical trauma. However, it is unclear whether primary OA is a distinct disease entity or has many causes, many of which remain unidentified. The difference between men and women is not due to differential exposure to identified risk factors. For example, although identified risk factors for OA of the knee such as obesity, previous knee injury, meniscectomy, and occupations which entail prolonged or repeated joint movement apply equally to men and women, the relative risk imparted by each factor is consistently higher in women (Cooper *et al.* 1994). The mechanism underlying this gender differential remains unexplained, although one hypothesis is that the tendency to develop OA in response to joint damage is an autosomal dominant trait with variable expression according to gender.

Rheumatoid arthritis (RA) is more than twice as common in females than males, and again the reason for the gender difference remains unknown. RA is an autoimmune process characterized by the presence of rheumatoid factors (autoantibodies directed against IgG) which can be detected in the blood of 80–90% of patients with the clinical syndrome. Autoantibodies are present in the blood of 5% of the population whereas the prevalence of clinical RA is about 2% and the prevalence of disabling RA is less than 1%. The factor which initiates the autoimmune process has not been identified, although the association with (HLA) haplotype DR4 suggests a genetic component.

The male excess of gout is more simple to explain. There is a very close relationship between the prevalence of gout and serum levels of uric acid, and women have lower levels of uric acid. A study of the prevalence of gout in 64 UK general practices in 1975 reported a prevalence of 2.6 per 1000 and an even higher male–female ratio (6:1) than recorded in the National Morbidity Survey (Currie 1979). The vast majority of cases were classified as 'primary' gout and only 10% could be explained by identifiable influences on purine metabolism; almost all of these 'secondary' cases were due to diuretic therapy rather than to myeloproliferative or identified genetic disorders. The 'attack rate' for gout is dependent on uric acid levels, with an annual rate of <1% in people with uric acid levels <6 mg/dl, increasing to over 90% in those with levels >9 mg/dl. However, there is no level which can be said to be diagnostic of the clinical syndrome and the level at which prophylactic treatment is recommended is a matter of judgement. The age–sex distribution of uric acid is similar to the distribution for ischaemic heart disease, with much lower levels in females from puberty until the menopause followed by a steady climb towards male rates thereafter. The lower levels of uric acid in women premenopausally are thought to be due to the uricosuric effect of oestrogen.

The male–female incidence ratio for ankylosing spondylitis (AS) is now thought to be about 4:1, with the highest prevalence in young men and a strong relation with HLA-B27 antigen (identified in about 90% of cases). Previous reports of sex ratios as high as 10:1 are almost certainly due to referral and ascertainment bias in hospital series (Carbone *et al.*

1992). The presentation of AS is similar in men and women, although the severity of the disease at diagnosis is greater in men. The HLA-B27 antigen is equally distributed between the sexes and is fairly common (population prevalence 8%), so it does not explain the gender difference. Recently, specific autoantigens have been identified in the serum of patients with AS which may increase our understanding of its pathogenesis, but at present the reason for its predilection for males remains uncertain.

Reiter's disease is similarly related to HLA-B27 and has an even higher reported male–female ratio (20:1). There is some evidence for the role of bacterial pathogens, and it has been reported that attack rates in patients HLA-B27 positive are 20–25% following exposure to specific enteric pathogens. Again, the HLA-B27 link does not explain the male excess.

Cerebrovascular disease

Cerebrovascular disease accounts for about 20% of male deaths from circulatory disease. The difference in mortality rates between men and women is much less striking than with ischaemic heart disease, although stroke incidence is still up to 30% higher in men until age 80 years. There is a familial predisposition to stroke but migrant studies indicate that environmental factors are also important. Not surprisingly, the identified risk factors for cerebrovascular disease are very similar to those for ischaemic heart disease. Both diastolic and systolic blood pressure are strong predictors of death from cerebrovascular disease and this seems to apply equally to cerebral infarction and intracerebral haemorrhage. The most recent report from the Framingham cohort study confirms that smoking is an independent risk factor and the risk of stroke increases with the number of cigarettes smoked (North *et al.* 1988). The risk for ex-smokers drops to the level of non-smokers after five years. Diabetes mellitus and obesity are also risk factors for cerebrovascular disease, although much of this association derives from higher blood pressures in the obese. The presence of cardiovascular disease – and in particular atrial fibrillation ($\times$ 5 risk) – increases risk at all levels of blood pressure. About 10% of strokes are preceded by transient ischaemic attacks and individuals with asymptomatic carotid bruits also have an increased risk of stroke. As with ischaemic heart disease, individual risks are cumulative.

Lung cancer and smoking

The vast majority of lung cancers can be attributed to smoking. There is a clear dose-response relationship between smoking and lung cancer (Box 1.3) which is modified by the duration of exposure and interaction with other pulmonary carcinogens such as asbestos and radon. Smoking explains nearly all the observed differences in lung cancer rates within and between populations and action to reduce smoking rates in the UK has led to a gradual decline in lung cancer.

In 1990, 31% of men aged 16 or over were smokers. Although this proportion has decreased steadily from 52% in 1972 and 42% in 1980, the rate of decrease appears to be flattening. The male population is now more or less divided into thirds – one-third never smokers, one-third ex-smokers, and one-third current smokers (Fig. 1.4). The proportion of never smokers has increased slightly more than the proportion of ex-smokers. Unfortunately, the highest smoking rate (38%) is amongst men aged 20–24 years; the proportion of men smoking declines gradually with age to 24% in those aged 60 or over.

Box 1.3 *Risk of lung cancer from smoking*

Four points summarize the risk of lung cancer from smoking:

- risk is directly related to the number of cigarettes* smoked i.e. the higher the consumption, the higher the risk
- risk is more dependent on duration of smoking than on consumption e.g. smoking 1 packet of cigarettes a day for 40 years is 8 times more hazardous than smoking 2 packets a day for 20 years
- risk is reduced by ceasing to smoke. After 10 or more years of giving up smoking, an ex-smoker has nearly the same risk as a non-smoker
- lower tar cigarettes appear to carry a lower risk of lung cancer than higher tar cigarettes.

* *Smoking cigarettes carries a much higher risk than smoking other forms of tobacco*

Source: Austoker, J. CRC Factsheet 11.4.1992

Fig. 1.4 *Percentage of current smokers, ex-regular smokers, and never smoked – Great Britain, 1972–90 (OPCS 1992)*

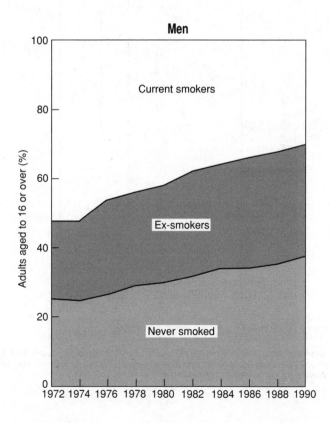

Smoking is strongly related to social status and disadvantage. In 1990, the smoking rate amongst male professionals was 16% against 48% in unskilled manual workers. High smoking rates in men are also associated with unemployment and being widowed, divorced, or separated. Although there is some dispute about the wisdom of encouraging smokers to change to a low-tar cigarette rather than encouraging them to stop completely, the tar profile of cigarettes smoked by men has improved: 75% of men are now smoking low or low to middle-tar cigarettes. As long as switching to a lower-tar brand does not encourage men to increase the number of cigarettes smoked (perhaps to main-

Fig. 1.5 *The relative risk (point estimate and 95% confidence interval) of lung cancer in non-smokers whose spouses smoke compared with non-smokers whose spouses do not smoke (Wald 1987)*

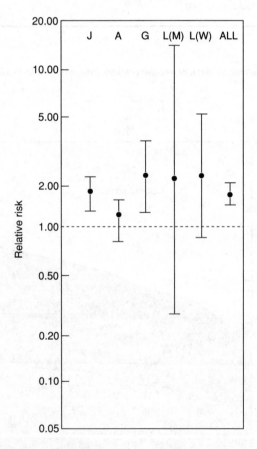

Results from four studies J=Japanese Study (Hirayama 1981), A=American Cancer Society Study (Garfinkel 1981), G=Greek Study (Trichopolous *et al.* 1983), L=Louisiana Study (Correa *et al.* 1983), M=men, W=women) and all studies combined (all).

tain their nicotine levels) or to feel that cigarette smoking is safe, it is likely that this will lead to some health benefit.

Breathing other people's tobacco smoke also causes cancer. This important possibility was first substantiated in 1983 with the results of four studies (Fig. 1.5) which show an increased risk of lung cancer of about 50%. Although initial uncertainty was expressed about the validity of using spouses' smoking history as a method of indicating exposure to other people's tobacco smoke, studies using biochemical markers of smoke exposure (e.g. cotinine) have supported these conclusions. Cotinine studies have also shown that exposure to tobacco smoke in an occupational environment can be of similar magnitude to exposure at home and can impart a similar risk. Although the risk of passive smoking may be significantly less than that of active smoking, informing non-smoking patients of this risk may be a very important mechanism for encouraging social and political change.

Bladder cancer

Bladder cancer is twice as common in men as in women, but the only well-established environmental risk factors are smoking and occupational exposure to chemical carcinogens at work. Occupational risks have been carefully monitored and the hazard reduced in recent years, and smoking is now the most important preventable cause of the disease (Ross *et al.* 1988). Various dietary factors have been discussed, including caffeine and analgesic intake, but the evidence is not conclusive. Similarly, a diet rich in vegetables and fruit (i.e. high in antioxidants) is thought to be protective but this relationship has yet to be confirmed. The only other important risk factor is physical irritation of the bladder, particularly by bladder stones and schistosoma infection, and perhaps long-term bacterial infection.

Prostatic cancer

The distinctive feature of prostate cancer is its rapidly increasing incidence with age and the very high prevalence of latent carcinoma (40%) found at autopsy (Noriwa and Kolomel 1991). International comparison and migrant studies suggest that environmental factors may play an important role, particularly in progression from latent to symptomatic disease. Diet is probably important. The incidence of prostate cancer appears to rise with the adoption of a western diet in countries like Japan and in Japanese migrants to western cultures. The two dietary elements which are of most interest are fat and antioxidants, especially carotenoids, but the difficult of undertaking dietary epidemiology means that there is still disagreement among experts on the effect of these factors. Most people would accept that a diet low in saturated fat and high in vegetables and fruit is likely to be protective.

Androgens are probably important in the aetiology of prostate cancer. Eunuchs do not get prostate cancer, castration has a palliative effect on cancer, and cancer risk is related to muscle mass. However, the results of case–control investigations of male and female sex hormones have been inconsistent. Definitive answers are unlikely without direct measurement of tissue concentrations in prostate tissue (in particular, dihydrotestosterone), but obviously such investigations are difficult in control subjects. Of interest in this context is the familial element to prostate cancer, with a twofold increase in risk among first-degree relatives of cases and an increase in trend of risk with the number of relatives affected. Obviously this does not prove a strong genetic component, as family members share common environments, but there does appear to be a concordance of serum testosterone levels among brothers, fathers, and sons. Certain aspects of sexual activity also appear to be indicative of a higher prostate cancer risk. These include early age of first intercourse and a history of venereal disease, but no infective agent has yet been identified.

There is a suggestion that vasectomy increases the risk of prostate cancer, perhaps because of increase in testosterone levels following this operation, although this is not certain. The two most recently published American follow-up studies do suggest an increased risk. In the health professionals' prospective follow-up study of 10 055 vasectomized men and 37 800 controls, the former had an overall increased risk of 66% and risk increased with time since operation (Giovannucci *et al.* 1993a). In the retrospective nurses' health study of 14 607 vasectomized husbands of nurses and age-matched

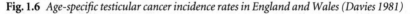

Fig. 1.6 *Age-specific testicular cancer incidence rates in England and Wales (Davies 1981)*

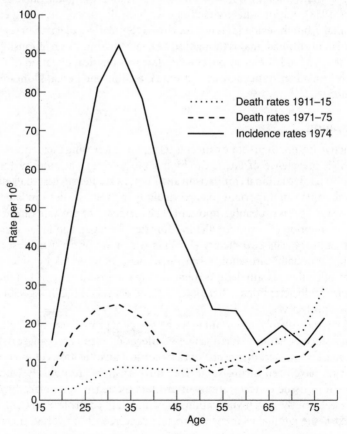

controls, the overall risk was 56% higher (Giovannucci *et al.* 1993*b*). It is still possible that the increase in risk reflects an unknown 'confounding' factor related to both vasectomy and prostate cancer, but this possibility cannot be eliminated without a randomized trial.

Testicular cancer

Testicular cancer is a relatively unimportant cause of death, resulting in less than 150 deaths in the UK in 1990. However, it is the most common type of cancer in young men and is increasing in incidence (Fig. 1.6). The majority of testicular tumours are malignant and about half are seminomas. The remaining 50% are predominantly ter-atomas and embryonal carcinomas which have a slightly younger age incidence. Cure rates are high with virtually all patients with stage 1 or 2 seminomas and 90% of patients with stage 1 teratomas surviving beyond five years. Cryptorchidism (undescended testes) is the most important risk factor. It imparts a risk of three- to fivefold and approximately 10% of cancers arise in patients with such a history. There appears to be an increased cancer risk in both ipsilateral and contralateral testes, suggesting that there may be an underlying prenatal cause. Other risk factors such as atrophic testes, inguinal her-nia, and hydrocele are infrequent and contribute very little to overall risk (Schottenfeld *et al.* 1980). There has been one report of increased incidence of testicular cancer in men who have had vasectomies although this has not been supported in further studies.

The fact that death rates from testicular cancer peak at ages 25–34 years has led to a demand for the promotion of testicular self-examination (TSE) in young men as a means of prevention. This is not generally recommended because of the low incidence of the disease, the low compliance with educational programmes, and the high success rates achieved by treatment. There is also very little evidence that diagnostic delay affects survival, particularly for seminomas. The only group in which instruction in self-examination might be justifiable are men with a history of cryptorchidism. Such men have a lifetime risk of developing testicular cancer of 2% if both testes were affected. The logistic difficulty of constructing a trial of TSE instruction in this high-risk group means that we shall probably never know for sure whether communicating this risk to patients will do more good than harm (Westlake and Frank 1987).

Accidents

Accidental death rates have been falling in the UK, but more steeply for women than for men. The downward trend for males appears to be flattening out and the rate may now be increasing (Fig. 1.7). One reason for the increase seen between 1989 and 1990 was the 3484 male deaths from motor vehicle traffic accidents – a 3% increase and the highest number of such deaths since 1984. There was also an 8% increase in male suicides (see below). Overall in 1990, road traffic accidents accounted for exactly half of the total of accidental deaths with home accidents contributing a further 25%, accidents at work and elsewhere 20%, and other transport accidents 4%. The rest of the 11 684 male deaths from injury and poisoning were due to suicide (2994), deaths undetermined whether acciden-tally or purposely inflicted (1337), and homicide (282).

The contribution of various road users to male mortality is shown in Fig. 1.8. The

Fig. 1.7 *Deaths from injury and poisoning: standardized mortality ratios by sex, 1971–80 (OPCS 1990)*

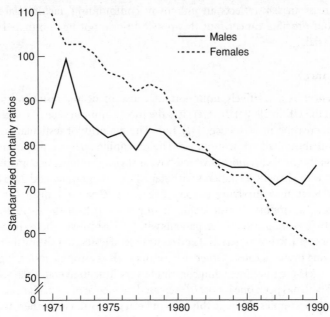

highest accident rate is, rather surprisingly, in the over-75s – mainly because of the very high rate of pedestrian accidents. Pedal cycle deaths are also highest in the elderly. The highest car and motorcycle accident rates are in the 15–24 age group. (Although these are overall death rates, it is important to realize that they are not related to actual road use. Very few over-75s ride motorcycles, hence the low motorcycle accident rate in this age group.)

The most common cause of death from non-transport accidents are falls, which accounted for 1441 male deaths in 1990; 48% of these occurred at home, 7% at work, 10% on the street, and the rest in other places. Falling from ladders or scaffolding was an important cause of death both at home and at work. Death by fire is relatively uncommon, causing 313 male deaths, 88% of which occurred at home. Death by drowning was even less common, accounting for 193 male deaths.

The epidemiology of accidental injury is part of the wider issue of environmental risk management and involves characterizing the environment in which risk-taking behaviour takes place as well as the human limits of risk appreciation. For example, Robertson (1991) points out that even at a moderate speed of 30 miles an hour a driver will take about 0.9 seconds to react to an emergency, during which time he or she will travel approximately 40 feet. A child darting into the street within that distance will therefore inevitably be struck. She therefore argues that intervention to reduce the incidence, severity, and eventual result of injury needs to be concentrated on a wide variety of factors and phases of the problem. Exclusive attention to 'accident prevention' is irrational, particularly in view of the limited ability of human beings to anticipate and react to hazardous conditions.

Fig. 1.8 *Road traffic accidents in males, 1990 (OPCS 1992)*

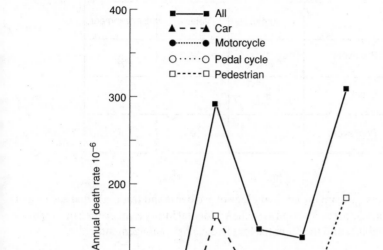

The best current model for assessing the epidemiology and scope for prevention of accidents is probably the matrix suggested by Haddon (1980) which is reproduced in a modified form in Fig. 1.9. This can be illustrated in relation to road traffic accidents, using examples taken by Robertson (1991). The key issue in cell 1 is use of alcohol – about half of fatally injured drivers have high blood alcohol concentrations. Cell 3 is also important and the separation of different sorts of road users, such as cars and bicycles, would fall into this cell. In cell 4, the concern is human tolerances to crash forces (the human body can tolerate rapid deceleration up to 35 times gravity with no injury and 45 times gravity with little injury if the load is distributed over sufficient body area, such as a safety harness). Cells 2, 5, and 8 are to do with vehicle design and might be summarized as owning a Volvo. Finally, an issue in cell 6 might be the provision of a central crash barrier to prevent crashed cars crossing the reservation and in cell 9, the adequacy of immediate medical response from the ambulance service.

The most important identifiable cause of road traffic accidents amenable to general practice intervention remains excess alcohol consumption. More than 20% of people killed on the road have a blood alcohol level over the legal limit and the total death toll from accidents caused by alcohol is even higher. This important issue is discussed further in Chapter 8.

Fig. 1.9 *Revised Haddon matrix for assessing aetiology and preventability of accidents*

	Human	Vehicle	Environment
Pre-event	1	2	3
Event	4	5	6
Post event	7	8	9

The overall message from the epidemiology of accidents and trauma is that each event is multifactorial and must be assessed as such. Accidental injury is misnamed in view of its statistical predictability and the potential for effective risk management.

Hernias

The vast majority of hernias in men are inguinal hernias, two-thirds of which are direct and one-third indirect. In women, femoral hernias are more common. The relative importance of anatomical predisposition and subsequent factors which increase intra-abdominal pressure is difficult to establish. Smoking has been cited as a risk factor. The overall prevalence in men of 'clinically obvious' inguinal hernias was estimated in one community study in Israel as 15%, but at ages 65–74 it was 31%, and age 75 and over it was 45% (Abramson *et al.* 1978). No UK-based community study has been done. The annual likelihood of strangulation of an inguinal hernia is less than 3% a year, but this is not constant. Risk is highest immediately after recognition and declines thereafter (Gallegos *et al.* 1991). It is often stated that strangulation is more frequent for indirect inguinal hernias, but the research data are inconsistent and interpretation is complicated by the tendency for earlier surgical intervention if an indirect hernia is suspected. The risk of strangulation from a femoral hernia is much higher – probably in the order of tenfold.

Suicide

Suicide is more common in men than in women and peaks in late middle age. At least half of suicides occur in people with a history of mental illness, particularly depression, although this does not explain the gender difference as clinical depression is more common in women. About 40% of people committing suicide have made contact with a health professional, often their general practitioner, in the preceding month. A recent editorial in the *Lancet* examined the question of whether suicide is preventable and concluded that the most effective strategy would be to improve long-term treatment and follow-up of patients with affective disorders (Lancet 1992). However, in his review Gunnel (1994) argued that no single intervention has been shown in a randomized trial to be effective, and the government target of a 15% reduction in suicide by the year 2000 will be difficult to achieve.

The lifetime suicide risk in patients with hospital-diagnosed affective disorders is about 15%, which gives an annual risk of about 0.3%. In the general population the key risk factors (other than age and sex) are physical illness, recent loss of a spouse or parent, and a family history of suicide. The risk of suicide is increased among unemployed men although it is unclear whether this is causal or simply an association with psychiatric illness. Interestingly, unemployment remains a risk factor for suicide among individuals with psychiatric disorders.

Depression is a strong predictor of suicide risk in alcoholics and the majority of alcoholics who kill themselves are also depressed. Other predictors of suicide in alcoholics are poor health, poor work record, and recent bereavement or marriage breakdown.

AIDS, HIV1, and sexual habits

The total number of AIDS cases and deaths reported in the United Kingdom, and their probable source of exposure, are summarized in Table 1.6. The majority of cases are in men (89%) and have resulted from homosexual intercourse (71%). The vast majority of cases diagnosed have come from the two Thames regions (9465) compared with 331 cases from West Midlands and 73 cases from Northern Ireland. Around three-quarters of the male cases are in the age range 25–44 years. The commonest presentations of the disease are pneumocystis carinii pneumonia (PCP) (38%) and Kaposi's sarcoma (15%).

Since 1990, anonymous surveys have been conducted on sentinel populations in England and Wales in order to monitor the prevalence of HIV infection. The highest prevalence has been amongst homosexual men – 13% in London and 5% outside London. Amongst drug users the comparable figures were 5% and 2%.

In view of the fact that anonymous monitoring data for HIV is available only for the last few years, prediction of trend is difficult. Of most concern is the high prevalence of infection amongst younger homo/bisexual men in London – a group in which there is also a high prevalence of other acute sexually transmitted diseases despite counselling on safer sex. The prevalence of HIV infection amongst injecting drug users appears to be stable, although some argue that official figures are unreliable and draw attention to rates of 10–15% discovered in local surveys. The prevalence of HIV in intravenous drug users is as high in women as it is in men. The public health challenge of AIDS remains the provision of effective health education. A recent editorial in the *British Medical Journal* about the inadequacy of sex education (Smith 1992) and the subsequent flurry of letters emphasizes that this task is not straightforward.

Gaining reliable information on the sexual habits of men is difficult. Probably the best available data relevant to a general practice population were gathered for the control group of the UK national case–control study of testicular cancer (Forman and Chilvers 1989). This study collected data on 480 male controls, aged 15–49 years, recruited from general practice age/sex registers (this reflected a response rate of 83%). Only about 5% of those interviewed never had heterosexual intercourse; eight (1.7%) had had homosexual intercourse, four of whom had had only one casual homosexual partner. Over half of the

Table 1.6 *AIDS cases and deaths by exposure category, United Kingdom to end March 1997 (Communicable Diseases Report, PHLS 1997)*

How HIV infection was probably acquired	Jan 82–Mar 97			
	Male	(Deaths)[6]	Female	(Deaths)
Sexual intercourse				
between men[1]	9967	7607	–	–
between men and women				
exposure to 'high risk' partner(s)[2]	48	36	176	119
exposure abroad[3]	936	550	699	376
exposure in the UK[4]	99	74	92	65
investigation continuing/closed[5]	28	10	20	7
Injecting drug use (IDU)	620	444	260	184
Blood				
blood factor treatment (e.g. for haemophilia)	624	554	6	5
blood/tissue transfer (e.g. transfusion) abroad/UK	54	38	76	58
Mother to infant	112	65	121	61
Other or investigation continuing/closed	126	99	18	12
Total	12614	9477	1468	887

[1] Includes 251 men who had also injected drugs
[2] Partner(s) exposed to HIV infection through sexual intercourse between men, IDU, blood factor treatment, or blood/tissue transfer
[3] Individuals from abroad, and individuals from the UK who have lived or visited abroad, for whom there is no evidence of 'high risk' partners
[4] No evidence of 'high risk' partners
[5] Closed – no further information available
[6] Includes 174 cases (160 males and 14 females) who have been lost to follow-up and presumed no longer to contribute to prevalent cases in the UK

men had intercourse over the age of 18 and over three-quarters had done so before the age of 20. Table 1.7 shows that sexual activity has increased over time. Of the men aged over 40, 71% had had only one regular partner and 48% no casual partners at all. However, in men aged 20–39 more than half had had more than one regular and more than one casual partner, despite having fewer years to accumulate this sexual experience. Twenty-nine men (6%) reported that they had had a sexually transmitted disease at least once and 12 reported more than one episode. The commonest infection reported was non-specific urethritis, followed by gonorrhoea and genital herpes.

Table 1.7 *Proportion (percentage) of men with specific numbers of regular and casual sexual partners (BMJ 1989)*

	Regular				Casual			
	0	1	2–5	6+	0	1	2–10	11+
Age at interview								
15–19	33	21	42	1	42	9	39	10
20–29	14	33	48	5	27	11	49	13
30–39	5	38	43	14	28	9	41	22
40–49	0	71	23	6	48	6	30	16
Total	10	40	42	8	31	9	42	17

By the age of 40, 13% of the men had had a vasectomy; this increased to 29% by the age of 50. There was no appreciable difference in vasectomy rate among social classes but it was higher in the south and midlands than in the north (18% vs. 12%). Of the 318 men who stated that they had at some time tried to father a child, 20% reported a period of six months or longer when they had attempted to do so and failed. However, only 7 (2%) had been unsuccessful in the long term.

Conclusion

Epidemiology is concerned with establishing cause rather than treatment, but the risk of premature death is of such magnitude that appropriate risk management is essential. The excess death rate in males may be partially preventable and general practitioners have an important role to play.

In four areas, risk-management strategies exist which could be carried out in general practice and are of proven value:
(1) helping men to stop smoking;
(2) identifying and treating high blood pressure;
(3) advising men to reduce alcohol consumption;
(4) advising and treating men with proven circulatory disease.

In other areas of risk management the evidence is much less clear. Any decision to change clinical practice will depend on the likely costs and benefits to both patients and practitioners and the doctors' own interests. For instance, advising men on the subject of taking more exercise or safe sex may produce substantial benefit for a few individuals at little additional cost.

Selective screening for male cancers is not yet feasible or desirable because of poor definition of high risk and the absence of appropriate screening tests.

References

Abramson, J., Gofin, J., Hopp, C., and Makler, A. (1978). The epidemiology of inguinal hernia. *Journal of Epidemiology and Community Health*, **32**, 59–67.

Allied Dunbar National Fitness Survey (1992). The Sports Council and Health Education Authority.

Berlin, J. and Colditz, G. (1990). A meta-analysis of physical activity in the prevention of coronary heart disease. *American Journal of Epidemiology*, **132**, 612–27.

Carbone, L., Cooper, C., Michet, C., Atkinson, E., O'Fallon, W., and Melton, L. (1992). Ankylosing spondylitis in Rochester Minnesota 1935–89. *Arthritis and Rheumatism*, **35**, 1476–82.

Cooper, C., Mc Alindon, T., Snow, S., *et al.* (1994). Mechanical and constitutional risk factors for symptomatic knee osteoarthritis. *Journal of Rheumatology*, **21**, 307–13.

Currey, H. and Hull, S. (1987). *Rheumatology for general practitioners.* Oxford University Press, Oxford.

Currie, W. J. (1979). Prevalence and incidence of gout in Great Britain. *Annals of Rheumatic Diseases*, **36**, 101–4.

DHSS/OPCS (1987). Hospital in-patient enquiry 1985. Series MB4 no. 26. HMSO, London.

Forman, D., and Chilvers, C. (1989). Sexual behaviour of young and middle-aged men in England and Wales. *British Medical Journal*, **298**, 1137–42.

Forman, D., Webb, P., and Parsonett, J. (1994). *H. pylori* and gastric cancer. *Lancet*, **343**, 243–4.

Gallegos, N., Dawson, J., Jarvis, M., and Hobsley, M. (1991). The risk of strangulation of groin hernias. *British Journal of Surgery*, **78**, 1171–3.

Giovannucci, E., Ascherio, A., Rimm, E., Colditz, G., Stamfer, M., and Willett, W. (1993*a*). A prospective cohort study of vasectomy and prostate cancer in US men. *Journal of the American Medical Association*, **269**, 873–8.

Giovannucci, E., Tosteson, T., Speizer, F., Ascherio, A., Vessey, M., and Colditz, G. (1993*b*). A retrospective cohort study of vasectomy and prostate cancer in US men. *Journal of the American Medical Association*, **269**, 878–82.

Gunnel, D. (1994). *Potential for preventing suicide*, Health Care Evaluation Unit, Bristol.

Haddon, W. (1980). Advances in epidemiology of injuries as a basis for public policy. *Public Health Reports*, **95**, 411.

Lancet (1987). The Drones Club. *Lancet*, **ii**, 1163.

Lancet (1992). Depression and suicide: are they preventable? *Lancet*, **340**, 700–1.

Lesko, S. M., Rosenberg, L., Shapiro, S. (1993). A case–control study of baldness in relation to myocardial infarction in men. *Journal of the American Medical Association*, **269**, 998–1003.

McCormick, A., Fleming, D., and Charlton, J. (1995). *Morbidity statistics from general practice. Fourth national study 1991–1992*. Series MB5 no. 3. HMSO, London.

Noriwa, A. and Kolomel, L. (1991). Prostate cancer: a current perspective. *American Journal of Epidemiology*, **13**, 200–25.

North, P. A., *et al.* (1988). Cigarette smoking as a risk factor for stroke – Framingham study. *Journal of the American Medical Association*, **259**, 1025.

Office of Population and Census Studies (1994). *Congenital malformations 1991.* HMSO, London.

RCGP/OPCS/DHSS (1986). *Morbidity statistics from general practice: third national study 1981–82.* MBJ no. 1. HMSO, London.

Robertson, L. S. (1991). Traumatic injury. In *Oxford textbook of public health* (ed. W. Holland, R. Detelo, and G. Knox), pp. 69–80. Oxford University Press, Oxford.

Ross, R. K., Paganini-Hill, A., and Henderson, B. E. (1988). Epidemiology of bladder cancer. In *Diagnosis and management of genito-urinary cancer* (ed. D. G. Skinner and G. Lieskovsky), pp. 23–31. WB Saunders, Philadelphia.

Schottenfeld, D., Warshauer, M. E., Sherlock, S., Zauber, A., Leder, M., and Payne. R. (1980). The epidemiology of testicular cancer in young adults. *American Journal of Epidemiology*, **112**, 232–46.

Silberberg, J. (1990). Estimating the benefit of cholesterol lowering: are risk factors for CHD multiplicative? *Journal of Clinical Epidemiology*, **43**, 875–9.

Smith, R. (1992). Promoting sexual health. *British Medical Journal*, **305**, 71.

Sparrow, J., O'Connon, G., and Weiss, S. (1988). The relation of airways response and atopy to the development of COAD. *Epidemiological Reviews*, **10**, 29–53.

Thomas, M., Goddard, E., Hicknam, M., and Hunter, P. (1994). *General Household Survey 1992* (GHS 23) OPCS. HMSO, London.

Veldhuyzen van Zanten, S. and Sherman, P. (1994). *H. pylori* infection as a cause of gastritis, duodenal ulcer, gastric cancer and dyspepsia: a systematic overview. *Canadian Medical Association Journal*, **150**, 177–85.

Webb, P. M., Knight, T., Greaves, S., Wilson, A., Newell, D., Elder, J., *et al.* (1994). Relation between infection with *H. pylori* and living conditions in childhood: evidence for person-to-person transmission in early life. *British Medical Journal*, **308**, 750–3.

Weinblatt, E., Shapiro, S., Frank, C., and Sage, R. (1968). Prognosis of men after myocardial infarction. *American Journal of Public Health*, **58**, 1329–47.

Westlake, S. and Frank, J. (1987). Testicular self-examination: an argument against routine teaching. *Family Practice*, **4**, 143–8.

PART I

Stages of life

CHAPTER TWO

The health problems of adolescent males

Ann McPherson and Aidan Macfarlane

There is a shortage of knowledge about adolescent health, although it is of great interest to health planners. More young females consult doctors than young males and GP consultations with adolescents are shorter than with adults. Appointments are usually made on the day of attendance and teenagers often feel uncomfortable with doctors and indeed vice versa. The delivery of primary care to adolescents can be improved and this chapter gives an upbeat account of adolescent health and highlights some unique aspects of male health.

Introduction

Adolescence is a period of rapid change – each loss of childhood representing a gain of adulthood. Loss of childhood – with its security blanket, the teddy bear, home-cooked meals, clothes bought, decisions made – means the adolescent gaining the independence to make personal decisions to buy his own clothes, eat what he wants and likes. Loss of a smooth face means both designer shadow and acne; loss of schoolfriends means gaining new friends, some of whom will present new risks at emotional, social, and health levels.

For their parents too there is a loss of involvement as adolescents feel an increased need for privacy and to 'do their own thing' in their own way. Parents may see the exchange of good home care for independent squalor as inexplicable and as failure. Adults who rarely learnt by being told what they should do when *they* were adolescents have to remember that tomorrow's adults will learn much by risk-taking, experimentation, and experience. Health professionals often have similar feelings to parents or guardians as it is often difficult to develop a rapport with, understand, and communicate with adolescents of both sexes.

For ease, adolescent males will be referred to as men and adolescent females as women.

Contact with the general practitioner

The main contacts the GP is likely to have with the adolescent will be over consultations concerning minor injuries and illnesses, sports injuries, and travel immunizations. Use of medicines and consultation rates seem to be clearly established at around 15 years of age with young males consulting less and taking less medicines than their female counterparts (Macfarlane *et al.* 1987). Most studies show that for all problems women consult more than men, but consultations are much more frequent for those problems labelled by GPs as 'trivial'. The only complaint that shows a reverse trend, with men consulting more than women, is in the category of accidents, injuries, poisoning, and violence.

Health concerns

Adolescent males are concerned about their health. In one study (Townsend *et al.* 1991), when 13, 15, and 17-year-olds were invited for a general practice health check, 73% attended, with a similar response rate in men and women. However, in another study (Donovan and McCarthy 1988), also in London, when the practice's 16-year-olds were called in for a health check, only 50% responded. Recent research suggests that the two areas that concern adolescents most in their relationships with GPs are confidentiality and being able to get telephone advice without giving their names. They wanted well-written information and most frequently expressed interest in sexually transmitted diseases, contraception, nutrition, acne, weight problems, and exercise (Macfarlane and McPherson 1996). The value of doing health checks on adolescents must be called into question, however, given the low prior probability of disease in this group. However, for practices wishing to target adolescent issues, there may be a receptive audience for whom they may make an important difference.

The common illnesses, as reported by adolescents themselves (Macfarlane *et al.* 1987) at a point in time, were coughs and colds (13%), hay fever (5%), skin problems (5%), and asthma (4%). Nearly three-quarters had taken medicines in the previous four weeks (40% of this was for headaches). Three-quarters of adolescents suffered from headaches and three-quarters again had fillings in their teeth. The commonest reasons for seeing their GP were for sore throats (7%), injuries (4%), gastrointestinal problems (4%), and skin problems (4%). Over a third of adolescents had visited their GP in the previous three months (90% of teenagers visit their GP during a year (Balding 1991)).

A similar study in Sweden which looked at the general health complaints of children aged 13–19 showed that they complained of acne (32.5%), sports injury or growth pain (32.4%), tiredness (29.3%), headache (28.4%), allergy or asthma (23.8%), stomach pains (22.8%), other pain (22.8%), sweating under arms or feet (16.1%), being too thin or fat (14.3%), and feeling low or in the dumps (13.3%) (Kohler and Jakobsson 1991).

Health promotion and the Health of the Nation targets

The UK government's document entitled Health of the Nation (HoN) contains targets that are very relevant to the health of adolescent males, although the document is not gender specific. The major HoN targets that are relevant to male adolescents are to:

(1) cut the smoking rate of 11–15 year-olds – from 8% in 1988 to 6% (60% of adults smokers started before the age of 16);
(2) cut the calories from fat from 40% to below 35% of total calorie intake(eating habits are embedded even as far back as the womb with the result of high cholesterol being laid down in the coronary arteries from an early age);
(3) cut deaths due to accidents in the under-15s by 33% – from 6.7 per 100 000 population in 1989 to no more than 4.5, and for the 15–24 age group by 25% – from 23.2 per 100 000 to no more than 17.4 (*the* major cause of death in young people);
(4) cut the pregnancy rate in under-16s by 50% – from 9.5 per 1000 girls aged 13–15 in 1989 to no more than 4.8 (pregnancy during the teens has a higher rate of prematurity and there are also a wide range of socio-economic consequences);
(5) cut the overall suicide rate by 15% – from 11.1 per 100 000 population in 1990 to no more than 9.4 (there is a steady rise in male adolescent suicides at the present time).

GPs, like other health professionals, will need to accept that the achievement of most of these targets will occur when individuals themselves and the government play their part and accept their respective responsibilities for their health. These responsibilities include the narrowing of social inequalities, banning advertising on smoking, and enacting legislation concerning cycle helmet-wearing. It also includes helping doctors understand adolescent males so that the concerns of this vulnerable group do not continue to be unmet.

The normal adolescent male

Growth

An updated set of centile charts for height and weight have been produced (Figs 2.1 and 2.2), based on recent data. This indicates that both the male and female population of young people are, at any particular age whilst still growing, taller than they used to be in the 1950s.

Pubertal changes

The frequency distribution of age at different pubertal criteria for males are shown in Fig. 2.3. It is usually considered wise to refer a young man for further investigation if he shows no signs of secondary sexual characteristics by the age of 14.

Penis size is often something that young men would like reassurance about but never

---

Box 2.1 *Age and penis sizes in adolescence*

Age	Range of penile lengths
10	4–8 cm
12	5–10 cm
14	6–14 cm
16	10–15 cm
18	11–17 cm

Fig. 2.1 *Boy's height 5–18 years*

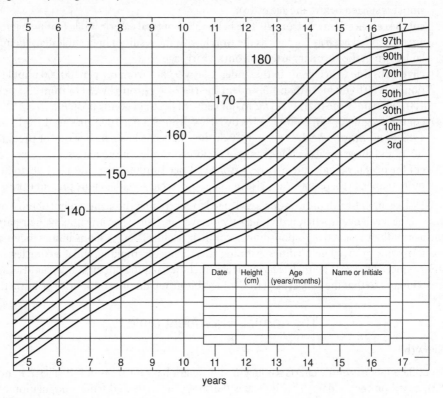

years

dare ask. Boys often use the agony columns of teenage magazines for such information as it seems to be a matter that is too sensitive for the normal information networks among their peers. Judiciously photocopied, the information in Box 2.1 may be invaluable for adolescent males and for those who advise them on sex and health education matters.

For most men and boys it was found that however small the non-erect penis was, penises were all roughly the same length when erect.

Sources of advice

Where do adolescent boys get their information from? Adolescents give parents as their best source of information about health, closely followed by friends and then television, books, and magazines (Challener 1990). There are many teenage magazines for girls, but there are few male equivalents. When asked, many teenage boys admit to reading these magazines even if they do not buy them. For example, *Just 17*, read by adolescents aged 13 onwards, has a boys' problem page. Significantly fewer young men that women see TV soaps as a source of information.

When a sample of adolescents were asked whom they first turn to for advice on health

Fig. 2.2 *Boy's weight 5–18 years*

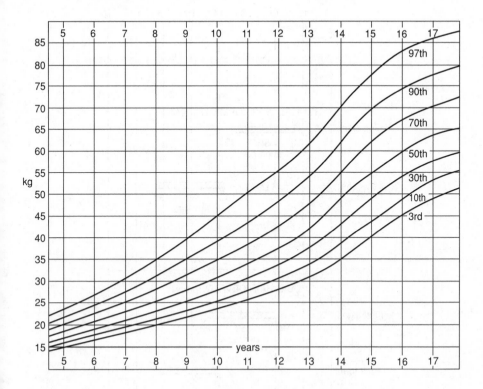

problems, 86% said they turned to parents (Macfarlane *et al.* 1987):

- but 70% of young men turned to their mothers first
- 7% of young men turned to their fathers
- 7% of young men consulted a doctor
- 2% of young men first consulted a friend.

The message from this study is that it is very important to ensure the parents are giving correct advice. Males see their mothers as primary sources of health advice with fathers playing a tiny role. Fathers may well be important role models in terms of lifestyle, even if their advice on health matters is not sought. It also highlights the small role friends play in giving health advice, which conflicts with the apparent influence of peer pressure which can, of course, be so harmful. As boys get older, the balance does appear to shift away from parents towards more private sources of information.

On sex

Around 40% of 15-year-olds quoted their friends as being the main source of information about sex with only 20% quoting their parents, whereas to the question 'Who *should* be the main source of information about sex', only 7% felt that it should be their friends and

Fig. 2.3 *Frequency distribution of age at different pubertal criteria for males*

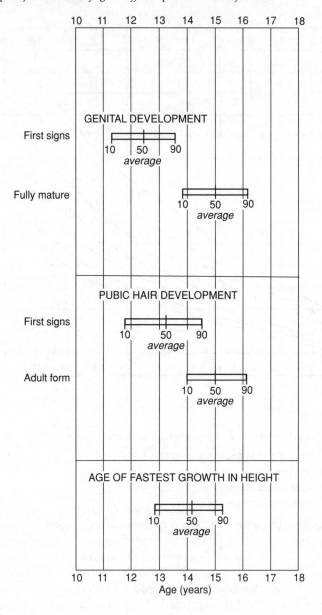

65% felt that it should be their parents (Epstein *et al.* 1989). It appears that informed discussion about sex is not particularly appealing to males. In discussing sex, males appear to be reticent with parents, friends, sexual partners, and medical professionals. When they do manage, they are most likely to discuss it with friends of their own age (75%) and least likely to talk to GPs or family planning clinics (6%) (Health Education Authority 1992). Not surprisingly then, it also appears that males are more ignorant of the facts about sex than women – at all ages.

What they *do* want advice from their GP about

Two studies show that more adolescents (both male and female) would like to discuss health-related subjects – sexually transmitted diseases, contraception, nutrition, fears about cancer – with a health professional (GP, school doctor, or nurse) than actually do (Challener 1990; Epstein *et al.* 1989). Is this because health professionals are seen as 'curing disease' rather than offering advice? Is it difficulty over accessibility? Is it shyness on the part of the teenager? These questions still need to be answered and the results responded to accordingly. However, as already pointed out, 90% of teenagers do visit their GP during a year (Balding 1991).

Exercise

The majority of male adolescents who take part in sports do so because they enjoy it rather than because it is 'healthy' (Macfarlane *et al.* 1987), and a further study (Townsend *et al.* 1991) showed that boys aged 13–15 exercised for a median of three hours per week and girls two hours per week. In males aged 16–19, in the month prior to being asked 40% had played soccer, 28% had cycled, and 24% had swum. Young women are less active – a quarter did gymnastics or aerobics, a quarter swam, and 14% cycled (*Social Trends* 1997). Nineteen per cent of men see themselves as very fit and 11% as unfit compared with 10% and 19% of women respectively. Thus 70% of young men see themselves as 'fit' and campaigns at encouraging sport have to take this into account.

Risk-taking (experience-gaining)

This is an area where inferences have to be drawn from data on, and experience of, different forms of adolescent behaviour. For example, although 47% of a sample of teenage cyclists wore a cycle helmet, only 18% *always* wore one (Joshi *et al.* In press). Males and females were no different in this, but those aged less than 15 were more likely to wear one than the over 15-year-olds. Helmet wearers were more likely to wear seat-belts in the back of cars and were less likely to smoke. When asked to rate themselves as a cyclist, males were more likely than females to rate themselves as 'reckless' and were less likely to wear helmets.

Another example (Health Education Authority 1992) is that men are less likely than women to see drug-taking as a health risk. For cannabis, 51% of men and 65% of women rated its regular use as being harmful to their health.

Major threats and worries

The two major threats to the health of adolescent males are poverty and ignorance, with the added threat of war in some countries. At present, every indicator seems to show that there is increasing poverty in the United Kingdom (Spencer 1996).

Health issues

General health

There is no difference by gender of perception of 'good' or 'bad' health amongst adolescents, with 95% feeling that their health is either very good or fairly good and only 5% as 'not very good'. However, in a survey, 33% of men and 42% of women aged 14–17 had time off school over a four-week period. Sixty-three per cent of men had taken some medicine over a four-week period – the main reason being for 'headaches' (Macfarlane *et al.* 1987). Further observations about health include:

(1) over three-quarters of adolescents of both sexes see themselves as responsible for their own health and understand that the way they choose to live will influence their health (Macfarlane *et al.* 1987);

(2) young men are less likely to worry about their health than young women (Bendelow and Oakley 1993);

(3) young men are significantly more likely than young women to see parents as being responsible for their health, particularly in relation to hereditary factors (Bendelow and Oakley 1993).

Deaths

In 1991, in the 15–24 age group, there were 806 male deaths compared with 314 female deaths per million population. Sixty-seven per cent of the male deaths were due to injury and poisoning compared with 47% of the female deaths (OPCS 1991).

Suicide

There are about five recorded suicides in children aged under 15 each year in the UK. However, there has been a marked increase in death in the 'undetermined and accidental due to poisoning' group in the last 30 years, and these may represent a significant increase in actual suicides in this age group. Rates of suicide in 15–19 year-olds are significantly higher for men than women (6/100 000 vs. 1.8/100 000 population) and are increasing in young males, amongst whom it is the second most common cause of death.

Whilst the reasons for the rising rates are unclear, increasing alcohol abuse, unemployment, and family breakdown have been suggested as being contributory. The commonest successful methods used are hanging, car exhausts, and self-poisoning, with those 'attempting' suicide going in for self-poisoning, using over-the-counter medications rather than prescribed medications for themselves or a parent.

Psychological disorders

Neurotic disorders, anxiety states, depression, and affective psychoses are all less common in males in general than in females. Adolescence is no exception to these findings. Drug dependence is the complete opposite with many more males being dependent on drugs than females. This difference is far more pronounced in the teenage years than at any other time in the life cycle (Fourth National Morbidity Study 1991–92).

Injuries

Injury, accidental or otherwise is the commonest cause of death for adolescent males. The mortality and morbidity rates in the 16–24 year age group are considerably higher for males than females. In the 17–20 age group overall, the car accident rate is four times higher than for people learning to drive later in life, and when an accident occurs they are nine times more likely to be at fault that another person involved.

In a study of 14–17 year-olds (Macfarlane *et al.* 1987), 24% had had an accident in the previous month – with no difference between the genders, though more men than women had sports and cycling-related accidents. In a study of adolescent cyclists in Oxfordshire (Joshi, 1994), 13% had experienced an accident that had necessitated a visit to either the emergency department or their GP.

The GP's role can really only be to reaffirm information about cycle helmets, safety belt wearing, drinking and driving, etc. – but four things to remember about teenagers are:

(1) they are slaves to peer pressure (to what their friends think and do);
(2) they are attracted to speed and danger;
(3) they need to explore their limits;
(4) they think they are immortal.

Weight and diet

Body image is very important to both males and females in the 16–19 age group. Nineteen per cent of males think they are overweight compared with 40% of females. In fact, using the body mass index (BMI), only 5% of 16-year-old men and 11% of 19-year-old men could be considered overweight. [However, BMI in this age group may not be a reliable measure.] Twenty-five per cent of males think they are underweight compared with 12% of females, and although GPs will occasionally see anorexic males, all eating problems are far more common in females of this age group (Health Education Authority 1992). It has been suggested that men are more commonly prone to compulsive exercise as a means of weight control, but there are no proper studies to substantiate this.

In almost all concerns about food, women rate higher than men with only 25% of men seeing a healthy diet as important to them and 38% seeing health foods as boring. Fifty-eight per cent of men believe that as long as they are reasonably active they can eat what they like. Only 7% of men have tried dieting, and only 4% of men are vegetarian (Health Education Authority 1992).

Skin

Seventeen per cent of boys and 31% of girls have skin problems – the commonest problem being acne. Warts and verrucas are the other common problems (Macfarlane *et al.* 1987). Skin problems are a common presentation to the GP in this age group, and while spots may be medically trivial they are very important to the sufferer. Indeed, the manner in which the doctor deals with such problems may determine the relationship the young man will have with the practice and any advice that is proffered.

Sexual abuse

It is almost impossible to get reliable data about the prevalence of sexual abuse in any population, and estimates continue to vary widely. As one example, in a questionnaire administered to 12–17 year-old adolescents attending nine London comprehensive schools, sexual abuse was reported by 16% of the 213 girls replying to the question and by 3% of the 167 boys (Epstein *et al.* 1989).

Sex

There are many studies about age of first intercourse, with considerable variation between them, but it would appear that around 28% (Welling 1994) of males have had full sexual intercourse by 16. Men are much more likely than women to perceive peer pressure as a reason for having sex. Men are less likely to have long-term relationships; they are likely to have more partners with 17% claiming (or boasting!) to have had four partners or more in the last year (Health Education Authority 1992).

Contraception

In a study of 16–18 year-old sexually active men, 60% claimed to have used a condom on the last occasion they had intercourse with 36% also mentioning that they knew their partner was on the Pill. Six per cent stated that neither they nor their partner used any form of contraception and 7% couldn't remember! Condom use appears to decline with age, from 77% usage at 16 to 47% at 19 years of age. It is more common amongst those in a casual relationship and from the upper social classes.

Some young men do not seem to make the connection between sexual intercourse and pregnancy, instead seeing intercourse as a conquest without responsibility; but the high number using contraception indicates a highly responsible attitude towards sexual intercourse.

Thirty-eight per cent of men felt embarrassed about buying condoms in shops in spite of the fact that (a) condoms were seen as the most effective protection against infection, and (b) 72% of young people agreed that it is too risky to have sex without a condom nowadays (Health Education Authority 1992). There is a need for greater availability of condoms via slot machines, and we would do well to copy the Scandinavian practice of having such machines placed in public streets rather than toilets in pubs and clubs. Similarly, manufacturers need to consider a range of pack sizes that can be dispensed from such machines rather than the traditional pack of three.

Smoking

While smoking in the adult population is falling steadily, smoking in children and young people is showing no clear downwards trend and there is evidence that it is rising in teenage girls (Balding 1997). Figures show that 10% of 11–15 year-olds smoke regularly, consuming an average of 50 cigarettes a week; 17 000 000 cigarettes are smoked each week by 11–15 year olds in England alone. Everyday, 450 children start smoking and 300 adults die from smoking-related diseases. There is no social-class gradient (unlike adults) for smoking in the young. The most common age for experimenting with the first cigarette is between 9 and 12. Regular smoking starts between the ages of 12 and 13; by 15 to 19 many smokers want to give up. Factors affecting cigarette consumption are affordability, tobacco advertising, others smoking in the family, friends who smoke, availability of supplies. The paper *Guidelines for health promotion, No. 33* suggests a number of anti-smoking strategies covering the NHS, education, mass media, sales of cigarettes to children, and pressure on the government (Faculty of Public Health Medicine 1993).

Drug use

Approximately half of the 16–19 year-olds in this country have been offered drugs, most often cannabis (39%), followed by acid (21%), amyl nitrate (19%), magic mushrooms (19%), ecstasy (17% and on the rise), and amphetamines (13%). Men (compared with women) are significantly more likely (37%) to have been offered class A drugs (heroine, crack, cocaine, ecstasy or acid) and 50% have been offered class B drugs (mainly cannabis). Actual experimentation with drugs is also higher amongst men (37%) and, not unnaturally, this rises with age. Over half the men studied (52%) agreed that most young people will try out drugs at some time in spite of the fact that 91% thought that taking drugs harmed their health (Health Education Authority 1992).

Alcohol use

From ages 16–19, regular consumption of alcohol is higher amongst men than women, the difference widening as they get older. At 16 years of age, 35% of men and 27% of women are regular drinkers and by 19 this has risen to 75% compared with 59%.

Alarmingly, drinking does appear to be an area of some ignorance as far as ill effects on health are concerned, with 75% of men aged 16–19 considering that drinking has no effects on health. As to the other dangers, 11% of men aged 16 have been involved in a physical fight after drinking, which rises to 20% at age 19. The proportion of men who have been in trouble with the police after drinking rises steadily from 5% at 16 to 12% at 19. Fifteen per cent of men aged 16–19 have ridden a bicycle after drinking alcohol, and 4% have driven a car whilst considering themselves to be 'over the legal limit'. Twenty-four per cent of men admitted to having a 'one night stand' after drinking alcohol, which was three times more common than with women (Health Education Authority 1992).

Confidentiality issues

Unless young people feel that confidentiality, if required, will be respected by all members of the primary health care team, it is unlikely that they will turn to this source for help and advice when they are in need.

The outcome of the Gillick rulings (Gillick vs. Wisbech and W. Norfolk AHA [1985] 3A 11 ER 402 HL) has been that if you consider that the young person can fully comprehend the issues concerning their health problem, then they should also be fully consulted, their views taken into account, and they should be able to provide their *own* choices re 'informed consent'. Although most of the discussion concerning this has been over giving contraceptive advice to girls under 16, the same basic rules apply to adolescent men. Most young men can be encouraged or persuaded that normally it is in their own best interests to discuss their health problems with their parents – if they have not already done so. There will, of course, be times when this is not appropriate, and this should not be a problem legally.

Conclusion

Despite the popular and often negative image of the adolescent male, he is someone who is well-informed and concerned on a wide range of health and environmental issues, investigative, thoughtful, and, on the whole, happy with his lot. The GP, however, may actually feel they have little to offer them, but if they (and perhaps a parent) manage to identify or exclude major pathology, avoid the alienation of face-to-face confrontations, listen carefully, understand the unintelligible, and maintain negotiations – much will have been achieved.

References

Balding, J. *et al.* (1997). *Young People in 1996.* 1997 Schools Health Education Unit. School of Education University of Exeter. Heavitree Rd Exeter EX1 2LU.

Balding, J. (1991). *Young people into the nineties. A nationwide study of 125 933 young people between the ages of 11 and 16.* Book 1.

Bendelow, G. and Oakley A. (1993). *Young people and cancer.* Social Science Research Unit, London.

Buckler, J. (1987). *The adolescent years: the ups and downs of growing up.* Castlemead Publications, London, England.

Challener, J. (1990). Health education in secondary schools – is it working? A study of 1418 Cambridgeshire pupils. *Public Health,* **104,** 195–205.

Donovan, C. F. and McCarthy, S. (1988). Is there a place for adolescent screening in general practice? *Health Trends,* **2,** 20, 64.

Epstein, R., Rice, P., and Wallace, P. (1989). Teenagers' health concerns: implications for primary health care professionals. *Journal of the Royal College of General Practitioners,* **39,** 247–9.

Faulds-Wood, L. (1993). *Accidents – how can we prevent them?* Report from 'Health of the Teenage Nation' meeting, Oxford, 1993. Available from National Adolescent Health Unit, Oxford Regional Health Authority, Old Road, Headington, Oxford, OX3 7LG.

Guidelines for Health Promotion, No. 33. Faculty of Public Health Medicine, 4 St Andrew's Place, London NW1 4LB. May 1993.

Hawton, K. (1996). Suicide and attempted suicide in young people. In *Adolescent Medicine.* Royal College of Physicians, London.

Health Education Authority (1992). *Today's young adults. 16–19 year-olds' looks at diet, alcohol, smoking, drugs, and sexual behaviour.* HEA, London.

Kohler, L. and Jakobsson, G. (1991). *Children's health in Sweden.* From Allmanna Forlaget, Kundt-janst, S-106 47 Stockholm, Sweden. ISBN 91 38 11230 2. Goteborg, Sweden.

Joshi, M., Beckett, K., and Macfarlane, A. (1994). Cycle helmet wearing in teenagers - do health beliefs influence behaviour? *Archives of Diseases in Childhood,* **71,** 536–9.

Macfarlane, A. *et al.* (1987). Teenagers and their health. *Archives of Diseases in Childhood*, **62**, 1125–9.

Macfarlane, A. and McPherson, A. (1995). Primary health care and adolescence. Editorial. *British Medical Journal*, **311**, 825–6.

Macfarlane, A. and McPherson, A. (1996). *The new diary of a teenage health freak.* Oxford University Press, Oxford.

OPCS (1982). *Second National Morbidity Study 1981–82.* HMSO, London.

OPCS (1991). *DH2 No. 18 Mortality statistics 1991.* HMSO, London.

OPCS (1992). *Morbidity statistics from general practice.* Fourth National Morbidity Study 1991–92. HMSO, London.

Preece, M. *Archives of Diseases in Childhood.* In press.

Social trends 27. 1997 edition. ISBN 0 11 620838–4. London, The Stationery Office.

Spencer, N. *Poverty and child health.* Radcliffe Medical Press, Oxford, 1996.

Townsend, J. *et al.* (1991). Adolescent smokers seen in general practice: health, lifestyle, physical measurements, and response to anti-smoking advice. *British Medical Journal*, **303**, 947–50.

Welling, K. *et al.* (1994). *Sexual behaviours in Great Britain. The national survey of sexual attitudes and lifestyles.* Penguin, London.

CHAPTER THREE

Adult life

David Jewell

Adulthood is the time when men are most absent from the doctor's office, and little is written about it in the medical literature. We want to redress this deficiency and a surprising number of chapters in the book concern themselves with disorders and diseases that occur in adult males. It is a time of many life events like marriage, fatherhood, divorce, and work-related problems. Men's emotions in this phase of life have come under scrutiny by both sexes and the consensus seems to be that adult males are quite afraid of their emotions. This has implications for the manner in which men deal with health symptoms and life crises. The language used to express depressive feelings has an emotional content that may well be rejected or denied by men, and this in turn has important implications for history-taking. The vulnerability of the adult single male to depression and suicide is highlighted in this chapter. Is there such a thing as the male menopause? The author is emphatic that there is not, making his arguments worth sceptical scrutiny.

Introduction

Men's adult years are those in which they are most obviously absent from the world of medicine and health care. The 1991–92 National Morbidity Survey reported consultation rates of 4.2 per year for women, compared with 2.7 for men (Royal College of General Practitioners, Office of Population Censuses and Surveys, Department of Health 1995). The difference between rates for men and women is particularly marked for those aged 25–44 (4.3 compared with 1.9), and much less for the age group 45–64 (4.3 compared with 3.0). The excess in the 25–44 age group might be thought to arise from consultations related to pregnancy and contraception. However, the consultation rates for women show an excess over those for men in all diagnostic groups except the category comprising accidents, injuries, poisoning, and violence; there is even a small excess in the category of diseases of the circulatory system. It is impossible to state whether this reflects a difference in illness behaviour or a true difference in the experience of illness. Although some information on illness behaviour in men and women exists in the field of mental health, the most frequently quoted study on symptoms perceived and reported to general practitioners was of women only (Morrell and Wale 1976). Similarly, while Wallace and Haines (1984) reported that men and women differed little in their feelings about the extent general practitioners were, or should be, interested in advice on smoking, alcohol, weight problems, and fitness, the qualitative study published by Stott and Pill (1990) which set out to elaborate Wallace and Haines's findings was conducted only on mothers. There is no escaping the conclusion that we know little about the different ways in which men experience health and illness or their relationships with health services.

Adulthood is a time when women's lives are subject to major life-event changes, demanding considerable adaptation. Superficially, men would appear to have much less to contend with. They have arrived at a stage of maturity where they hope to be able to realize their potential at work, where they have confidence in their health, and a clear sense of their physical and mental identity. However, it would be wrong to see this period as one of serene stability. In an essay on the young adult years, Rindfuss (1991) pointed out that men aged 18–30 are at their period of maximum fertility and migration, with the highest rates of marriage, remarriage, and divorce. The group contains 15% of the married population and contributes 32% of divorces. While most men in this age group are working, their first jobs may be unstable and comparatively poorly paid, and they may lack the economic and political power that many men are assumed to enjoy. They share with women the problem of role diversity and transition between roles. Throughout the adult years men face the problems which surround the world of work, either too much of it or not enough, both of which are discussed elsewhere in this book (see Chapters 5 and 6). At the end of this stage in their lives, as they approach retirement and the consequent loss of economic power, they may have to confront a decline in physical and mental health. Men's mental health itself presents a puzzle. While there is a consistent excess of depression among adult women, suicide, which is usually seen as an indicator of depression, shows a consistent excess among men.

Men's absence from the consulting room when compared with women might imply that such life changes have no expression in their health. This chapter will discuss the health consequences of the life events that occur in men's adult years, and which appear to be largely unseen by clinicians. It will also discuss the puzzle of suicide and depression.

Men as husbands

The conventional view of marriage is that men's health is enhanced by marriage while that of women is diminished. The influence of marriage on men's health is well-documented, using a wide variety of evidence. At the 'hard' end, there is data on the effects on mortality. In a study of mortality in a group admitted to hospitals in Baltimore with myocardial infarction, married men had better survival than the non-married group. The mortality for the hospital period, adjusted for factors that included age, sex, race, smoking history, and history of previous ischaemic heart disease, was 19% in married men compared with 26% in single men. Married men continued to have significantly better survival rates for 10 years after discharge from hospital (Chandra et al. 1983). Similar findings were reported in a 10-year longitudinal study of middle-aged Dutch men recruited from the general population for a cardiovascular screening programme (Mendes de Leon *et al.* 1992).

The non-married group comprises three components of never married, divorced, and widowed men, and one would predict different effects among these groups. For instance, any apparent worsening in health might result from the effects of loss following divorce and widowhood and not affect men who have never married. This is illustrated in a secondary analysis of men born in Gothenburg between 1915 and 1925 who participated in a primary coronary heart disease prevention. During a follow-up period of 11 years the all-cause mortality rate was 9% for married men compared with 20% for divorced men (Rosengren *et al.* 1989).

Being widowed has for long been recognized as a risk factor for premature death. Colin Murray Parkes has pointed out that in Heberden's mortality returns for London in 1657 the simple term 'griefe' was an acceptable cause of death (Parkes 1972). Parkes himself followed up a sample of 4000 widowers aged 55 or over for a total of nine years. There was a rise in mortality of 40% among the widowers. This excess occurred in the first six months after bereavement, after which time mortality quickly fell to the expected rate. Two-thirds of the excess mortality was caused by ischaemic heart disease (Parkes *et al.* 1969). A similar increase in mortality was observed over a slightly longer period in a study following a sample of the UK 1971 census over 10 years. Here, excess mortality was seen in malignant and respiratory disease as well as ischaemic heart disease, but the largest excess was found among deaths due to violence and accidents (Jones 1987). The relationship is supported by the finding that those men who remarry after bereavement are less likely to die than those who remain single. However, this may be evidence for a selection bias, that the healthy men are more likely to remarry than the unhealthy (Helsing *et al.* 1981).

Finally, there is the group of never-married men. In the Dutch study discussed above, the single men had higher relative risks of both total mortality and coronary mortality than both divorced and widowed men (Mendes de Leon *et al.* 1992). The adjusted risks were 2.3 for total mortality and 2.9 for coronary mortality (compared with 1.7 and 2.2 for all the non-married men).

There are three different mechanisms by which marriage could be bringing such benefits to men. Either it is through selection, implying that healthy men are more likely to marry than less healthy ones, or through marriage bringing with it emotional and psychological benefits that influence physical health, or through married men following more healthy lifestyles. As mentioned above, some, but not all, of the excess mortality of divorced men in the study by Rosengren *et al.* (1989) was explained by an excess of alcohol intake and smoking in the non-married group. Horwitz and White (1991), in a prospective study of men and women aged 21–24, showed that the group that had not married by the age of 24 contained a higher proportion of problem drinkers at the age of 21. In other words, marriage was being delayed in those with alcohol problems, supporting the selection hypothesis. However, the same study found no such relationship for depression, with no evidence that less depressed people were more likely to be married at the age of 24. A different conclusion is suggested in a meta-analysis of 12 longitudinal studies, where being never married or becoming single was associated with increased alcohol consumption, but where becoming married was accompanied by a drop in alcohol consumption at all ages (Temple *et al.* 1991).

That marriage seems to make men happier is also widely accepted. For instance, Gove *et al.* (1983) showed that being married was associated with higher scores on measures of satisfaction with home life, general mental health, overall happiness, and satisfaction with life overall. Marital status was a powerful predictor of mental health; better than age, race, or childhood background. Of the non-married groups, the widowed men had the lowest scores on all scales. A similar finding was reported in a study using a psychological screening questionnaire, in which married men were found to have lower rates of minor affective disorder than single men (Bebbington *et al.* 1991).

Such data therefore support the popular view of marriage as working to men's advantage. However, the evidence fails to support the view that this is at the expense of women's health. For instance, data from the United States for 1966–68 showed that mortality was lower for the married compared with the single in both men and women (Kobrin and Hendershot 1977). Similarly, in a study on men and women in northern Norway using an abbreviated version of the General Health Questionnaire, the married of both sexes had lower rates of psychological distress than the single (Hansen and Jacobsen 1989). The findings quoted above, linking marital status with mental health, applied to both men and women (Gove *et al.* 1983). The quality of the marriage, assessed by the men and women participating in the survey, was a powerful predictor of the happiness on all scales. This is not surprising since one would expect marital happiness to be a component, rather than a determinant, of overall life satisfaction and home life satisfaction. However, the authors noted that marital *quality* was a more powerful predictor of happiness for women, whereas marital *status* was the more powerful predictor for men. What matters for women is how good the marriage is, whereas for men it is being married at all.

Men as fathers

The gap between the popular perception of marriage as bad for women, and the reality, can be at least partly explained by the effect of children on the marriage. There is substantial evidence that child-rearing significantly increases the risk to women of depression (see below). Such findings echo the evidence from Brown and Harris's classic study of depression among women, which found that having three children under the age of five years was a strong predictor for developing depression (Brown and Harris 1978).

This raises the question whether having children has any effect on the health of fathers. The existence of couvade, in which the partners of pregnant women experience some of the physical symptoms of pregnancy, is widely known. The anthropologists who studied it in primitive societies interpreted its existence in a number of ways. For instance, in matriarchal societies it was seen as a means whereby fathers staked a claim to the future offspring. Alternatively, the phenomenon can be seen as rituals shared by father and mother in order to make statements in a society where laws of inheritance are unclear (Lewis 1982).

Although such examples represent an extreme, they may shed light on the experience of men in western societies. In different studies, 48–65% of expectant fathers report troublesome symptoms over the course of pregnancy, with the numbers falling substantially after delivery (Ferkeitch and Mercer 1989). Nausea, indigestion, fatigue, and backache figure prominently among the symptoms reported, and therefore they could be taken to comprise modern-day couvade. Mostly, these studies have not been rigorous in comparing the partners of expectant mothers with those of non-expectant women. One study which compared the gastrointestinal symptoms of husbands of pregnant women with those of non-pregnant women concluded that 11% of men suffered from symptoms, predominantly loss of appetite, nausea, and vomiting which could be ascribed to the pregnancy. In the same study it was also reported that parity had no effect; symptoms occurred at the same rate in second as in first pregnancies (Trethowan and Conlon 1965). They concluded that the symptoms were somatic expressions of anxiety associated with pregnancy. More recently, Masoni *et al.* (1994) has compared 73 husbands of pregnant women with those of non-pregnant women. In this case there was an excess of nausea in the pregnancy group, but all other symptoms were less common than in the non-pregnant group. Ninety-two per cent of the men showed emotional involvement in the pregnancy and 37% reported fear or anxiety, although such anxiety is not a consistent finding in all studies (Ferkeitch and Mercer 1989; Scott-Hayes 1982).

Three cautionary notes are important here. First, any anxiety that occurs in the course of pregnancy could be linked to circumstances around pregnancy, such as the sense of increasing financial and general responsibility, as much as to the medical events of pregnancy (Lewis 1982). Second, as Scott-Hayes points out, those who voluntarily agree to participate, as happened in her own study, may be a self-selecting group with positive attitudes to pregnancy and the results may be difficult to extrapolate to an unselected population. Third, men who, together with their wives, found a first pregnancy very stressful may avoid further pregnancies, distorting the parity effects reported.

Generalizing at all loses the variety of experience felt by different men. Not surprisingly, in a study exploring men's own perceptions of their 'careers' as partners of pregnant women, Lewis found a range of responses (1982). Many shared the euphoria felt by their partners. Others reported their wives as moody or difficult; when this happened they either saw themselves providing stability or reported that some of their wives' moodiness rubbed off on them.

The last aspect of fatherhood which needs to be noted are the more general effects that children have on men. For instance, Ferkeitch and Mercer (1989) noted a reduction in the overall sense of health in their sample. Similarly, a study of 96 couples reported a reduction in marital satisfaction from shortly before to three months after birth (Tomlinson 1987). The differences noted were small but consistent, and they did affect men and women equally.

The overall picture is not that men's health is substantially altered by fatherhood; there is no suggestion of a major burden of hidden or unrecognized illness. The impression indeed is that the health problems reflect the subordinate, at times insignificant role that men play in bringing up children. This, in turn, is reflected in the way that children are seen in surgery with their mothers so much more often than with their fathers. If this is changing, so that men take a more substantial part in their children's upbringing, then general practitioners will need to be sensitive to subtle influences on men's health as well as make the services accessible under such circumstances.

Men's friendships

If the evidence on marriage and health points to marriage exerting a powerful, beneficial effect on men's health, then a similar beneficial effect might be produced by other important social relationships. One American study which followed a sample of men aged 35–69 found that those reporting themselves to be more actively involved in social relationships were significantly less likely to die during the follow-up period of 9–12 years. The association was consistent across a variety of different social measures, including marriage, relationships with friends, and involvement in voluntary organizations. Passive or solitary leisure activities, such as watching television or listening to the radio, were associated with a higher rate of death, although exercise may be a strong confounding variable where this is concerned (House *et al*. 1982). A similar Swedish study followed a group of men born in 1933, and aged 50 at recruitment, for seven years. Significant life events in the year before recruitment to the study were significantly associated with mortality, but this only applied to men who were categorized as having low levels of emotional support (Rosengren *et al*. 1993). Again the paper makes no distinction between emotional support from marriage partners or from others. It is a pity that this distinction was omitted from the study since the conventional view is that men get little emotional support from their friendships, as discussed below. Nevertheless, it does demonstrate how friendships could provide a protective effect. Curiously, and despite so much that has been written about male friendship, these were the only two references directly linking friendship and health that came out of extensive literature searches in the course of writing this chapter.

In the debate about gender and behaviour in the 1990s, about female and male values, and 'new men', the field of male friendships represents a fascinating microcosm. A modern convention has developed that relationships between men are less intimate, and therefore less close, than those between women. Seidler (1992), for instance, drawing largely on his own feelings, talks about men being afraid of their own emotions. This in turn he relates to the protestant work ethic which rewards independence and competitiveness. Men are brought up, largely in the absence of their fathers, afraid to express vulnerability and ask for support.

Wellman (1992) studied a group of men and women in Toronto in order to find out in more detail what happens within their family and friendship networks. When emotional support was considered it was true that the women all looked to their female friends for this, and for the men their female friends were more likely than their male friends to provide it. However, almost all men received emotional support from at least one male friend. The word 'intimacy' has different meanings for men and women. Among male college students it meant shared activity, whereas for women it meant being together and talking (Caldwell and Peplau 1982).

Similar arguments surround group behaviour. Here, the stereotypes are the traditional settings of men's and women's friendships: women's in more intimate domestic settings, and men's in the more public settings of work, clubs, pubs, and bars. In primitive societies, exclusively male groups may operate to help men to consolidate their power and to socialize the younger men into a power structure that simultaneously excludes women. Equivalent groups in contemporary societies can work in the same way if, as has been suspected for certain male groups, real work is done during apparently harmless but closed social gatherings.

How far these differences between men and women affect health and health care is open to speculation. There is a lot of information about the ways in which people handle symptoms and decide whether to consult a doctor. Most will discuss their symptoms with family and friends in order to assess the seriousness and risks of a particular symptom and, perhaps not surprisingly, at least one study has reported that men use lay networks less than women when they have to make decisions about their health (Meininger 1986). An earlier study of myocardial infarction found that when husbands were suffering from chest pain, it was often their wives who took the decision to call a doctor (Finlayson and McEwen 1977).

Apart from the protective effect of close relationships on mortality discussed above, the most likely way in which the subject of male friendships will influence primary care concerns the 'preconsultation pathway', or the process of discussing and dealing with symptoms between their appearance and the decision whether or not to consult a doctor. Brown and Harris (1978) established that women who were at risk of becoming depressed when there were trigger events could be partially protected if, among other protecting factors, they had a close confiding relationship with one other person. If it is assumed that when this happens intimate discussion is providing the protection, then it is likely that married men will receive such support from their wives, and that single men may be particularly vulnerable. Research highlights the adverse effect of life events on males and emphasizes the vulnerability of single, emotionally unsupported males to psychological and physical illness.

Depression

In 1995, the numbers of deaths from suicide and self-inflicted injury were 2787 men and 783 women (Office for National Statistics 1997). More striking than the numbers is the trend with time. In a review of the figures for suicide deaths in England and Wales between 1911 and 1990, Charlton *et al.* (1992) showed that the male excess has been consistent over the whole of the period. The rate for both men and women dropped at the time of both world wars, with the drop more marked in men, and there was a drop for both sexes again between 1961 and 1975. Since 1975, however, there has been a striking divergence, with the rates for women continuing to fall while the rates for men have risen (Fig. 3.1). Both the absolute rates and the recent rise are most clearly shown in men aged 15–29, and in those living in deprived areas (Gunnell *et al.* 1995; McLoone 1996). In the Scotland, the suicide rate in 1991–93 in deprived areas was double that in the most affluent areas (McLoone 1996). Within Bristol and district, rates for suicide were strongly linked to rates for admission to hospital following parasuicide (Gunnell *et al.* 1995). A survey in the south west of England showed rates for parasuicide to be lower among men but less than might be expected with men contributing 45% of all admissions to hospital (Gunnell *et al.* 1996). The rise of male suicide in the United Kingdom is also seen in most other European countries: only in West Germany was the rate for those aged 25–44 falling in the years 1970–91 (Charlton *et al.* 1993).

In attempting to identify more closely specific risk factors within the broader picture, Charlton *et al.* (1993) have pointed out that vets, pharmacists, dentists, doctors, and farmers are particularly at risk. Mortality from suicide is slightly higher among men from class I than among those from other employed groups; the rate is highest among the unoccupied group. However, the relationship between suicide and unemployment is not

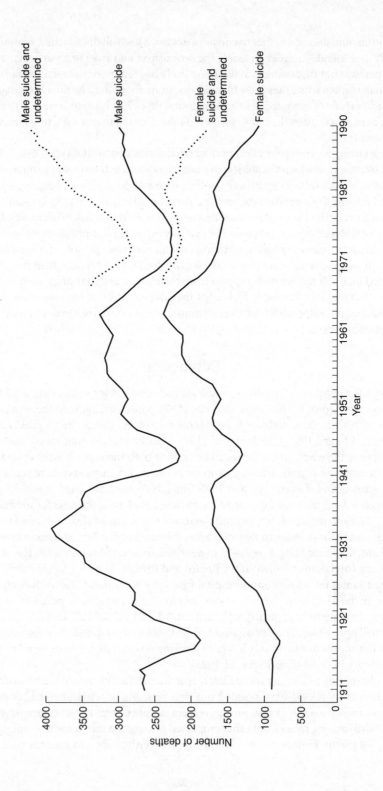

Fig. 3.1 *Number of suicide deaths by sex, 1911–90, England and Wales. (Three-year moving average.)*

consistent; the rate among young men rose consistently from 1974 to 1990 despite both a rise and a fall in unemployment rates. The effect of marital status is consistent with what has been discussed above; rates are highest for widowed and divorced men, lowest for married men, and intermediate for single men. (Although in the period 1972–1989 the rates for widowed and divorced men fell substantially, they remained substantially higher than those for the other two groups). The authors suggest that part of the overall increase in the numbers of male suicides in recent years may be the result of larger numbers of young men remaining single, although they point out that the census figures on which these conclusions are based do not distinguish between those cohabiting and those living alone. Finally, they point out the link between alcoholism and suicide and the large increase in all alcohol-related deaths for men aged 25–44 in the period 1968–1990.

Whether any of the findings about suicide point to strategies for its prevention was the subject of a recent review (Gunnell and Frankel 1994). High-risk groups can be identified: those with past or recent psychiatric hospital admissions or contact with the psychiatric services, those with a history of parasuicide, and sufferers from HIV and AIDS in addition to the groups discussed above. Nevertheless, many suicides do not fall into any of these groups, and from the perspective of general practitioners those who commit suicide are so infrequent that they will be difficult to identify among the larger group. The small numbers also make it extremely difficult to carry out research in this area. One interesting experiment carried out on the Swedish island of Gotland appeared to demonstrate benefit from a simple educational intervention for general practitioners, but this has not yet been replicated elsewhere (Rutz *et al.* 1989). The authors concluded that the most gain might accrue from measures taken to limit the availability of means for committing suicide, for instance by reducing harmful emissions from car exhausts. The only specific recommendation made for general practitioners was for them to pay particular attention to the recognition and treatment of depression, and to their psychotropic prescribing, limiting the quantities dispensed and being aware of the drugs most often taken in overdose.

In contrast to the excess of suicide among men, there is a well-established excess of depression among women. All studies of depression that compare the prevalence of depression in men and women report an excess in women, with a mean female to male ratio of 2.1:1 (Paykel 1991). The same proportion has been reported as far back as 1916 in Amsterdam, in places as diverse as India, Iraq, and New Guinea, and applies to both treated cases and community surveys (Weissman and Klerman 1977). Various reasons for this have been suggested. First, there is the possibility that it is a genuine difference mediated by biology, intrinsic in the genetic make-up of the sexes. Second, there is the possibility that men's and women's experience of depression is identical, but that women report their depression more and seek help for it more frequently than men. In modern terms it may be preferable for men to acknowledge symptoms of 'stress' rather than 'depression'. A third possibility is that it is socially mediated, brought about by the different life experience of men and women. The popular answer is that both men and women experience distress. Women internalize their distress and express it as depression; men externalize theirs and express it as aggression and social problems such as alcoholism and crime (Paykel 1991).

As far as biological differences are concerned, the evidence does not support explanations either in genetic or hormonal terms. Hormonal differences would support some empirical observations; the association between depression and premenstrual tension and the existence of post-partum depression are well-known. However, these have never been linked to specific hormonal patterns and neither oral contraception nor the menopause is associated with any increase in depression.

Whether women are more willing than men to seek help at the same level of distress can be tested by looking at those studies which have compared rates of depression as presented to doctors and those which have surveyed whole populations, measuring either diagnostic caseness or levels of depressive symptoms. Generally, the female preponderance is found in both presenting populations and in community surveys. This suggests that, at least for the symptoms covered in such surveys, there is no difference in the way that symptoms are handled either by men and women themselves or by doctors, once they have been recognized.

The evidence for social causes is more persuasive than that for biological causes. In a comprehensive review of studies that had surveyed rates of depressive states at different ages, Jorm (1987) showed that there were no differences in prevalence between men and women in youth, adolescence, and old age, but a substantial difference in middle years. The estimated prevalences were for men 8% in childhood, 17% in their twenties, and falling to 11–12% from age 40 onwards. For women the equivalent figures were 8% in childhood, 26% in their twenties, and 17% in their forties. The excess among women has been found in one study to be closely linked to parity, suggesting that it is the strains associated with motherhood which are most to blame (Bebbington et al. 1991). Similar conclusions are indicated by a study examining rates of admission for affective psychosis to mental hospitals in the north western region (Gater et al. 1989). This found that the difference in admission rates between men and women could be entirely explained by the effects of parity. Different evidence which supports social causes, but in an apparently inconsistent direction, is supplied by Silverstein and Perlick (1991), looking at the difference in rates for cohorts of men and women born at different times. Here it was found that the preponderance of depressed women was greatest in those cohorts reaching adolescence at the time of greatest employment opportunities for women, although the differences did not become apparent until the cohort was aged 30 or more. The conventional wisdom is that work has some sort of protective effect against developing depression. However, one study has suggested that whether working outside the home is associated with more or less depression depends very heavily on the amount of social support available to the women (Parry 1986).

One means of identifying more precisely the contribution made by life experience is to study men and women whose life experience is largely similar. Two such studies have recruited men and women from a single occupational group. Jenkins (1985) studied a group of civil servants, aged 20–35, working in the Home Office. No difference was found in the rates of depression or in the rates of recovery measured 12 months later. Wilhelm and Parker (1989) conducted a careful study among a group of teachers in training and five years later. They had hypothesized that this period would see a major diversion in the roles adopted by men and women, and hence a change from equal to unequal rates of depression. In the event there was little difference between the sexes from the beginning to the end of the study. The authors admitted that the five years after training might not have been long enough for large sex-role differences to appear, but also wondered whether this particular occupational group might have attracted an atypical group of nurturing men who were more vulnerable to depression than other men. Both of these papers can be criticized for the short timescale covered by their studies. Also, by studying such similar groups they may have controlled for so many factors and made it impossible to identify any emerging differences. Equally, they can be taken to support the idea that the major part of the discrepancy is a consequence of child-rearing.

The extent to which men and women interpret symptoms differently, both to themselves and to others, including their doctors, is an interesting, unresolved question. As stated above, epidemiological studies suggest that there is no difference, but this is hard to believe when considering depression at the level of individuals. Deborah Tannen (1991) has written about the different ways in which men and women use language, pointing out, for instance, that men see conversations much more as arenas to establish their place in the hierarchy than women do. Since all depressive symptoms are processed by language and since the language has a large emotional content, many of the symptoms, for instance crying or fatigue, may be rejected or denied by men. More broadly, depression may be seen as a syndrome of being an inactive victim and distinctly unmale. This follows the traditional view that men are brought up not to express emotional weakness. O'Brien (1990) has described the state of 'internal inattentiveness', by which she means that men start by consciously ignoring their own emotions and eventually arrive at a point at which they are not even aware of them. A large nationwide study did find that women reported more negative-feeling states that their husbands, and they also reported more positive-feeling states. However, contrary to one of the original hypotheses, they did not report more symptoms about their husbands than the men did about themselves (Briscoe 1982). In a smaller study of college students, Robbins and Tanck (1991) found that men and women did not differ in the rates of recording depressed feelings, but that the men were more likely to attribute them to academic concerns and the women to relationship problems.

The interest for those concerned with the health of men, in a subject which is so consistently shown to be more important for women, lies in two questions. First, if it is true that part of the discrepancy results from denial on the part of men or the transformation into other syndromes such as 'stress', then does this amount to problems that could be better recognized and more effectively treated? Bringing about such changes may well be outside the remit of doctors since much would depend on challenging ideas of what are acceptable male symptoms. Nevertheless, given that there has recently been a campaign to make general practitioners in the United Kingdom more aware of depression in general, there may be a need to identify more specifically the ways in which depressed men may present to their doctors. If internal inattentiveness is operating then doctors may need to pay more attention to the physical symptoms and less to the feelings associated with depression. Second, there are many examples in this book where problems currently affect men much more than women, but where the difference between them is diminishing. There is a suggestion that the sex difference in depression is also diminishing (McLanahan and Glass 1985). If the current difference is a result of women's responsibility for child-bearing and rearing then two possible explanations emerge. First, does it mean that men are taking on a more equal role in child care? This is difficult to accept as a major explanation. The idea of the new man who shares equal responsibility for domestic chores with his partner seems to be more of a myth than a reality. While there is almost universal agreement that this is the desirable aim, there is little concrete evidence that it is actually happening. The second explanation is that the shift reflects changes in the job market, a combination of women being protected by going out to work in larger numbers than previously and men suffering more from the effects of unemployment. Such changes may in the future more substantially affect men from lower socio-economic groups as their work becomes increasingly casualized and part time.

Middle age

Ageing for both men and women means a loss of physical strength and fitness, and for some the bloom of their youthful good looks. Accompanying such obvious image problems are the more subtle losses: the abandonment of ambitions and fantasies which sustain the struggle to succeed. In women, such changes in middle age may coincide with the biological climacteric, so the equivalent problems associated with ageing in men have been termed the male menopause. However, the comparison is misleading. The menopause is primarily a biological phenomenon, signifying the end of reproductive life and the accompanying hormonal changes, which in turn carry particular medical implications. In men there are no such changes. There appears to be no limit to men's reproductive life span. While testosterone levels do decline with age, the change is gradual and overall not marked. Mean levels of plasma testosterone at the age of 75 are two-thirds of those at the age of 25 (Vermeulen 1991). Nor is it clear that the decline causes any specific symptoms. Some hold the view that the drop in testosterone is responsible for the observed increase in body fat and decrease in bone and muscle mass. This view is contrasted with that of Bowskill and Linacre (1976) who collected case studies of men with major life problems in their forties. They argue persuasively that men are vulnerable to such pressure at this age because it is then that they have to stop assuming that their lives will always get better and start coming to terms with the process of ageing. Nevertheless, the accounts in their book represent only isolated examples and there is no sense that they represent a generalizable syndrome. A major study of health and lifestyles, while confirming the gradual increase in the incidence of minor symptoms for men and women as they age, did not show any particularly dramatic change in the age groups 45–54 and 55–64, and men's scores on the General Health Questionnaire changed little between the ages of 18 and 74 (Cox *et al.* 1987).

More recently, there has been interest in dehydroepiandrosterone (DHEA), synthesized in the adrenal gland, and its sulphate (DHEAS), synthesized in the liver. The concentration of this steroid is at a maximum in young men, falling to a level approximately 20% of the peak value by the age of 70 (Weksler 1996). Again the physiological effects are not clear, but this has not stopped it being widely consumed, and in the US it can be obtained by mail order without a prescription. One randomized trial treating male and female volunteers of various ages with DHEA and placebo reported an increase in a sense of well-being, but it was not clear how this was defined or measured. No change in libido was reported (Morales *et al.* 1994). If there is no generalizable entity, and therefore no treatment for its effects, is there any purpose in retaining the term in the medical vocabulary – will it help men to label this period in their lives as the male menopause? For men, it is difficult to see how characterizing a vague period in their life and giving it greater prominence than other phases in this way is likely to be any help to them. There is no obvious way in which it can represent freedom from anything, and on the other hand it may become an unnecessary obstacle to leading a rich and fulfilling life in late-middle and old age. For doctors, it is unlikely that thinking of a man as going through the male menopause will help to understand patients' unique predicaments and may prejudice the judgement of what is going on and what should be done about it.

Conclusion

The adult years reflect more starkly than any other stage of life the central themes of men's health. Over this period in their lives both the differential morbidity from heart disease and the comparative absence from the world of medicine and health care are greater than at any other time, and at the end of this chapter the reasons are no clearer than they were at the beginning. The evidence from depression ought to supply some clues, but here too the findings are mixed and inconclusive. The evidence does not support the idea that men consciously deny depressive symptoms, although there is the possibility that subconsciously they label them differently and channel them in different directions. Given the only conclusive part of the findings on depression and the strong evidence of how far men suffer from undertaking their duties as breadwinners (see Chapter 5), we might suggest that the sacrifices which men make to their careers are balanced by those that women make to their families.

How should general practitioners respond to men in their adult years? First, it is important to remember the reality of excess morbidity as the context within which adult men consult their doctors. It would be tempting to conclude that new consultations with men should be considered more likely than those with women to be presenting serious physical disease, but no evidence exists to support this. It is as likely that men's and women's illness behaviour leads to an equal mismatch of many self-limiting illnesses presented to doctors and much unrecognized or undeclared serious physical disease. Second, it is single men, and particularly the recently widowed, who seem to be at highest risk of having poor health, and if general practitioners can bring about any change they should pay particular attention to this group. Third, they should all be alive to the need to recognize hidden depression in men and women, but that for reasons of culture, language, 'internal inattention', and the way in which depression has been constructed as a disease entity it may be harder to discover in men than in women. In the longer term the important question is whether men's health would be improved by encouraging them to become more sensitive to their own symptoms and emotions and, if so, how health professionals might help to bring that process about. The proposition ought to be true, but as yet there is no evidence to support either the first part of the question or to start experimenting with the second.

References

Bebbington, P. E., Dean, C., Der, G., Hurry, J., and Tennant, C. (1991). Gender, parity and the prevalence of minor affective disorder. *British Journal of Psychiatry*, **158**, 40–5.

Bowskill, D. and Linacre, A. (1976). *The 'male' menopause*. Frederick Muller, London.

Briscoe, M. (1982). Sex differences in psychological well-being. In *Psychological medicine* (monograph supplement 1). Cambridge University Press, Cambridge.

Brown, G. W. and Harris, T. (1978). *Social origins of depression: a study of psychiatric disorder in women*. Tavistock Publications, London.

Caldwell, M. and Peplau, L. A. (1982). Sex differences in same-sex friendships. *Sex Roles*, **8**, 721–32.

Chandra, V., Szklo, M., Goldberg, R., and Tonascia, J. (1983). The impact of marital status on survival after an acute myocardial infarct. *American Journal of Epidemiology*, **117**, 320–5.

Charlton, J., Kelly, S., Dunnell, K., Evans, B., and Jenkins, R. (1993). Suicide deaths in England and Wales: trends in factors associated with suicide deaths. *Population Trends*, **71**, 34–42.

Charlton, J., Kelly, S., Dunnell, K., Evans, B., Jenkins, R., and Wallis, R. (1992). Trends in suicide deaths in England and Wales. *Population Trends*, **69**, 10–6.

Cox, B. D., Blaxter, M., Buckle, A. L. J., Fenner, N. P., Golding, J. F., Gore, M., *et al.* (1987). *The health and lifestyle survey*. Health Promotion Research Trust, London.

Ferkeitch, S. L. and Mercer, R. T. (1989). Men's health status during pregnancy and early parenthood. *Research in Nursing and Health*, **12**, 137–48.

Finlayson, A. and McEwen, J. (1977). *Coronary heart disease and patterns of living*. Croom Helm, London.

Gater, R. A., Dean, C., and Morris, J. (1989). The contribution of childbearing to the sex difference in first-admission rates for affective psychosis. *Psychological Medicine*, **19**, 719–24.

Gove, W., Hughes, M., and Style, C. B. (1983). Does marriage have positive effects on the psychological well-being of the individual? *Journal of Health and Social Behavior*, **24**, 122–31.

Gunnell, D. J., Brooks, J., and Peters, T. J. (1996). Epidemiology and patterns of hospital use after parasuicide in the south west of England. *Journal of Epidemiology and Community Health*, **50**, 24–9.

Gunnell, D. J. and Frankel, S. (1994). Prevention of suicide: aspirations and evidence. *British Medical Journal*, **308**, 1227–33.

Gunnell, D. J., Peters, T. J., Kammerling, R. M., and Brooks, J. (1995). Relation between parasuicide, suicide, psychiatric admissions and socioeconomic deprivation. *British Medical Journal*, **311**, 226–30.

Hansen, V. and Jacobsen, B. K. (1989). Mental distress and social conditions and lifestyle in northern Norway. *British Medical Journal*, **299**, 85–8.

Helsing, K. J., Szklo, M., and Comstock, G. W. (1981). Factors associated with mortality after widowhood. *American Journal of Public Health*, **71**, 802–9.

Horwitz, A. V. and White, H. R. (1991). Becoming married, depression, and alcohol problems among the young. *Journal of Health and Social Behaviour*, **32**, 221–37.

House, J. S., Robbins, C., and Metzner, H. L. (1982). The association of social relationships and activities with mortality: prospective evidence from the Tecumseh community health study. *American Journal of Epidemiology*, **116**, 123–40.

Jenkins, R. (1985). Sex differences in minor psychiatric morbidity. In *Psychological medicine* (monograph supplement 7). Cambridge University Press, Cambridge.

Jones, D. R. (1987). Heart disease mortality following widowhood: some results from the OPCS longitudinal study. *Journal of Psychosomatic Research*, **31**, 325–33.

Jorm, A. F. (1987). Sex and age differences in depression: a quantitative synthesis of published research. *Australian and New Zealand Journal of Psychiatry*, **21**, 46–53.

Kobrin, F. E. and Hendershot, G. E. (1977). Do family ties reduce mortality? Evidence from the United States, 1966–1968. *Journal of Marriage and the Family*, **39**, 737–45.

Lewis, C. (1982). 'A feeling you can't scratch?': the effect of pregnancy and birth on married men. In *Fathers: psychological perspectives* (ed. N. Beail and J. McGuire), pp. 43–70. Junction Books, London.

McLanahan, S. S. and Glass, J. L. (1985). A note on the trend in sex differences in psychological distress. *Journal of Health and Social Behavior*, **26**, 328–36.

McLoone, P. (1996). Suicide and deprivation in Scotland. *British Medical Journal*, **312**, 543–4.

Masoni, S., Maio, A., Trimarchi, G., De Punzio, C., and Fioretti, P. (1994). The couvade syndrome. *Journal of Psychosomatic Obstetrics and Gynaecology*, **15**, 125–31.

Meininger, J. C. (1986). Sex differences in factors associated with use of medical care, and alternative illness behaviours. *Social Science and Medicine*, **22**, 285–92.

Mendes de Leon, C. F., Appels, A. W. P. M., Otten, F. W. J., and Schouten, E. G. W. (1992). Risk of mortality and coronary heart disease by marital status in middle-aged men in the Netherlands. *International Journal of Epidemiology*, **21**, 460–6.

Morales, A. J., Nolan, J. J., and Yen, S. S. C. (1994). Effects of replacement dose of dehydroepiandrosterone in men and women of advancing age. *Journal of Clinical Endocrinology and Metabolism*, **78**, 1360–7.

Morrell, D. C. and Wale, C. J. (1976). Symptoms perceived and recorded by patients. *Journal of the Royal College of General Practitioners*, **26**, 398–403.

O'Brien, M. (1990). The place of men in a gender-sensitive therapy. In *Gender and power in families* (ed. R. J. Perelberg and A. C. Miller), pp. 195–208. Tavistock, London.

Office for National Statistics (1997). *Mortality statistics, cause. Review of the Registrar General on deaths by cause, sex and age, in England and Wales, 1995.* Stationery office, London.

Parkes, C. M. (1972). Bereavement. Studies of grief in adult life. Tavistock Publications, London.

Parkes, C. M., Benjamin, B., and Fitzgerald, R. G. (1969). Broken heart: a statistical study of increased mortality among widowers. *British Medical Journal*, **1**, 740–3.

Parry, G. (1986). Paid employment, life events, social support, and marital health in working-class matters. Journal of Health and Social Behaviour, **27**, 193–208.

Paykel, E. S. (1991). Depression in women. *British Journal of Psychiatry*, **158** (suppl. 10), 22–9.

Rindfuss, R. R. (1991). The young adult years: diversity, structural change and fertility. *Demography*, **28**, 494–512.

Robbins, P. R. and Tanck, R. H. (1991). Gender differences in the attribution of causes for depressed feelings. *Psychological Reports*, **68**, 1209–10.

Rosengren, A., Wedel, H., and Wilhelmsen, L. (1989). Marital status and mortality in middle-aged Swedish men. *American Journal of Epidemiology*, **129**, 54–64.

Rosengren, A., Orth-Gomer, K., Wedel, H., and Wilhelmsen, L. (1993). Stressful life events, social support and mortality in men born in 1933. *British Medical Journal*, **307**, 1102–5.

Royal College of General Practitioners, Office of Population Censuses and Surveys, Department of Health (1995). Morbidity statistics from general practice. Fourth national study 1991–1992. HMSO, London.

Rutz, W., Von Knorring, L. and Walinder, J. (1989). Frequency of suicide in Gotland after systematic postgraduate education of general practitioners. *Acta Psychiatrica Scandinavica*, **80**, 151–4.

Scott-Hayes, G. (1982). The experience of perinatal paternity and its relation to attitudes to pregnancy and childbirth. In *Fathers: psychological perspectives* (ed. N. Beail and J. McGuire), pp. 23–42. Junction Books, London.

Seidler, V. S. (1992). Rejection, vulnerability, and friendship. In *Men's friendships* (ed. P. M. Nardi), pp. 15–34. Sage, Newbury Park, California.

Silverstein, B. and Perlick, D. (1991). Gender differences in depression: historical changes. *Acta Psychiatrica Scandinavica*, **84**, 327–31.

Stott, N. C. H. and Pill, R. M. (1990). 'Advise yes, dictate no.' Patients' views on health promotion in the consultation. *Family Practice*, **7**, 125–31.

Tannen, D. (1992). *You just don't understand: women and men in conversation.* Virago Press, London.

Temple, M. T., Fillmore, K. M., Hartka, E., Johnstone, B., Leino, E. V., and Motoyoshi, M. (1991). The collaborative alcohol-related longitudinal project. A meta-analysis of change in marital and employment status as predictors of alcohol consumption on a typical occasion. *British Journal of Addiction*, **86**, 1269–81.

Tomlinson, P. S. (1987). Spousal differences in marital satisfaction during transition to parenthood. *Nursing Research*, **36**, 239–43.

Trethowan, W. H. and Conlon, M. F. (1965). The couvade syndrome. *British Journal of Psychiatry*, **111**, 57–66.

Vermeulen, A. (1991). Androgens in the aging male. *Journal of Clinical Endocrinology and Metabolism*, **73**, 221–4.

Wallace, P. G. and Haines, A. P. (1984). General practitioners and health promotion: what patients think. *British Medical Journal*, **289**, 534–6.

Weissman, M. M. and Klerman, G. L. (1977). Sex differences and the epidemiology of depression. *Archives of General Psychiatry*, **34**, 98–111.

Weksler, M. E. (1996). Hormone replacement for men. *British Medical Journal*, **312**, 859–60.

Wellman, B. (1992). Men in networks. Private communities, domestic friendships. In *Men's friendships* (ed. P. M. Nardi), pp. 74–114. Sage, Newbury Park, California.

Wilhelm, K. and Parker, G. (1989). Is sex necessarily a risk factor to depression? *Psychological Medicine*, **19**, 401–13.

CHAPTER FOUR

Later life

Charles Freer

Men who survive have to come to terms with the consequences of old age. Old age is seen as being a period of multiple losses: employment and the financial independence it brings, loved ones, fitness, and freedom from illness. As a consequence of the earlier differences in mortality, men beyond the age of 65 are increasingly outnumbered by women and can become truly less visible with time. However, as this chapter points out, it is beguilingly easy for younger men and women to adopt an unrealistic negative view of old age. The experience of older men can be both positive and enriching. The challenge for doctors is to resist the tendency towards ageism and be prepared to do the simple things that help to make this possible.

Introduction

Arguably, the most significant change in contemporary society is the ageing of the population. However, the preponderance of females in the growing number of older people has resulted in very little particular attention to men and their health in later life. For example, a 1990 text on social gerontology has only three index references to men (solely in relation to retiring) compared to 39 for women (covering nine topic headings) (Bond and Coleman 1990).

The paucity of literature on the implications of growing older for men is compounded by the invariably cross-sectional nature of research in this area. Longitudinal studies are now underway, but even these are likely to find it difficult to capture the effects of rapid changes in the health status, beliefs, attitudes, and expectations of succeeding cohorts of people growing older.

What follows is guided by the available literature, but also has an anecdotal element from a predominantly general practitioner perspective.

Sociodemographic trends

Declining mortality rates in the very young and the older age groups have led to significant changes in life expectancy. Between the 1961 and 1981 censuses, the population aged

65 years and over increased from 11.8% to 15%, with the largest increase occurring in the very old. The number of over 85-year-olds is projected to increase by 42% by the year 2025 (Victor 1991). These trends are to be found in all countries, including those in the Third World, and it is only differences in changes in fertility rates which will determine the age structure of the populations. In Britain, a reduction in fertility has meant that today, for the first time in history, many adults have more older than younger relatives.

The place of older men in society is influenced by the greater life span enjoyed by women, a feature that has persisted with the increasing number of older people. For every 100 men in the 65–69 year-old age group there are 121 women, with the equivalent figure rising to 325 for over 85-year-olds (Bond and Coleman 1990). The exact reasons for these differences have been difficult to establish but are undoubtedly contributed to by the hormonal protection women have from atherosclerosis and lifestyle factors, particularly smoking. The changing role of women and changes in female smoking habits are thought likely to reduce the gender ratio of future older populations.

Mortality and morbidity trends

The higher mortality rates experienced by men in earlier age groups as compared to women reduce the number of male survivors into very old age, but those who do survive suffer much less chronic ill health than their female counterparts. In part, this can be explained by the fact that the diseases causing morbidity and mortality are quite different. This subject is discussed in more detail in Chapter 1.

In the last 10–15 years there have been prolonged and heated debates about the impact of longer life on health and ageing (Bury 1988). The appealing notion of a 'rectangular survival curve' has, however, found little support and while there has been a definite decrease in mortality in later life, this has been accompanied by increasing levels of morbidity from non-fatal diseases such as arthritis (Verbrugge 1984).

Challenges of later life – myths and realities

The prevailing stereotype of growing old is a negative one. For many, being 'old' is seen as reaching pensionable age, and with this can come many feelings of loss – loss of job, loss of being useful and a contributor, loss of family, and the likely future loss of health and, eventually, life. Certainly, this tends to be the view held by younger adults concerning the health and status of older people but in fact does not reflect the actual experiences of older people themselves (Age Concern England 1977; Harris *et al.* 1975). There is now widespread evidence to support a much more positive view of growing older in modern society and this will be considered with respect to some of the events and experiences likely to concern men as they reach later life.

Retirement

Since an important and legitimizing role for many men is work, it is not surprising that there is a widespread assumption that retirement creates major problems for them. In fact, although the thought of retirement can undoubtedly create uncertainty and stress, there is evidence that the majority of men adjust to retirement with minimum difficulty (Maas and Kuypers 1974; Phillipson 1990). Unfortunately, the pattern of most working men retiring at the age of 65 no longer prevails. An increase in early retirement and the serious persistent problems of long-term unemployment (discussed in detail in Chapter 6) mean that this adjustment is not one that is confined to later life.

Coping with retirement can be improved by effective preparation and some employers recognize the responsibility for organizing this. In Britain, the Pre-Retirement Association has created an important resource to assist in the design of pre-retirement education. Unfortunately, for many, however, if experienced at all, this type of employee benefit comes as too little too late. General practitioners can make an important contribution in this field, not least by challenging some of the myths about health in later years.

There are some potentially positive trends for retired men. Despite high levels of current unemployment, there are in some jobs and areas a shortage of younger recruits because of changing demographic patterns. In addition, older people can bring not only the skills of a lifetime's experience but also the ability to cope with some jobs and hours difficult for younger people with families. The renewed importance of volunteers and voluntary organizations in contemporary Britain is also creating opportunities for older people to contribute their talents in unpaid but fulfilling ways. It is likely that in the future we will see much less of the 'one job for life' pattern with increasing numbers of individuals pursuing a series of different jobs throughout their lifetime and making individual choices about the age of retirement. Changes in career patterns have been stressful for many, particularly in mid-life, but in the long term these trends may provide more opportunities for more men to find challenging work in later life.

Fitness

The physiological changes in ageing lead to changes in function and performance, but it is likely that for many the decline in fitness cannot be accounted for by ageing alone – the so-called fitness gap (Gray 1988). Of those aged 65–74, 92% can walk half a mile and 96% can climb stairs (Mulley 1995). This may be one area where men are in better health than women: in a survey of people aged 75–84 in Dutch residential homes, women were more likely to fall over than men (Van Weel et al. 1995). While older men today show increasing levels of fitness, no doubt the result of earlier improvements in lifestyle, it is important that older people are aware of the continuing benefits of health promotion in later years since it is likely that they are less convinced than younger age groups of their ability to influence their health (Victor 1991).

Health problems

Health problems increase with age and, as discussed earlier, survival into later life is likely to be accompanied by increasing levels of morbidity. However, many surveys have consistently shown that the majority of older people are well (Coleman 1983; Hunt 1978; Office of Population Censuses and Surveys 1982), and there is no evidence of a significant decline in happiness or life satisfaction with age (Palmore and Maddox 1977). Men in fact show lower levels of morbidity than women in later years, in part because of the continuing high mortality rates among men in late middle age from cardiovascular disease, meaning healthier survivors in later life. Like fitness, it is reasonable to assume that continuing improvements in lifestyle in all age groups will yield greater benefits in the future, although this has to be tempered by the knowledge that the causes of mortality differ from those responsible for morbidity.

One problem that can contribute to a rather pessimistic view of health status in later years is the tendency with the traditional medical model to measure the prevalence of disease in contrast to the more important, functional status. Many older people with diseases such as arthritis and heart disease manage to cope and live full and satisfying lives. While morbidity studies in older people tend to show higher levels of degenerative diseases, the more positive view of the functional approach is illustrated in the study by Luker and Perkins (1987) which found that over 90% of older people rated their health as being fair to good, with 80% being able to use public transport and only a minority requiring assistance with mobility.

Economic status

The health of any population can be directly linked to its economic status and while poverty remains an important problem for a group of older people, the majority of people retiring today have higher incomes and levels of home ownership than previously. The consequences of socio-economic differences on health persist in old age. A recently published follow-up of 18 000 male civil servants recruited to the first Whitehall study reported that employment grade continued to be a predictor of mortality after retirement. The absolute difference in death rates between the lowest and highest employment grades increased with age (Marmot and Shipley 1996).

Coping with adjustments and changing roles in later life

Like most aspects of life for older people, there is mixed, sometimes conflicting, evidence of positive and negative features. In part, this will be a reflection of the heterogeneity to be expected in any population group, but there remain contradictions. For example, as mentioned above (Palmore and Maddox 1977), there is no evidence for significant decline in happiness or life satisfaction with age, yet the prevalence of depression is higher for over 65-year-olds than in other age groups and while the rate for men is approximately half that of women, the suicide rate for men is considerably higher, as it is in younger men (Victor 1991).

A major and distinctly positive trend has been in the role and contribution of older people, including men, in contemporary society. The image of a sick, passive, and dependent age group has been radically weakened. The growing numbers of fitter, more articulate, and better-resourced retirees have transformed the potential for many to create and control their lives and activities. Initially, this was particularly reflected in the social and leisure field but as discussed above has now been extended into work in later life through either paid employment or voluntary work. The changes from a passive recipient role to an active contributory one has been a major influence in improving morale and status for not only current older people but those approaching later life. Finally we are witnessing increasing consumerism from this age group with the rights and needs of older people being represented by a growing number of national and international lobbying groups.

Long-term care

Only a small percentage of over-65s – 5% – are unable to remain living in their own homes, but this level increases to 20% for the over 75-year-old age group. Survival rates in this age group mean that men form the minority of residents. Only a small number of married couples are to be found in long-term care. This imbalance can clearly create difficulties for men who are likely to find it difficult to fit into the social dimensions of the home.

However, it does appear that many of the male residents of nursing homes have significant mental health problems or physical disabilities, secondary to cerebrovascular disease or Parkinson's disease. There is an absence of available statistics from recent trends but it does appear that in the last few years there has been an increasing percentage of men in nursing homes, who, while younger than female residents, are severely disabled as a result of strokes.

The last 10 years have witnessed a dramatic shift in long-term care from the NHS to the private sector, but in general this has led to an increased quality of life for these residents (Bowling and Formby 1992).

Death

A difficult but intriguing area is the attitude of older people to death. The literature on this is reviewed by Coleman (1990) but as with other topics tends to be mainly from the United States.

While there are undoubtedly some individuals who appear to have difficulty coping with the thought of death, perhaps showing signs of what could be called 'pre-bereavement grief', the prevailing view is that most older people express less fear than might be expected at the prospect of facing death. This view is supported by the evidence of the numbers of people interested in making advance directives about how they would like to be treated in the event of terminal illness. In a survey in Massachusetts, 93% of outpatients and 89% of the general public expressed positive views about advance directives (Emanuel *et al.* 1991). A later survey, after the passing of a national Act of Congress, found that 72% of patients discharged from hospital had made some form of advance care planning, although in approximately two-thirds of these the arrangements were informal and unwritten (Emanuel *et al.* 1993).

Changing family and marital relationships

Married couples live longer and remain healthier than single people, with husbands accruing greater benefits in both respects than their wives (Hess and Soldo 1985).

Men and women have important and interesting contrasts in their views of expectations of marriage. Among today's older couples, the majority of husbands entered marriage viewing it as a source of benefits, mainly material, through the housekeeping role their wives played. In addition, however, and this remains true today, men have an important need for a confidante. Women on the other hand tend to share their confidences with a wider circle of friends and the majority of today's older wives saw marriage as a means to achieving status and a legitimate role in life.

There are a number of factors which can affect the quality of the marital relationship as couples grow older. The literature that exists produces conflicting results, in part because many of the factors are capable of having both positive and negative effects. Furthermore, these factors can be confounding. For example, the presence or absence of adequate financial resources can be critical whatever the status of the underlying relationship.

Role changes

The traditional role of the provider husband with a wife at home changes suddenly when the husband retires from employment and spends more time at home. Of course some men, and perhaps this is an increasing trend, have always participated in the household routine but, if not, there can be problems with role conflict or even role reversal. With the changing position and attitudes of women in modern society and, in particular, their involvement with jobs and careers, the effects on marriages will be more complex and varied. Age differences in marriages can sometimes mean that women continue to work while the retired husband takes on the homemaker role. In addition, the increasing trend for women to return to work or embark on new careers later in life may mean that some husbands will be unable or unwilling to cope with or support their wives in this at a time when they are keen to settle down and adopt a retired lifestyle.

Economic

Financial problems can produce and aggravate difficulties in a marriage but overall there is evidence of increasing financial security for older couples, bringing with it opportunities for luxuries such as travelling and holidays, all of which can enhance the quality of their relationship.

Children

The effect of children growing up and leaving the home has received frequent attention, mainly in respect of the effect on women through the 'empty nest syndrome'. It can also contribute to the mid-life problems of men as described in Chapter 3. For some couples, it may set the scene for increasing difficulties as both find it difficult to rebuild a satisfying relationship without the involvement of children. For others, however, it can create opportunities to return to the type of relationship that prevailed early in the marriage.

It is widely believed that families no longer look after their elderly relatives as they did in previous decades and generations. It is true that there have been important social changes with greater mobility of the population and a reduction in the extended family. This has meant more older people living on their own, but most studies have shown that families, especially daughters, remain the most important support for frail, older people (Luker and Perkins 1987; Shanas 1979). In the UK, 62% of retired people were visited by their children at least once a week and one-third lived under the same roof (Mulley 1995). In one study of elderly Asians in the Midlands, only 4% of over 75-year-olds were living alone and 58% were living in households of three or more generations (Donaldson 1986).

Health and disability

Arguably, the greatest fear for individuals and couples is the possibility of serious health problems. Much will depend on the pre-existing relationship and dependency status. For example, disability in a partner who has always been the more dependent is likely to be much less disruptive than when the stronger partner is no longer able to take the lead role. Men may have particular difficulty in fulfilling the carer role and, in her study of very elderly people, Wenger (1986) found that men tended to complain of the physical strain of nursing, lifting, and housekeeping while women found most difficulty with the social and emotional needs of caring.

There is a prevailing belief that disabled men receive more support than their female counterparts; in fact there is very little gender difference, with frail, older people of either sex living on their own receiving much more support than couples with high levels of disability (Arber and Gilbert 1989).

Successful partnerships

It is difficult to know what makes for a long and successful marriage. American research which looked at couples who had been together for over 40 years expected to find support for the view that in the successful marriages there was a sharing of lifestyles and interests (Maas and Kuypers 1974). Surprisingly, they found the opposite. The lifestyles of husbands and wives in these long and happy marriages were more likely to develop independently of each other. One important observation was that in happy marriages there appeared to be a feeling of equality in the relationship. The ability of couples to cope with the possible stresses and difficulties of later life is likely to depend very much on how they develop coping strategies over the years and the ability of the couple to work together through crises.

Sexuality

It is a cliché that younger people find the idea of old people and sex difficult to deal with. However, the major survey of sexual behaviour in Britain, planned in 1986 and published in 1994, did not study anyone over the age of 60 (Wellings *et al.* 1994). Previous evidence has reported differently: one longitudinal study of men and women born in Gothenburg in 1901–2 reported rates of coital activity of 52% in men at aged 70, falling to 13% at age 81 (Nilsson 1987). In a similar survey from North America, reporting similar rates of sexual activity, the major reason for stopping was reported as the death of a spouse (Pfeiffer *et al.* 1968). Old people remain at risk of sexually transmitted disease (Rogstad and Bignell 1991).

Divorce

While the divorce rate among older people remains small and has only shown small increases (Henwood and Wicks 1985), the rapid increase in younger couples mean that many families of older people will be disrupted by divorce. It is also likely that in the future more retired people will have themselves experienced divorce. The low rate of divorce is more likely to be explained by pre-existing social and cultural attitudes to marriage and the financial disincentives to divorce than a high prevalence of happy relationships. Many older couples have persisted with the type of relationship that would be unlikely to survive today with younger couples. These unhappy marriages can be further aggravated in the later years by the addition of health problems to one or both partners.

Remarriage

For both divorced and widowed men, remarriage remains popular. It is much commoner for men than women for a number of reasons – the greater availability of unmarried women than unmarried men, the fact that men tend to marry women younger than them, and not least the need for men as opposed to women to have a confidante.

Older people tend to select partners that remind them of their previous spouse (McKain 1969) and often someone known to them and their wife for many years. Despite the social changes of recent decades there is still some stigma attached to remarriage in older people, and it is interesting that some children who have assumed liberal attitudes for themselves remain uncomfortable with their widowed parent's remarriage, and not just because of concern about the risk to any future inheritance.

Widowhood

There is no reason to assume that the loss of a spouse is any less devastating for older men than women, but it is not clear from the available literature whether men or women find widowhood more difficult (Troll *et al.* 1979). The small number of widowers below the age of 75 means that this group has received very little detailed research attention. It is likely however that men, who are more likely than women to see their spouse as part of themselves, experience a sense of loss (Glick *et al.* 1974) while women are more likely to report a feeling of abandonment through the loss of status and role that marriage brings to them.

The effect of widowhood will depend on a number of factors – the status of the marital relationship, the level and direction of dependency in the marriage, the age of the man, and the pre-existing coping strategies of the husband. For some men, the importance of marriage will grow after retirement and thus loss of the spouse will be even greater. Furthermore, in contrast to women who have formed many more intimate relationships with relatives and friends and who find a ready-made empathic support group in the many widows around them, men are likely to be much less prepared and supported in widowhood. While pre-existing membership of clubs, for example working men's clubs, golf clubs, bowling clubs, etc. can reduce the risk of social isolation, many senior citizens' clubs deter men because of the preponderance of female members.

In their detailed examination of risk groups among older people, Taylor and colleagues (1983) found no evidence to show that the recently widowed were significantly disadvantaged by comparison with other older people (cf. Parkes 1969 and Jones 1987, cited in Chapter 3).

Never married

Those who have never married tend to develop lifestyles and coping strategies which prepare them for older life and in general seem to be more content than widowed older people.

Living alone

There is a widespread assumption in the professional literature that living alone is an important risk factor for older people despite little evidence to support this view (Freer 1988). Loneliness on the other hand is an important problem among older people that can be seen equally in individuals living with their families.

For those men recently widowed, living alone will undoubtedly aggravate their feelings of isolation and perhaps rejection, but with the effect of family, social, and medical support, most can gradually resolve their bereavement and grief and readjust to a new lifestyle. In the longer term, living alone may for many older people be an important source of autonomy and privacy.

Ageism

Unfortunately, the inevitable concentration of health professionals on ill-health aspects of ageing helps to reinforce the widespread negative image of growing older held by society. General practitioners, for example, are unlikely to see healthy older people whom research has shown to be low or non-attenders (Ebrahim *et al.* 1984; Williams 1984). Furthermore, there remains a concern that doctors not infrequently collude with the older patients to attribute problems to their age. A further contribution to ageism is the tendency to see older people as a homogeneous group, denying the heterogeneity which is as valid for older people as other age groups.

As discussed earlier, there is widespread evidence that the majority of older people are well, contented, and happy. Until both health professionals and lay people realize that ageing is a quite distinct process and separate from disease, it will be difficult to alter the general view that growing older is a downhill path rather than one more stage in the life cycle; and that like earlier stages, such as middle age or adolescence, it is likely to have both positive and negative features but also the potential for the start of a new and fulfilling stage of life.

General practitioners, through their high contact rate with older people, have valuable opportunities to counter ageism. This would be more likely to happen if doctors were able to place less emphasis on the disease model which still underpins much of medical education and replace this with a more functional and psychosocial orientation. Moreover, greater concentration on the healthy and positive lifestyles that can be achieved by older people with chronic diseases would improve their outlook and be likely to reduce their dependence on lay and professional carers.

Conclusion

It would be wrong to swing from an overly gloomy picture of life in later years to an unjustifiably optimistic one. In attempting to counter ageism, a balanced view will be necessary to represent the interests of the small but significant group of older people, as in other age groups who have health, social, and economic problems. However, it is encouraging to see the emphasis shift from burden to challenge (Wells and Freer 1988), and an informed view of the existing evidence will help to encourage the belief that men in later life can continue to enjoy a satisfying lifestyle while contributing to the lives of those around them.

References

Age Concern England (1977). *Profiles of the elderly.* Vol. **1**. *Who are they? Standards of living and aspects of life satisfaction.* Age Concern England, Mitcham.

Arber, S. and Gilbert, N. (1989). Men: the forgotten carers. *Sociology,* **23**, 111–8.

Bond, J. and Coleman, P. (ed.) (1990). *Ageing in society: an introduction to social gerontology.* Sage Publications Ltd, London.

Bowling, A. and Formby, J. (1992). Hospital and nursing home care for the elderly in an inner city health district. *Nursing Times,* **88**, 51–4.

Bury, M. (1988). Arguments and ageing: long life and its consequences. In *The ageing population: a burden or a challenge?* (ed. C. Freer and N. Wells), pp. 17–32. MacMillan, London.

Coleman, P. (1983). Cognitive functioning and health. In *Ageing: a challenge to science and society.* Vol. **3**. *Behavioural sciences and conclusions* (ed. J. Birren, J. Munnichs, H. Thomae, and M. Marois), pp. 57–67. Oxford University Press, Oxford.

Coleman, P. (1990). Adjustments in later life. In *Ageing in society: an introduction to social gerontology* (ed. J. Bond and P. Coleman), pp. 101–4. Sage Publications, London.

Donaldson, L. J. (1986). Health and social status of elderly Asians: a community survey. *British Medical Journal,* **293**, 1079–82.

Ebrahim, S., Hedley, R., and Sheldon, N. (1984). Low levels of ill health among elderly non-consulters in general practice. *British Medical Journal,* **289**, 1273–6.

Emanuel, E. J., Weinberg, D. S., Gonin, R., Hummel, L. R., and Emanuel, L. L. (1993). How well is the Patient Self-Determination Act working? An early assessment. *American Journal of Medicine,* **95**, 619–28.

Emanuel, L. L., Barry, M. J., Stoeckle, J. D., Ettelson, L. M., and Emanuel, E. J. (1991). Advance directives for medical care – a case for greater use. *New England Journal of Medicine,* **324**, 889–95.

Freer, C. (1988). Old myths: frequent misconceptions about the elderly. In *The ageing population: a burden or a challenge?* (ed. N. Wells and C. Freer), pp. 3–15. MacMillan, London.

Glick, I., Wess, R., Murray Parkes, C. (1974). *The first year of bereavement.* John Wiley and Sons, New York.

Gray, J. (1988). Living environments for the elderly: Part 1. In *The ageing population: a burden or a challenge?* (ed. N. Wells and C. Freer), pp. 203–16. MacMillan, London.

Harris, L., *et al.* (1975). *The myth and reality of aging in America.* The National Council on the Aging, Washington, DC.

Henwood, M. and Wicks, M. (1985). Community care, family trends and social change. *The Quarterly Journal of Social Affairs,* **37**, 1–9.

Hess, B. and Soldo, B. P. (1985). Husband and wives network. In *Social support network and care of the elderly* (ed. W. Sauer and R. Coward), pp. 67–92. Springer, New York.

Hunt, A. (1978). *The elderly at home.* HMSO, London.

Luker, K. and Perkins, E. (1987). The elderly at home: service needs and provisions. *Journal of the Royal College of General Practitioners,* **37**, 248–50.

Maas, H. and Kuypers, J. (1974). *From thirty to seventy*, p. 76. Jossey Bass, San Francisco.

McKain, W. (1969). *Retirement marriage*. University of Connecticut, Agriculture Experiments Station, Connecticut.

Marmot, M. G. and Shipley, M. J. (1996). Do socio-economic differences in mortality persist after retirement? 25-year follow-up of civil servants from the first Whitehall study. *British Medical Journal*, **313**, 1177–80.

Mulley, G. P. (1995). Preparing for the late years. *Lancet*, **345**, 1409–13.

Nilsson, L. (1987). Sexuality in the elderly. *Acta Obstetrica et Gynecologica Scandinavica*, Suppl. **140**, 52–8.

Office of Population Censuses and Surveys (1982). *General Household Survey 1980*. HMSO, London.

Palmore, E. and Maddox, G. (1977). *Sociological aspects of aging in behaviour and adaptation in later life* (2nd edn) (ed. E. Pfeiffer and E. W. Busse). Little and Brown, Boston.

Pfeiffer, E., Verwoerdt, A., and Wang, H.-S. (1968). Sexual behaviour in aged men and women. I. Observations on 254 community volunteers. *Archives of General Psychiatry*, **19**, 753–8.

Phillipson, C. (1990). The sociology of retirement. In *Ageing in society: an introduction to social gerontology* (ed. J. Bond and P. Coleman). Sage Publications Ltd, London.

Rogstad, K. E. and Bignell, C. J. (1991). Age is no bar to sexually acquired infection. *Age and Ageing*, **20**, 377–8.

Shanas, E. (1979). Social myth as hypothesis. The case of the family relations of old people. *Gerontologist*, **19**, 3–9.

Taylor, R., Ford, G., and Barber, J. (1983). *The elderly at risk: a critical review of problems in screening and case finding*. Age Concern England, Mitcham.

Troll, L., Miller, S., and Atchley, R. (1979). *Families in later life*, p. 39. Wadsworth, Belmont, California.

van Weel, C., Vermeulen, H., and van den Bosch, W. (1995). Falls: a community perspective. *Lancet*, **345**, 1549–51.

Verbrugge, L. (1984). Longer life but worsening health? Trends in health and mortality of middle-aged and older persons. *Milbank Memorial Fund Quarterly*, **62**, 475–519.

Victor, C. (1991). *Health and healthcare in later life*. Open University Press, Milton Keynes.

Wellings, K., Field, J., Johnson, A. M., and Wadsworth, J. (1994). *Sexual behaviour in Britain. The National Survey of Sexual Attitudes and Lifestyles*. Penguin Books, London.

Wells, N. and Freer, C. (ed.) (1988). *The ageing population: a burden or a challenge?* MacMillan, London.

Wenger, G. (1986). A longitudinal study of changes and adaptations in the support networks of the Welsh elderly over 75. *Journal of Cross-cultural Gerontology*, **1**, 277–304.

Williams, E. (1984). Characteristics of patients over 75 not seen during one year in general practice. *British Medical Journal*, **288**, 119–220.

PART II

The life men lead

CHAPTER FIVE

Men at work

Delia Skan and Ken Addley

If all the year were playing holidays, to sport would be as tedious as to work.

Shakespeare, *Henry IV*, Part 1

General practitioners are likely to come across work related illness more often nowadays because of the rapid increase in small businesses which cannot afford their own full-time medical advisor. This chapter is written by two occupational physicians both of whom used to be GPs. They highlight the importance of history taking, social class and common illnesses in men at work. The reluctance of men to consult is again pointed out. However the type of illness is dictated by the type of work more than by gender. Alcohol appears again as it relates to work. Some employers are adopting enlightened attitudes to both alcohol abuse and to psychological problems in the workplace.

In many countries of Western Europe, women outlive men. Many reasons have been put forward to explain the reduced longevity of men and studies have stressed the importance of differences in behaviour such as cigarette smoking, alcohol consumption, and occupational hazards (Skelton 1988). Social class also exerts a powerful influence on health with the majority of illnesses showing an inverse relationship between social class and standardized mortality rates. In men the death rate in social class V is double that in social class I (Skelton 1988). The relationship between work and health is complex. Manual workers have a relatively poor health status, some of which may be attributable to adverse working conditions, but research has also shown that they suffer more financial problems, more stressful life events, more feelings of disempowerment in the workplace, and less social support (Griffiths 1996). The workplace has the potential to impact positively on health in the broadest sense or, conversely, take away from it, if workplace risks exist and ill health and accidents ensue.

Sickness absence

Sickness absence increases as socio-economic status decreases. Furthermore, the physically demanding nature of many tasks which semi- and unskilled workers undertake may dictate the necessity for absence when physical fitness is minimally impaired. The term 'sickness absence' is defined 'as absence from work which employees attribute to sickness and which the employer accepts as such' (Taylor 1983). Many factors other than illness and injury contribute to sickness absence and the existence of gender differences of both a qualitative and quantitative nature has long been recognized. Data from the 1987–1991 Labour Force Survey provided an analysis of gender and occupational influences on sickness absence (Clarke *et al.* 1995). Men have lower rates of sickness absence than women, but a higher percentage of men report health problems which limit their work. Women have a relatively greater proportion of short-term sickness absence. Sickness absence is high in the younger age groups and highest in the older age groups. These groups differ in the relative length of sickness absence; young workers have a high percentage of short-term absence whereas the trend in older workers is towards more long-term absence. Several reasons have been put forward to explain the gender differences, including the different responsibilities, commitments, and job types between men and women, even in the same occupational order. Moreover, women undertake a greater proportion of caring and have more family and domestic responsibilities than men.

Accidents at work

Health losses attributable to work, whether caused by accidents or ill health, are notoriously difficult to quantify. However, the total cost of work-related ill health and accidents in Great Britain has been estimated to be between 2–3% of the gross domestic product (GDP) or between £11 and 16 billion each year (Davies and Teasdale 1994).

The dictionary defines an accident as 'an unforeseen and unplanned event or circumstance'. The attribution of events to chance as the definition implies suggests that accidents cannot be prevented. In reality, the majority of harmful events occurring in the workplace are the result of known, identifiable, and controllable hazards and as such are preventable. Accidents cause losses to the individual, his family, the employer, and to society as a whole.

From 1 April 1993 to 31 March 1994 in Great Britain almost 167 400 injuries were reported to enforcement authorities. Of these:

(1) 151 900 were to employees, of which 245 were fatal;
(2) 3900 were to the self-employed, of which 51 were fatal;
(3) 11 700 were to members of the public, of which 107 were fatal (Health and Safety Commission 1995).

Injury rates in males are consistently higher than those in females. This reflects the pattern of employment whereby men are more likely to work in higher-risk occupations. The gender difference is greatest for fatal injuries. In 1993–94, the male rate (2.2 per 100 000 employees) exceeded that in females by a factor just greater than 20 (Health and Safety Commission 1995). Seventy-two per cent of all non-fatal injuries to employees occurred in men. For 1993–94, rates for fatal and major injuries were highest in the construction industry with energy and water supply showing the highest rates for injuries necessitating an excess of three days' absence from work. Since 1986–87, falls from a height have consistently been the most common cause of death. They accounted for 25% of fatalities in 1993–94. Slips, trips, and falls made up just over one-third of non-fatal major injuries in the same period. The most common age group of employees who were fatally injured was 45–54 years. Major non-fatal injuries in men occurred most commonly in the 25–34 age group. The occupations in which excess male deaths due to occupational injuries occur include those related to transport and the construction industry, particularly roofers and glaziers (Coggon *et al.* 1995).

Suicide

The occupations with greatest risk of suicide for both men and women are mostly in social classes I and II and include several professions related to medicine. Access to effective means is reported as being an important factor in suicide mortality (Table 5.1).

Table 5.1 *Job groups with the highest PMR* from suicide. Men aged 20–64. England and Wales 1979–80, 1982–90 (Coggon et al. 1995)*

Job group	Deaths	PMR	95% CI
Veterinary surgeons	32	431	294–609
Pottery decorators	8	340	147–671
Dentists	32	227	155–321
Pharmacists	40	227	162–310
Doctors	124	198	165–236
Farmers	983	161	151–172
Foresters	33	159	109–224
Driving instructors	50	158	117–209
Chemical engineers and scientists	64	155	119–198
Health professionals	34	151	105–212

* *PMR = proportional mortality ratio. A PMR is calculated by measuring the proportion of deaths in the general population from a particular cause. This proportion is then applied to the number of deaths in the occupation group under investigation to produce an expected number of deaths from a particular cause. The ratio of the actual number of deaths to the expected number is multiplied by 100 to give the PMR. If the observed number of deaths is greater or less than expected, the PMR will be greater or less than 100.*

A review of suicides for the period 1982–1992 found that poisoning by motor vehicle exhaust gas and hanging accounted for 24% and 23% respectively of male suicides.

Poisoning by solid or liquid substances was the method used by men in health-related professions, veterinary surgeons, chemical scientists, and engineers, all of whom have access to drugs or other harmful agents, and was also the method used by almost half of female suicides (Kelly *et al.* 1995). Firearms accounted for 38% of suicides in farmers, 21% in veterinary surgeons, and 15% in forestry workers.

Work-related ill health

The relationship between work and ill health was recognized some 300 years ago by Bernardino Ramazzini, the author of the first comprehensive textbook on the subject of occupational diseases (Ramazzini 1713). His recommendation that doctors ask 'What is your occupation?' is still as relevant today if doctors are to recognize work-related ill health, advise patients on fitness for work, and prescribe safely.

In previous centuries, the link between work and ill health was so clear that the name of the disease frequently incorporated the job title – thus *Billingsgate hump* – a fibrolipomatous bursa over the lower cervical spine caused by carrying fish boxes, *woolsorters' disease* – anthrax, *knife-grinders' rot* – silicosis, and *brass founders' ague* – metal fume fever. Attribution of an illness to occupation in the past may have been relatively easy but now the link between work and many commonly encountered conditions such as asthma, musculoskeletal problems, and psychological symptoms is more obscure. The disappearance of the classical occupational diseases and the emergence of those in which the link with work is subtle makes the question of attribution more difficult. Furthermore, work may contribute to, rather than cause, ill health. For example, a cold workplace may exacerbate angina or late-onset asthma. The advantage of the term 'work-related ill health' is its inclusion of the latter category. The term means 'any illness, disability, or other physical problem which reduces temporarily or permanently the functioning of an individual and which has been caused in part or whole by the working conditions of that individual' (Davies and Teasdale 1994).

The effective treatment and management of patients depends on the accuracy of the diagnosis. Symptoms related to hazardous workplace exposures may affect any organ system and occupational diseases may mimic common medical conditions. As in the case of accidents, the majority are preventable. The occupational history, regarded as the cornerstone of the practice of occupational medicine, is the key to exploring a work-related cause or contribution to ill health. It is equally important in the setting of general practice, in which approximately 7% of consultations in people of working age are related to occupational ill health. It comprises the following (Goldman 1994):

(1) a short list of current and past jobs, with a brief description where possible, including potential hazards and materials used;

(2) inquiry into exposure to fumes, chemicals, dust, loud noise, or radiation, either at present or in the past;

(3) with reference to the main complaint:
   (a) any temporal relationship to work activities
   (b) any relationship to job titles and history of exposures
   (c) other contributing factors.

The patient should also be asked if co-workers are similarly affected and his opinion sought regarding the relationship of the illness to work and the basis of his opinion.

The diagnosis of an occupational disease may have implications for both the patient and his employer. In the patient's case it may affect current and future employment and eligibility for benefit. For the employer it may highlight a previously unknown workplace risk which requires assessment and control. Furthermore, it may have legal implications for both, and should the disease cause or contribute to death, doctors must inform the coroner. Wrongly attributing a disease to a workplace risk may result in an unnecessary change of work, causing hardship for the patient and his family.

The organ systems at greatest risk in the workplace are those in direct contact with the working environment: the lungs, skin, musculoskeletal system, and the ear. It is now also recognized that specific aspects of some working environments may adversely affect the psyche. Such data as exist on the incidence of occupational diseases are derived from a number of different sources which vary in their coverage, comprehensiveness, and reliability.

Occupational asthma

Occupational asthma is asthma induced by sensitization to an agent inhaled at work (Newman Taylor and Pickering 1994). An estimated 1000 new cases of occupational asthma occur each year in Britain. Although there are over 200 known respiratory sensitizers, six main groups account for over half the cases (Ross *et al.* 1995). These and the work activities associated with them are shown in Table 5.2. The highest risk arises in spray painting of cars and coaches as a consequence of exposure to isocyanates, constituents of many so-called two-pack paints.

Gender differences are apparent when data based on new cases of assessed disablement under the Industrial Injuries Scheme are analysed. In the five-year period ending in 1994, cases of occupational asthma due to isocyanates in males outnumbered those in females by a factor just greater than 10. For asthma caused by flour/grain dust and hardening agents, males predominated whereas the sexes were almost equally represented in asthma caused by both soldering flux and animals/insects.

Typically, in occupational asthma symptoms identical to those of late-onset asthma develop within a few months of exposure to a respiratory sensitizer. In rare instances, cases arise several years after symptom-free exposure (Health and Safety Executive 1994). In some cases, symptoms persist after exposure has ceased (Venables *et al.* 1987). In the early stages the occupational history will reveal a temporal relationship with work, with symptoms occurring during the week and abating at weekends and holidays. As the condition worsens this pattern tends to disappear and symptoms may extend into weekends. Isocyanates and some other agents may cause a late or dual response with symptoms after work, typically cough and wheeze, occurring in the evening or night. In the case of the higher molecular weight respiratory sensitizers, such as rat urine, nasal and eye symptoms may antedate the development of respiratory symptoms. The occurrence of a wheeze which is work-related may not be related to exposure to a workplace sensitizer. Rather, cold, dust, or fume in the working environment may cause acute airways narrowing in individuals with airway hyperresponsiveness.

Table 5.2 *Substances responsible for most cases of occupational asthma (Ross et al. 1995)*

Group	Example	Activities
Isocyanates	MDI, TDI, HDI	Spray painting, foam manufacture
Flour/grain	Flour, barley, wheat, maize, rye	Baking, milling, handling grain
Solder flux	Colophony fumes	Soldering, electronic work
Laboratory animals	Urine, dander from laboratory animals	Laboratory animal work
Wood dusts	Iroko, Western red cedar	Woodworking
Glues/resins	PA, TCPA, TMA, MA, MTPA	Curing of epoxy resins

MDI = diphenylmethane di-isocyanate
TDI = toluene-2,4-di-isocyanate
HDI = hexamethylene-di-isocyanate
PA = phthalic anhydride
TCPA = tetrachlorophthalic anhydride
TMA = trimellitic anhydride
MA = maleic anhydride
MTPA = methyltetrahydrophthalic anhydride

Occupational asthma may present diagnostic difficulties, but in the majority of cases the diagnosis can be made from the following:

(1) exposure at work to an agent recognized as causing occupational asthma;
(2) a history of work-related symptoms that have developed after an initial symptom-free period of exposure;
(3) reliable, self-recorded, serial peak-flow readings which show consistent deterioration during periods of work and improvement during absence from work;
(4) where applicable and relevant, specific evidence of an immunological response to the inhaled agent (RAST testing or skin-prick testing). In some rare instances, inhalation testing with the putative agent is necessary (Newman Taylor and Pickering 1994).

Once a diagnosis of occupational asthma is confirmed, prompt removal to an area where there is no exposure is necessary. Despite this move, some workers will continue to suffer. The likelihood of recovery is greatest in workers with the least duration and intensity of exposure, and who have no further exposure to the agent. Hence the importance of early diagnosis.

Asbestos-related diseases

It is estimated that between 3000–3500 people die each year in the United Kingdom as a consequence of asbestos exposure (Department of Health 1995). 'Asbestos' is the collective term applied to a group of fibrous mineral silicates, the inhalation of which causes a number of respiratory diseases, the most important being asbestosis, diffuse pleural thickening, pleural plaques, mesothelioma, and lung cancer.

Asbestosis is defined as pulmonary interstitial fibrosis which occurs following the inhalation of asbestos fibres. It occurs after prolonged, direct, and often intense exposure to respirable asbestos (Craighead and Mossman 1982). Recent figures indicate that four out of five new cases relate to dates of first exposure prior to 1960. The interval between exposure and certification of the disease is 17.5 years and the median age at first diagnosis is over 65. Breathlessness on effort is the most important symptom and, typically, is insidious in onset. Cough is a feature of the later stages but does not occur in all cases. Bilateral end-inspiratory crackles, audible at the bases, are the earliest sign of the disease. They may ante-date symptoms, abnormalities on lung-function testing, and radiography (Brown 1994).

Mesothelioma is a malignant neoplasm of the pleura or peritoneum. In provisional figures for the three-year period 1989–91, males comprised 86% of all mesothelioma deaths. The ratio of pleural to peritoneal sites is in the order of 10:1 in males and 5:1 in females. The number of male deaths is expected to continue to rise for the next 15–25 years to reach an estimated peak of between 1300 and 3300 annual deaths (Peto *et al.* 1995). Mesothelioma has a mean latent period of between 35 and 40 years. Cigarette smoking is not a risk factor. Cases in spouses of workers, occurring as a consequence of domestic exposure to dust carried home on clothing, have been described. Breathlessness on exertion and pain are the presenting symptoms in the majority of pleural cases, with lassitude and malaise occurring later. The disease is invariably fatal. For pleural tumours the average survival time between diagnosis and death is 16 months.

Asbestos exposure increases the risk of lung cancer, particularly amongst those who also smoke (Selikoff and Lee 1978). The features of lung cancer caused by asbestos are identical to those in which asbestos has not been involved. The true incidence is difficult to estimate but it is likely that the number of cases occurring annually is at least equal to the number of cases of mesothelioma (Health and Safety Commission 1995). Lung cancer occurring in the presence of asbestosis and/or bilateral diffuse pleural thickening is a prescribed indus-trial disease. The prevention of these diseases falls into the following categories:

(1) Educational strategies to ensure that employers and employees are aware of sources of exposure and risks;

(2) the use of engineering controls, such as substitution of less toxic substances, enclo-sure, ventilating systems, and other measures;

(3) the use of personal protective devices (respirators) to minimize the inhaled dose of the agent;

(4) the use of administrative procedures to remove those at increased risk or already suf-fering from the condition from areas of exposure.

Of the above measures, the first is the most important as it tackles the problem at source.

Noise and vibration

Noise-induced hearing loss and the Hand–Arm Vibration syndrome are almost exclu-sively male diseases. In the case of hearing loss caused by noise, early symptoms are absent though a temporary tinnitus or deafness following work suggests that noise exposure is excessive. The hearing loss which, initially, is maximal at the higher frequencies involves the speech frequencies if excessive exposure continues. In patients presenting with hearing difficulty it is important to consider both occupational noise exposure and non-occupational factors such as age, family history, recreational noise, trauma, concurrent and past diseases, antibiotic therapy such as streptomycin, neomycin, other amino-glycosides, and other ototoxic drugs.

The Hand–Arm Vibration syndrome (previously called Vibration White Finger) describes a constellation of symptoms caused by the use of hand-held vibrating tools such as chain saws, percussive metal-working tools, and grinders. Early symptoms include periodic tingling of the fingertips accompanied by numbness and blanching as a consequence of spasm of the digital arteries. As the blood supply returns to normal a painful, throbbing sensation is felt. The interval between exposure and disease, i.e. the latency, is related to the vibration dose, which is a function of time and magnitude of the vibration. Early recognition is important as there is some evidence that following removal from vibration, the vascular symptoms may improve though the neurological symptoms do not. Prevention of both these conditions relies on controlling workplace exposures and educating workers. Detection of disease at the earliest possible stage is also important.

Dermatitis

Skin disorders are the most common occupational disease, comprising 40% of all reported cases (Wang 1978). Each year, an estimated 50–70 000 cases of occupational dermatitis are seen by family doctors. Dermatitis, either irritant or contact-allergic, comprises 80–90% of all occupational dermatoses, with irritant dermatitis (representing 80% of all cases of dermatitis) predominating.

The presentation of irritant and contact-allergic dermatitis may be similar with the development of itchy lesions on the hands, wrists, or arms. The thinner skin on the dorsum of the hands is particularly vulnerable. Redness and small blisters are early manifestations, cracking and thickening indicating chronicity. Patch testing will provide confirmatory evidence of a diagnosis of contact-allergic dermatitis, but as tests to confirm an irritant reaction do not exist, reliance is placed on the history and knowledge of workplace exposure.

If an occupational skin disease is suspected, a full occupational history should be obtained and evidence of changes in work practices sought. The patient should be asked how and when the rash presented and if any temporal relationship with holidays or time off exists. Details of medication used should be noted and the patient's own opinion on the likely cause sought. He should be asked if fellow workers are affected. A past medical history, specifically of an allergic diathesis or skin disorder, should be sought and, finally, relevant hobbies should be noted (Shama 1994).

Gender differences in dermatitis exist. The prevalence of irritant-contact dermatitis is higher in women, and high-risk occupations differ between men and women (Table 5.3) (Smit *et al.* 1995). Early diagnosis is important as is prevention. Methods of prevention include substitution with a safer substance, enclosed systems of work, splash guards, and ventilation controls for airborne substances. Personal protection includes appropriate gloves, good personal hygiene, and the use of barrier and conditioning creams.

Table 5.3 *Major occupational activities causing dermatitis as identified from case series (Smit et al. 1995)*

Men	Women
Engineering/metal work	Hairdressing
Food handling	Nursing
Construction	Food handling
Rubber industry	Cleaning
Painting	Dental work
Agriculture	

Back pain and other musculoskeletal conditions

Back pain, like other musculoskeletal conditions, is common, with nearly half of adults of working age experiencing low back pain in any six-week period (Verbrugge and Ascione 1987). In 1993, an estimated 150 million days of incapacity were attributable to back pain and in the same year it accounted for approximately 14 million GP consultations (Clinical Standards Advisory Group 1995). Some cross-sectional studies have shown that physically heavy work and heavy repetitive lifting while twisting increase the risk of both back pain and disc degeneration (Riihimäki 1995). There is little evidence of biological differences in back pain between men and women although women report a slightly higher frequency of back pain than men, consistent with the pattern of reporting of other symptoms. The Labour Force Survey identified miners, nurses, and those involved in transport and material moving, construction, and processing to be particularly at risk (Hodgson *et al.* 1993).

Earlier estimates of the rate of recovery of back pain were over-optimistic. Although 50% of attacks of acute back pain settle more or less completely within four weeks, some 15–20% continue to show symptoms for at least one year. The Clinical Standards Advisory Group has developed management guidelines for back pain which include useful advice on the management of painful backache in primary care. These emphasize the importance of distinguishing simple backache from nerve-root pain and serious spinal pathology. In the case of simple backache, early activity is encouraged and rest recommended only if essential (1–3 days). The guidelines advise the prescription of simple analgesics such as NSAIDs. Physical therapy is recommended if symptoms persist for more than a few days (Clinical Standards Advisory Group 1995). Attacks which do not settle within six weeks are at risk of becoming chronic. The longer the duration of absence, the lower are the chances of ever returning to work. The likelihood of return to a previous job is reduced to 50% if the duration of absence is six months.

A close liaison between the GP and the workplace, particularly the occupational physician, should ensure the best vocational and medical rehabilitation.

Work-related upper-limb disorders (WRULDs)

Upper-limb disorders and their connection with work are subjects of considerable controversy. A variety of non-specific labels indicating aetiologies that have not been convincingly proven have been applied to these conditions, including cumulative trauma disorder and repetitive strain injury (RSI), (Hadler 1989). These conditions were originally described in Australia during the 1980s when tens of thousands of office workers suffered from various complaints relating to the upper limb. Mechanization, the automation of work, and the introduction of personal computers were blamed for the epidemic, but it has also been suggested that loose diagnostic criteria also played an important part (Miller and Topliss 1988). Food processing, packaging, inspection, and repetitive assembly work are examples of tasks in which the risk of WRULDs is high.

Soft-tissue disorders represent the bulk of musculoskeletal disorders of the upper limb. Typically, patients complain of localized discomfort and tenderness, with exacerbation of symptoms with motion of the painful region. The dominant hand is primarily affected. Whilst no specific pathology is identifiable, tendonitis, tenosynovitis, epicondylitis, peritendonitis crepitans, De Quervains syndrome, and carpal tunnel syndrome are distinct clinical entities included in the group heading of WRULDs. The prognosis is excellent although symptoms may take months to remit.

In the United Kingdom, the Health and Safety Executive (HSE 1990) has defined WRULDs as:

(1) inflammation or trauma of the tendon, muscle-tendon junction, or surrounding tissue, particularly the tendon sheath. This may be temporary or chronic;

(2) inflammation of the tissue of the hand caused by constant bruising or friction of the palm – known as 'beat conditions';

(3) compression of the peripheral nerves serving the upper limb, including the hand. Many of these, such as carpal tunnel syndrome, arise in the general population but can be aggravated by work;

(4) temporary fatigue, stiffness, or soreness of the muscles comparable to that following unaccustomed exertion, but where no pathological condition exists and rest aids recovery.

Both work and leisure activities may contribute to the development of upper-limb disorders. Risk factors can be divided into three groups: those related to awkward, prolonged, static, or extremes of posture; excessive and highly repetitive movements and force; and the nature of the work itself, including job demands, lack of autonomy, insecurity, and other psychological factors.

As management of these conditions is difficult, prevention must be the primary aim. Preventive strategies are based on the application of ergonomic principles to machine design, workstations, and performance. Organizational matters are also important in any preventive strategy. The use of alternative computer technology may allow continued work with computers. These include: roller-ball systems, touch screens, voice-activated systems, and ergonomic keyboards. Consideration should also be given to reduced hours of work and increased work variety. In severe cases, redeployment may be necessary.

Occupational cancer

Cancer exacts a huge toll in terms of human suffering and economic costs. The proportion of cancers which might be attributable to occupational exposure to hazardous substances is not known, but it has been estimated that between 2–8% of cancer deaths each year could be avoided by the elimination of all workplace carcinogenic risks (Doll and Peto 1981). These estimates apply to the United States, and if applied to Britain, would imply the occurrence of some 6000 deaths per year as a result of work-related cancers, with margins of error suggesting a minimum of perhaps 3000 and a maximum of 12 000.

There is considerable difficulty in proving a causal link between a particular chemical and cancer in humans. Epidemiological data may be limited, latent periods are long, and the mechanisms involved incompletely understood. For haematological malignancies the latent period is in the range of 4–5 years, while in solid tumours periods of at least 10 or 20 years and even up to 50 years are quoted (Frumkin 1994). Carcinogenesis in experimental situations is a multi-step process comprising three stages: initiation, promotion, and progression. Initiation is seen as a process in which an irreversible potential for malignancy is induced in a target cell. Only when the cell is further acted upon by a promoter does this potential become manifest. It is accepted that many carcinogens can, of themselves, induce the entire sequence of events leading to the development of malignant neoplasms. These are known as complete or solitary carcinogens (Waldron 1990).

Where there is suspicion that cancer may be related to an occupational cause, it will be necessary to take a full occupational history detailing occupations and exposures since work commenced. In only a very small percentage of cancers is there a clear occupational link. For asbestos-related lung cancer and mesothelioma the link is well-established. Cancer of the nose and nasal sinuses has been associated with hardwood dust and male cabinet makers have a relative risk eight times that in the general population. Other associations include bladder cancer and exposure to aromatic amines in the rubber industry, lung and nasal cancer in nickel manufacture, angiosarcoma of the liver and exposure to vinyl chloride, and skin cancer and exposure to mineral oil. Table 5.4 provides a list of industrial processes causally associated with human cancer. A comprehensive listing is contained in the International Agency for Research on Cancer monographs (IARC 1987).

Exposure to industrial carcinogens constitutes only a small proportion of the total risk of cancer. Industry can help to reduce the total risk, not only by ensuring that workers are protected from the risks of industrial carcinogens but also by ensuring that they can work in an atmosphere free from both tobacco smoke and harmful concentrations of natural radon.

Work-related psychological and behavioural ill health

Stress

Stress is an integral part of life. The right amount enhances life, improves motivation, imagination, decision-making skills, and use of time thereby leading to a sense of fulfilment. If the amount of stress is less than this optimal level, monotony and boredom

Table 5.4 *Industrial processes causally associated with human cancer (IARC 1987)*

Exposure	Human target organ*
Aluminium production	Lung, bladder, (lymphoma, oesophagus, stomach)
Auramine manufacture	Bladder
Boot & shoe manufacture & repair	Leukaemia, nasal sinus, (bladder, digestive tract)
Coal gasification	Skin, lung, bladder
Coke production	Skin, lung, kidney
Furniture & cabinet making	Nasal sinus
Hematite mining – underground with exposure to radon	Lung
Iron & steel founding	Lung, (digestive tract, genitourinary tract, leukaemia)
Isopropyl alcohol manufacture – strong-acid process	Nasal sinus, (larynx)
Magenta manufacture	Bladder
Painters (occupational exposure as)	Lung, (oesophagus, stomach, bladder)
Rubber industry	Bladder, leukaemia, (lymphoma, lung, renal tract, digestive tract, skin, liver, larynx, brain, stomach)
Strong inorganic acid mists, including sulphuric acid	Larynx, lung

* *Suspected target organs in parenthesis*

occur. Conversely, if stress levels are excessive, performance decreases. If an organization is to thrive, the right amount of stress is necessary. Minor psychological morbidity is relatively common in the working population, with a prevalence of between 270–370 per 1000 employees being quoted in some studies (Jenkins 1993). Stress is considered to be the second most common cause of absence lasting more than 21 days and is the overall cause of 30–50% of all absenteeism (Health and Safety Executive 1988).

Society has put particular pressures on men and created a situation in which they may have difficulty in admitting health problems, be they physical or psychological. As a consequence they are less able than women to recognize emotional distress and seek help (Griffiths 1996). The male patient will then tend to play down problems of stress at work or bottle up feelings associated with it until it becomes unbearable.

Stress can be simply defined as the negative changes seen in individuals as a result of an imbalance between pressures placed upon them and their ability to cope. The effects of job-related stresses can be moderated by social support, family situation, and financial status. There are well-recognized factors in the workplace that can create the environment in which stress may arise. These include:

- poor management support
- lack of effective communication
- job insecurity
- work overload or underload
- low control over work or working conditions
- personality conflict and other relationship difficulties
- role ambiguity and poor job satisfaction.

It will be recognized that these conditions respect no occupational boundaries. Stress may also be caused by factors in other areas of life, including domestic, marital relationships, and physical health. Some studies have highlighted the importance of personality type, with the type-A individual (competitive, aggressive, ambitious, difficulty in relaxing, and showing poor time management) being thought to be more susceptible. It has been further postulated that stress reactions are made up of, or determined by, four elements (Beech *et al.* 1992):

(1) the basic disposition or temperament of an individual;
(2) the ability of an individual to cope with pressure;
(3) the nature of the stressors;
(4) the presence of a type-A personality.

Individuals vary in their capacity to deal with pressure and what one may find stressful another may regard as a challenge. When workers are experiencing effects of pressure it may manifest itself as:

(1) behavioural changes:
    (a) increased accidents at work
    (b) poor productivity
    (c) increased absenteeism
    (d) erratic time-keeping
    (e) poor working relationships
    (f) excessive smoking,
    (g) excessive drinking of coffee
    (h) alcohol and drug abuse;
(2) physical changes:
    (a) tiredness and lethargy
    (b) dyspepsia and peptic ulceration
    (c) headaches and muscle tension;
(3) psychological changes:
    (a) unhappiness
    (b) impatience and irritability
    (c) labile emotions
    (d) anxiety
    (e) depression.

It is important both for individuals themselves to recognize these features and for general practitioners to be aware that patients seen out of the context of their working environment may have problems that are being caused by, or made worse by, negative occupational influences.

How can general practitioners help patients cope with work stress? First, they should encourage the individual to bring their problem to the attention of the employer through contact with the line manager, welfare officer, or occupational health department if one exists. This is fundamental if organizational sources are to be addressed. Second, individuals should be encouraged to appraise their situation realistically – is it as bad as they think? Third, they should not take too much on themselves and should not dwell on overtly negative aspects over which they have no control. Finally, patients should be encouraged to look for the positive aspects of work.

The tendency in the past was to focus only on the stressed employee. Now a greater emphasis is placed on identifying and preventing organizational practices which undermine mental well-being. These primary preventive strategies complement employee-focused initiatives. Stress-management workshops aim to raise awareness of the nature of stress and its manifestations. They are useful in teaching relaxation skills and allow the development of a personal action plan to combat stress.

Promotion of general fitness can be useful and workers should be encouraged to take exercise regularly, to take alcohol only to the recommended limits, to stop smoking, and eat a sensible, balanced diet. Some may benefit from learning relaxation techniques or using many of the alternative therapies now available, such as reflexology, yoga, transcendental meditation, and shiatsu (Hatchwell 1995). Others may need counselling or psychiatric treatment if their symptoms warrant it. Occasionally, suicidal behaviour may be exhibited. Occupational health services work alongside management in developing strategies aimed at combating stress. They also provide counselling support and advice on rehabilitation for employees who suffer from stress.

Post-traumatic stress disorder (PTSD)

This complex condition is of relevance to the theme of men and work although not exclusive to work situations or to males. PTSD is a condition which can occur after a traumatic event or critical incident with which the individual who experienced the event cannot cope. Occupations considered to be at risk include the emergency services (McCloy 1992) – police, fire, and ambulance. In addition, people in many occupations may be involved in a single, unexpected incident of sufficient horror to have the potential to provoke PTSD, e.g. a major accident at work or a robbery with extreme violence. Usually, feelings of terror, bewilderment, intense fear, and a sense of helplessness have been present during the course of the incident.

The diagnostic criteria for post-traumatic stress disorder using the fourth edition of the Diagnostic and Statistical Manual–DSM IV (American Psychiatric Association 1994) are:
(1) exposure to a traumatic event in which both of the following were present:
  (a) the individual experienced, witnessed, or was confronted with an event or events that involved actual or threatened death or serious injury, or a threat to the physical integrity of self or others

(b) the individual's response involved intense fear, helplessness, or horror;
(2) the traumatic event is persistently re-experienced;
(3) persistent avoidance of stimuli associated with the trauma and numbing of general responsiveness (not present before the trauma);
(4) persistent symptoms of increased arousal (not present before the trauma);
(5) duration of the disturbance (symptoms in criteria 1, 2, and 3) is more than one month;
(6) the disturbance causes clinically significant distress or impairment in social, occupational, or other important areas of functioning.

Research, particularly among Vietnam veterans, has shown that early and appropriate intervention can prevent up to 80% of detrimental long-term effects, including PTSD (McHenry 1995). The intervention takes the form of a defusing or critical-incident debriefing. This allows those exposed to ventilate their feelings, usually those of inadequacy, anger, grief, and resentment. Often this occurs in a group situation. Normally one follow-up session will be all that is required, although for some, further individual or group counselling may be needed. It is estimated that up to 20% of those involved in traumatic incidents may develop PTSD despite the preventive procedures outlined above, and for them psychiatric and psychological support is required (Duckworth 1991). A new technique known as Eye Movement Desensitization and Reprocessing (EMDR) is a therapeutic procedure that has been shown to be effective in treating the traumatic impact of critical incidents (Montgomery and Ayllon 1994; Vaughan *et al.* 1994).

Alcohol and substance abuse

Even though this topic is dealt with in a chapter on its own, there are specific problems related to alcohol in the workplace. Employees with a substance-misuse problem can be defined as those whose regular or intermittent use of a substance or a mixture of substances repeatedly interferes with their work or the work of others, their job performance or their ability to work, or their relationships with colleagues or clients (Chick 1994). It is thought that 4% of the population in England and Wales and over 8% in Scotland are consuming alcohol to excess, thus affecting their health, employment, and social and domestic life (Smith and Lipsedge 1995). Drink-related absenteeism is estimated to cost British industry about £960 million a year, with sickness and absence due to hangovers accounting for at least 8 million lost working days per year (Health Education Authority 1994). In a 1991 OPCS survey, 4% of men and 2% of women admitted that a hangover caused them to stay away from work at least once in the past year (Goddard 1991).

The acute effect of alcohol is depression of the central nervous system. The associated impairment of higher mental functions is manifest as impaired judgement, reduced reaction times and impaired perception, balance, and coordination. The ability to operate machinery, drive, and to make decisions is compromised. Relatively low levels of alcohol can cause impairment. Effects on decision-making skills have been shown at blood alcohol levels as low at 25–50 milligrams per decilitre. At blood alcohol levels of 60 milligrams per decilitre, the risk of involvement in an accident increases twofold compared with drivers who have not taken alcohol. Blood alcohol levels of 100 milligrams per decilitre and 150 milligrams per decilitre are associated with a six- and 25-fold increase in accident risk respectively. Workers who chronically abuse alcohol are likely to escape detection and may only be identified because of abnormal liver function tests or a raised mean corpuscular volume (mcv) in the absence of other causes.

Mortality rates from hepatic cirrhosis are highest in the alcohol manufacturing and retail industries. Research has shown that brewery workers have a higher average intake of alcohol on recruitment compared to other factory workers. They also increase their consumption to a greater extent during the next two years (Hore and Plant 1981). Selective recruitment and exposure would therefore appear to contribute to alcohol-related risks in the brewing industry. Other occupations at risk include seamen and fishermen, the armed services, and the construction industry. Alcohol-related problems also occur in the professions, including insurance, finance, law, journalism, and medicine.

Frequently, an alcohol or drug problem is first identified in the workplace. Features indicative of problem drinking include poor time-keeping and absenteeism. Where excessive weekend drinking occurs, Monday is the commonest day for absence (Addley 1989). Companies who pay employees on Thursday will find that Friday will be the commonest day. Other presentations include accidents, withdrawal fits, illness, or a drink/drive conviction. Signs such as tremor, red conjunctivae, smell of alcohol on the breath, irritability, and aggressiveness may be significant. Prolonged lunch breaks during which alcohol is consumed and delay on returning home in the evenings due to drinking en route may also be seen.

Denial in the workplace is common. A manager is often best placed to intervene at an early stage when an alcohol or drug-related problem occurs. The employee should be offered an alcohol recovery programme and the inevitability of disciplinary action explained unless improvement occurs. Close liaison between the occupational physician and the general practitioner is essential.

Many employers have now introduced alcohol policies. These cover the following areas:

(1) alcohol or drug problems are to be regarded as a health matter with the corollary that the employee is expected to pursue and comply with treatment;

(2) any disciplinary action which is required is postponed while the employee seeks treatment;

(3) the firm will grant sick leave if this is required for treatment purposes;

(4) information about compliance or success of treatment may be communicated to the employer. If there is evidence of relapse at work this will be passed to the treatment agency if the employee is still being dealt with under the policy;

(5) when all efforts of help have failed, the ultimate sanctions of disciplinary action or termination of employment on health grounds remain (Chick 1994).

The use of cannabis in the United Kingdom is widespread, particularly in males aged 15–25 in whom the level of usage is estimated to be around 12% (Smith and Lipsedge 1995). Cannabis use impairs memory, concentration, judgement, and ability to carry out perceptual tasks. The effects on memory may persist for some weeks after a period of abstinence. The impaired performance consequent on these effects has implications for safe driving and the operation of machinery. It is particularly detrimental to jobs involving trains, planes, buses, and taxis as well as occupations which involve the operation of, or monitoring of, safety systems, such as air traffic controllers and signal operators.

It is now becoming more acceptable for UK companies to introduce drug-screening programmes. These usually take the form of pre-employment, post-incident, and random sampling or a combination of all three (McHenry 1994). Specific groups of workers, such as train drivers, can be screened under legislation – Transport and Works Act 1992 – using a sample of breath, blood, or urine for alcohol and the latter two to test for other drugs.

Conclusion

Work and health are fundamental elements that interact in our lives. Work provides a sense of purpose, social contacts, status, income, and a sense of belonging. Both accidents and ill health caused by work reflect a breakdown in control measures and as such are preventable.

A knowledge of occupational health is essential for the family doctor. It enables the recognition of the earliest manifestation of work-related diseases and informs judgement on prescribing and fitness for work. An interest in occupational medicine allows family doctors to broaden their preventive and educational roles and to have a positive impact not only on the health of their own patients but also on others who may be exposed to workplace risks to health. Finally, doctors in all branches of medicine have become increasingly aware and concerned about work-related aspects of their own health, and family doctors being employers have additional health and safety responsibilities in respect of those they employ.

In recent years the pattern of employment has changed, with part-time work and self-employment showing a rapid increase and small businesses increasing in number. These trends are reflected in the reduced provision of comprehensive occupational services by employers. This lack of specialist occupational medical advice increases the likelihood of general practitioners being asked to advise on occupational health matters. If specialist assistance is required, this can be obtained from doctors of the Employment Advisory Service based at local Health and Safety Executive offices, who can, where necessary, assess risks to health first-hand through a workplace visit.

Where occupational health services exist, a close liaison between the family doctor and the occupational physician is particularly useful for early and appropriate rehabilitation after illness, if retirement on medical grounds is under consideration, and when workplace risks are suspected to be harming health. The respective roles of general practitioner and occupational physician are complementary. Both have, as their aim, workplaces in which accidents and ill health are eliminated and in which work forms part of a satisfying life, actively contributing to health.

References

Addley, K. (1989). Change in Sunday licensing laws and the effect on Monday absenteeism. A short report on a small poultry processing plant. *Ulster Medical Journal*, **58** (21), 137–9.

American Psychiatric Association (1994). *Diagnostic and statistical manual of mental diseases*. APA, Washington, DC.

Beech, H. R., Burns, L. E., Sheffield, B. F. (1992). Occupational stress and stress reactions. In *A behavioural approach to the management of stress: a practical guide to techniques.* John Wiley and Sons, Chichester.

Brown, K. (1994). Asbestos-related disorders. In *Occupational lung disorders* (ed. W. R. Parkes), pp. 411–504. Butterworth Heinemann, London.

Chick, J. (1994). Substance abuse and the workplace. In *Hunter's diseases of occupations* (ed. P. A. B. Raffle, P. H. Adams, P. J. Baxter, and W. R. Lee), pp. 602–11. Edward Arnold, London.

Clarke, S., Elliott, R., and Osman, J. (1995). Occupation and sickness absence. In *Occupational health decennial supplement* (ed. F. Drever), pp. 217–31. HMSO, London.

Clinical Standards Advisory Group (1995). *Back pain.* HMSO, London.

Coggon, D., Inskip, H., Winter, P., and Pannett, B. (1995). Occupational mortality by cause of death. In *Occupational health decennial supplement* (ed. F. Drever), pp. 62–76. HMSO, London.

Craighead, J. E. and Mossman, B. T. (1982). The pathogenesis of asbestos-associated disease. *New England Journal of Medicine,* **306,** 1446–55.

Davies, N. V. and Teasdale, P. (1994). The costs to the British economy of work accidents and work-related ill health. HSE Books, Suffolk.

Department of Health (1995). *On the state of the public health 1994.* HMSO, London.

Doll, R. and Peto, J. (1981). *The causes of cancer.* Oxford University Press, Oxford.

Duckworth, D. H. (1991). Information requirements for crisis intervention after disaster at work. *Stress Medicine,* **7,** 19–24.

Frumkin, H. (1994). Occupational cancers. In *A practical approach to occupational and environmental medicine* (ed. R. J. McCunney), pp. 187–98. Little, Brown, and Co., Boston.

Goddard, E. (1991). Drinking in England and Wales In The Late 1980's, OPCS, London.

Goldman, R. H. (1994). Suspecting occupational disease. In *A practical approach to occupational and environmental medicine* (ed. R. J. McCunney), pp. 301–20. Little, Brown, and Co., Boston.

Griffiths, S. (1996). Mens' health: unhealthy lifestyle and an unwillingness to seek medical help. *British Medical Journal,* **312,** 69–70.

Hadler, N. (1989). The roles of work and of working in disorders of the upper extremity. *Baillière's Rheumatology,* **3,** 121–41.

Hatchwell, P. (1995). Stress management and therapy. Part 1. Mainstream and complementary techniques. *Occupational Health Review,* **56,** 26–30.

Health Education Authority (1994). Drinkwise in the Workplace: Getting the Message Across. Health Education Authority, London.

Health and Safety Commission (1995). *Annual report 1994–1995.* HSE Books, Suffolk.

Health and Safety Commission (1995). *Health and safety statistics 1994/1995.* HSE Books, Suffolk.

Health and Safety Executive (1988). Mental health at work (IND (G) 59 (L)). HSE Books, Suffolk.

Health and Safety Executive (1990). *Work-related upper limb disorders – a guide to prevention.* (HS(G)60). HSE Books, Suffolk.

Health and Safety Executive (1994). *Preventing asthma at work: how to control respiratory sensitisers.* HSE Books, Suffolk.

Hodgson, J. T., Jones, J. R., Elliott, R. C., and Osman, J. (1993). *Self-reported work-related illness. Research paper 33.* HMSO, London.

Hore, B. D. and Plant, M. A. (ed.) (1981). *Alcohol problems in employment.* Croom Helm, London.

International Agency for Research on Cancer (1987). *IARC monographs on the evaluation of carcinogenic risks to humans: an updating of monographs, Vol. 1–42.* (Suppl. 7). IARC, Lyon.

Jenkins, R. (1993). Defining the problem: stress, depression and anxiety – causes, prevalence and consequences. In *Promoting mental health policies in the workplace* (ed. R. Jenkins and D. Warman). HMSO, London.

Kelly, S., Charlton, J., and Jenkins, R. (1995). Suicide deaths in England and Wales 1982–1992: the contribution of occupation and geography. *Population Trends,* **80,** 16–25.

McCloy, E. (1992). Management of post-incident trauma: a fire service perspective. *Occupational Medicine,* **42,** 163–6.

McHenry, C. (1994). Drug testing in the workplace. *Occupational Health Review,* **47,** 9–13.

McHenry, C. (1995). Stress in the police service: preventing the long-term effects of trauma. *Occupational Health Review,* **56,** 17–20.

Miller, M. H. and Topliss, D. J. (1988). Chronic upper limb pain syndrome (repetitive strain injury) in the Australian workforce: a systematic cross-sectional rheumatologic study of 229 patients. *Journal of Rheumatology,* **15,** 1705–12.

Montgomery, R. W. and Ayllon, T. (1994). Eye movement desensitisation across subjects: subjective and physiological measures of treatment efficacy. *Journal of Behavioural Therapy and Experimental Psychiatry,* **3,** 217–30.

Newman Taylor, A. J. and Pickering, C. A. C. (1994). Occupational asthma and byssinosis. In *Occupational lung disorders* (ed. W. R. Parkes), pp. 710–74. Butterworth Heinemann, Oxford.

Peto, J., Hodgson, J. T., Matthews, F. E., and Jones, J. R. (1995). Continuing increase in mesothelioma mortality in Great Britain. *Lancet,* **345,** 535–40.

Ramazzini, B. (1713). *De morbis artificium diatriba.* In *Hunter's diseases of occupations* (ed. P. A. B. Raffle, P. H. Adam, P. J. Baxter, and R. Lee). Edward Arnold, London.

Riihimäki, H. (1995). Back and limb disorders. In *Epidemiology of work related diseases* (ed. J. C. McDonald), pp. 207–38. BMJ Publications, London.

Ross, D. J., Sallie, B. S., and McDonald, J. C. (1995). SWORD 1994: surveillance of work related and occupational respiratory disease in the United Kingdom. *Occupational Medicine,* **45**(4), 174–8.

Selikoff, I. J. and Lee, H. K. (1978). *Asbestos and disease.* Academic Press, New York.

Shama, S. K. (1994). Occupational skin disorders. In *A practical approach to occupational and environmental medicine* (ed. R. J. McCunney), pp. 248–64. Little, Brown, and Co., Boston.

Skelton, R. (1988). Man's role in society and its effect on health. *Nursing, 3rd series,* **26,** 953–6.

Smit, H., Coenraads, P. J., and Emmett, E. (1995). Dermatoses. In *Epidemiology of work related diseases* (ed. J. C. McDonald), pp. 143–64. BMJ Publications, London.

Smith, G. and Lipsedge, M. S. (1995). *Stress, alcohol, and drug abuse.* In *Fitness for work: the medical aspects* (ed. R. A. F. Cox, F. C. Edwards, R. I. McCannon, pp. 398–412. Oxford University Press, Oxford.

Taylor, P. J. (1983). Absenteeism: definition and statistics. In *Encyclopaedia of occupational health and safety.* International Labour Organisation, Geneva.

Vaughan, K., Wiese, M., Gold, R., and Tarrier, N. (1994). Eye-movement desensitisation: symptom change in post-traumatic stress disorder. *British Journal of Psychiatry*, **164**, 533–41.

Verbrugge, L. M. and Ascione, F. J. (1987). Exploring the iceberg: Common symptoms and how people care for them. *Medical Care*, **25**, 481–6.

Venables, K. M., Topping, M. D., Nunn, A. J., Howe, W., and Newman-Taylor, A. J. (1987). Immunologic and functional consequences of chemical (tetrachlorophthalic anhydride) induced asthma after four years of avoidance of exposure. *Journal of Allergy and Clinical Immunology*, **80**, 212–18.

Waldron, H. A. (1990). *Lecture notes on occupational medicine.* Blackwell Scientific Publications, Oxford pp. 133–144.

Wang, C. L. (1978). *The problem of skin disease in industry.* Office of Occupational Safety and Health Statistics, US Department of Labour.

CHAPTER SIX

Problems of not working

Norman Beale

The recent past has seen the return of mass unemployment, a phenomenon that most commentators thought had vanished along with crystal radio sets, cobbled streets, and cloth caps. Work has always been the traditional arena in which men function, gaining self-respect, social contact, and a rhythm to their lives as well as the wages to support themselves and their families. In this chapter, the author discusses the effects on men's health of not having a job, and leaves little room for disagreement.

'Lying in harbour rots good ships and good men' is a maxim attributed to Lord Nelson. Like all successful military leaders he had an innate grasp of the male psyche. He understood that idle men are soon unhappy. The sooner he could put to sea and divert his sailors with activity, however repetitive or unpleasant, the fewer the disciplinary problems for him and his officers. Unfortunately, national economies cannot be run along the lines of nineteenth-century battleships.

Only a few decades ago, people worked for about 47 hours per week, for about 47 weeks a year, and for about 47 years (100000 hours) (Smith 1987). Life expectancy may have risen during this century but 'work expectancy' has dropped. On average, people now only work for 50000 hours in a lifetime (37 hours × 37 weeks × 37 years) (ibid). Faced with this trend, the most equitable outcome would be for everyone to work, each for a smaller proportion of their time. However, the equation is being allowed to balance, in many societies and certainly in the UK, by restricting available work to a depleted majority. The 'employed' continue to enjoy a busy and satisfying lifestyle while a deprived minority have to cope with the difficulties of being 'unemployed' (Dean 1993).

Although this is a book written mostly by men about men, it is not male chauvinism to assert that men are more exposed than women to the traumas of unemployment in societies like ours. Having a job, 'bringing home the bacon', remains the central role in the lives of most adult men.

The assumption that unemployment is a male problem is so ingrained that authors of the relevant literature usually assume all the jobless to be men or forget to state, unambiguously, the gender of their study subjects. But accepting assumptions as fact is a common fallacy in the context of unemployment. It is essential to discuss terminology and sociology before looking to see what we know of how not working can affect men's health.

The definitions of unemployment

At its simplest, being unemployed means being out of work, but this assumes we know what we mean by 'work'. Defining the term less circuitously is not easy. The most respected sociologist in this field has suggested that the unemployed are '. . . all those who have not got a job but who would like to have one or who, when they have no job, are dependent on some financial support . . .' (Jahoda 1982).

It is customary to distinguish different types of unemployment, but the terms are often inadequate and ambiguous. The terms may describe the nature of the experience itself, for instance 'frictional unemployment', when workers are between jobs, or 'long-term unemployment', usually defined as lasting more than a year. Alternatively, it may refer to the cause, such as 'structural unemployment', being the phenomenon which has recently been so familiar of unemployment which results from a decline in particular industries.

The meaning of work

The loss of a job does not simply equate with loss of income. It was Freud who suggested that work is a person's strongest tie to reality (Freud 1930). Redundancy can provoke an identity crisis parallel to those associated with other life changes (Higgs 1984). The reasons for this are found outside the wage packet. The so-called 'latent functions' of work have been described authoritatively by Jahoda (1979):

(1) the imposition of a time structure on the waking day – 'traction';
(2) shared experiences and contacts outside the home – 'social life';
(3) linking an individual to goals transcending his own – 'sense of purpose';
(4) personal standing and identity – 'status'.

These hidden advantages of work help to explain the strong motivation most people feel to seek a new job even if working conditions are poor and even if they fall into the 'poverty trap' of having, finally, less disposable income than if they remained idle and relied on benefit payments.

Not all work is preferable to unemployment (Gallie et al. 1994) but having a job is certainly a symbol of maintained health. Continuous employment will appear to confer well-being via the 'healthy worker effect' (McMichael 1976). Over time, the rigours of a job will weed out those not healthy enough to maintain an acceptable level of performance. The remaining workforce will be, in Darwinian parlance, the 'fittest survivors'. In fact, Warr (1987) has developed a 'vitamin' analogy. He sees work as one of the primary environmental features that can affect (mental) health. A certain intake of the vit(al)amine called 'work' is necessary to maintain well-being, but after attainment of optimal levels no further benefit is derived from additional quantities which may even be detrimental.

People who work too hard have acquired the label 'workaholics' and this fits very well with Warr's proposal.

Unemployment: a recurring problem

Although it was not the first, the best-known period of high UK unemployment was during the 1930s. The problem was solved, fortuitously, by the outbreak of war. But by then there were those who were determined to effect such profound changes in economic policy that the dole queues would never be seen again (Beveridge 1944). After the war, 'Keynesian' economics – the creation of jobs by encouraging state investment, government capital projects, and high consumer spending – formed the basis of policy in the UK. The ideal of full employment was realized. The creed was so strongly held by the 1960s that fears that the unemployment rate might rise above half a million provoked emergency cabinet meetings (Howard 1979). However, unemployment crept up again during the 1970s and increased dramatically during the 1980s (Fig. 6.1). The 'new' economics fostered by the administration that came to power in 1979 – '... unemployment ... (is a) ... price well worth paying' (Hansard 1991) – resulted in the UK unemployment total being consistently above 2.5 million for more than a decade.

Fig. 6.1 *UK registered unemployment (Employment Gazettes, 1973–1993)*

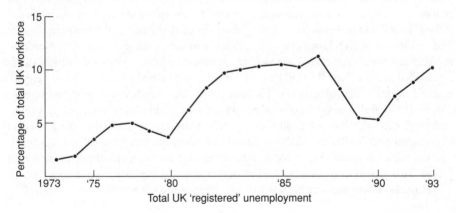

Total UK 'registered' unemployment

The unemployed

When jobs are plentiful the unemployed tend to be a small group of vulnerable individuals who repeatedly lose short-lived jobs. The situation changes as unemployment rates climb. Economic recession leads to mass redundancies and people with previously stable jobs find themselves coping with the cruel realities of unemployment, often for the first time.

The actual number unemployed in Britain is a contentious issue since it is in the political arena and there is no universally agreed definition of unemployment. The figure based on the largest denominator is the 'registered unemployed' – those claiming benefit at UK benefit offices on the day of each monthly count. Not all the jobless will want to register for work; on the other hand, studies consistently report that no more than 2% of the unemployed could be classified as 'shirkers' or 'scroungers' despite a high profile generated by the media (Porter 1989). There is also a small satellite of the potential workforce who are unemployable because they are severely disabled. But the unemployment 'register' is now also a doubtful index for a more significant reason. The mechanism of the monthly count remained essentially the same for the whole of the post-war period until 1979. Since October of that year there have been 34 adjustments in the way in which the Department of Employment calculates the official total. At least 20 of the changes have reduced the declared number, effecting a cumulative decrease of 1.5 million (Taylor 1990), a trend that government ministers pretended to see as fortuitous (Cole 1995).

There is now the prospect that the monthly unemployment 'figures' will be consigned to history as 'workfare' is introduced. In schemes of this sort the unemployed are obliged to 'earn' their benefits in some form of compulsory training or community work. Whether or not this will help those with no paid employment (in the present sense), it has obvious attractions for politicians since it will further obfuscate the size of the problem (Smith 1993).

The unemployed (classified by their last occupation) are not found equally across the social-class spectrum (see Table 6.1). Until the last decade there were dramatic differences between socio-economic groups in this respect. However, the new wave of unemployment associated with the economic recession of the early 1990s has uniquely affected skilled clerical and professional workers who have been shed from the financial and service sectors. All social classes are having to learn to cope with job insecurity. Nevertheless,unemployment has always been a more significant problem among the unskilled and low-skilled groups (Sinfield 1981) whose higher standardized mortality ratios were recognized in the 1940s (Morris and Titmuss 1944). The health/wealth gradient remains (Arber 1987) and it is very unlikely, therefore, that unemployed men will have been endowed with the best of health even while working. In fact, the 'Black Report' (Townsend and Davidson 1982) concluded that when unemployment levels climb, the link between low social class, poor health, and sparse employment opportunity is reinforced. This view is now corroborated by new evidence using data from successive General Household Surveys over the last 20 years (Bartley and Owen 1996).

The experience of unemployment

'He was standing there as motionless as a statue, cap neb pulled over his eyes, gaze fixed on the pavement, hands in pockets, shoulders hunched, the bitter wind blowing his thin trousers tightly against his legs. . . . He was an anonymous unit of an army of three million for whom there was no tomorrow.' (Greenwood 1933). The images of unemployment in the 1930s are still familiar, but the factors that influence the experience of unemployment now differ from those in the pre-war period. They have been summarized recently by Jahoda (1982):

Table 6.1 *Social class distribution at ages 16–64 of men who were seeking work in 1981 compared with that of all men (Moser et al. 1984)*

Social class:	All men aged 16–64	Men seeking work aged 16–64	
		No	As % of all men in that class
I	8248	181	2.2
II	32687	926	2.8
III non-manual	17339	793	4.6
III manual	53346	4531	8.5
IV	25347	2543	10.0
V	9131	1895	20.8
[I–V]	[146098]	[10869]	[7.4]
Armed forces	2030	79	3.9
Inadequately described	5199	3718	71.5
Unoccupied	10336	6	0.1
All men aged 16–64	163680	14675	9.0

- material improvements
- increased life expectancy
- the National Health Service
- redundancy payments and other benefits
- extended compulsory education
- increased expectation of work after high employment
- increased communication and awareness
- decreased work ethic
- fewer dirty or dangerous jobs
- more women at work.

There has also been a disintegration of the closely-knit, working-class communities of earlier decades, with erosion of the mutual social and economic support they offered (Hoggart 1957). And the latest upsurge of unemployment has exposed how mortgaged ownership of property can provoke an immediate financial crisis for those who lose their jobs; redundancy may rapidly be compounded by house repossession.

Each of a large number of observers has studied in depth a few families suffering 'modern' unemployment (Fagin and Little 1984; Fryer and Ullah 1987; Marsden 1982; Seabrook 1983; Sinfield 1981). Except for Fagin's study, such qualitative reports have concentrated on the social consequences of unemployment and there is little doubt that financial privation is still the dominant experience of the unemployed despite the creation of a social security 'safety net'. A study in 1978 (Moylan *et al.* 1984) showed that unemployed men had earned, while working, far less than national averages. Half of them drew wages in the bottom fifth of the national earnings distribution. Despite this, a third of the cohort were living on less than half of their former incomes now that they were unemployed. They had been poor when working; now they were even more impoverished. It was no surprise when it was found that very few of them had any savings.

Much of the experience of unemployment is governed by benefits legislation. In the UK for instance, there are redundancy payments for those employees dismissed when their labour is no longer required. There is also, from October 1996, a job-seeker's allowance, available to all ex-employees who cannot find a new job. There are conditions that restrict their availability and the job-seeker's allowance will be means tested after six months. In all cases, the unstated assumption is that they should help people between jobs; they were never intended to support people through long periods of unemployment.

However, the unemployed face pressures other than financial; they have to fill their free time. There is a popular notion that the unemployed in the 1930s loitered on street corners whereas they now loll at home all day in front of a television or video recorder. But in Brighton in 1982, 200 men who had been unemployed for at least six months only watched TV for an hour longer per day than employed counterparts and did not sleep more (Miles 1983). There was some role reversal. The married men performed domestic chores for four hours per day (controls for one hour) and did more shopping. Their lives were not as inactive as prejudice would suggest but none of them felt that they were using their time creatively.

The so-called 'phased response pattern' to unemployment – shock – optimism – money worries – boredom – declining self-respect – pessimism – fatalism – (Harrison 1976) resembles the more familiar one associated with bereavement (Murray-Parkes 1972). However, there is no evidence that all men who lose jobs experience these distinct stages in the order proposed by Harrison (Archer and Rhodes 1987). There can be no doubt that repeated rejection will result in the unemployed feeling unwanted and stigmatized. An unknown proportion of those made redundant are provoked to create their own paid employment by forming small businesses, individually or in partnerships. Many such enterprises are, however, doomed to failure and only serve to delay entry into the job market.

Government training programmes – advertised as an attractive alternative to idleness – have not been popular and have had a mixed press. At best they can teach suitably motivated individuals new skills, but they can also raise a man's hope of another job without increasing his chances of actual re-employment; promise without fulfilment.

At an emotionally taxing time, moral and economic pressures will result in cumulative pressures on a man to get a new job, but there is evidence that the likelihood of fresh employment declines with time (Colledge and Bartholomew 1980; Krahn *et al.* 1985; Moylan *et al.* 1985). The resulting vicious spiral generally produces a feeling of helplessness and unemployment is, for most people, a 'profoundly corrosive experience' (Harrison 1976). If unemployment is an acknowledged personal, social, and economic burden, would we not expect it to damage health? Surprisingly, the morbidity of being unable to find a job is one of the least explored territories of social medicine.

Research on unemployment and health

Nineteenth-century Poor Law reforms (1834) were framed, like their medieval predecessors, by legislators who attributed unemployment to personal failings; anyone with motivation could find work. The steep and inexorable rise in unemployment in the 1920s and 1930s forced a change in attitude. It was no longer tenable that the unemployed were suffering self-inflicted wounds and exposed the need for research on the health and social consequences of unemployment.

Testing hypotheses

Although most case-history reports on unemployment and health reinforce the view that there is a strong, inverse relationship, very few of them have increased our understanding of the complex mechanisms involved (Bartley 1994). In essence, we still have no real measures of three possible hypotheses:

(1) that unemployment causes ill health (the causal hypothesis);
(2) that deteriorating health leads to unemployment (selection hypothesis);
(3) that unemployment and morbidity are both linked to common background factors (association hypothesis).

Fig. 6.2 *The hypotheses of the relationship between unemployment and health*

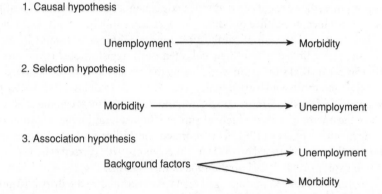

1. Causal hypothesis

Unemployment ⟶ Morbidity

2. Selection hypothesis

Morbidity ⟶ Unemployment

3. Association hypothesis

Background factors ⟶ Unemployment
Background factors ⟶ Morbidity

The literature on unemployment and health is widely dispersed and difficult to organize. But if testing the causal hypothesis (1) is taken to be the gold standard of unemployment/health research, it becomes possible to assemble investigations in a hierarchy that should represent increasing value.

Aggregate studies

Studies which compare population statistics, such as mortality or suicide rates with national economic indicators like unemployment, involve large numbers of unidentified individuals (Brenner 1971, 1979; Bunn 1979; Forbes and McGregor 1984; Franks *et al.* 1991; Furness *et al.* 1985; Hawton and Rose 1986; Platt and Kreitman 1984). The findings are not all consistent and such trend studies cannot isolate the specific influence of unemployment from other secular changes. For instance, there is a clear linear relationship between the unemployed rates of the then 14 English regional health authorities and the number of prescriptions per person annually dispensed (Griffin 1993). Although those regions with the highest levels of unemployment faced the highest drugs bills, other factors such as overall social deprivation could partly account for these findings.

Cross-sectional studies

Taking a 'group snapshot' of the workforce and contrasting images of the active and inactive members is probably the easiest type of study to perform, and the effect of unemployment itself is more discrete. Such cross-sectional studies lack the design elegance to discriminate cause and effect but they can be very useful in examining the influence of third variables such as social class (Payne *et al.* 1984), employment commitment (Jackson *et al.* 1983), duration of employment and age (Fryer and Warr 1984; Jackson and Warr 1984), social support (Ullah *et al.* 1985), and the prevailing unemployment rate (Jackson and Warr 1987), whatever the direction of causality. The unified conclusions suggest that a man suffering the worst psychological effects of unemployment will be aged 40–49, have few close relatives or friends to support him, be endowed with a strong work ethic, and be out of work in a community where the unemployment rate is relatively low and where having no job carries a high degree of social stigma.

Longitudinal studies

In 'follow-up' studies, data are collected at repeated sequential assessments of identified individuals. For instance, the Office of Population Censuses and Surveys (OPCS) based its longitudinal study on a 1% sample of the 1971 census. Employment status in census week was subsequently linked to routinely collected death registrations. It was already apparent after five years that subjects in work during the census had a lower standardized mortality (SMR) than those who were unemployed (Fox and Goldblatt 1982). After further follow-up, the findings were more convincing and supported by a regional analysis in which SMRs of the unemployed were higher in areas of high unemployment (Moser *et al.* 1984). The next census figures (1981) corroborated the earlier findings (Moser *et al.* 1987), as did parallel research based on the Danish census of 1970 (Iversen *et al.* 1987) and by Martikainen's study (1990) based on the 1980 Finnish census.

Between 1978 and 1980, 7735 middle-aged men were recruited to the British Regional Heart Study – a prospective survey of the ecological and personal risk factors in cardiovascular disease. Because of the rising interest in unemployment shortly after the initiation of the BRHS, entry data were reanalysed with respect to employment status of the recruits (Cook *et al.* 1982). Those who were unemployed but felt fit for work (1.9% of the sample) were found to have a significant 60% excess of ischaemic heart disease over their employed peers. The project continues to provide us with useful data. Study men who, by the mid 1980s, had lost their stable jobs faced a doubling of their expected risk of mortality in the first five years after their redundancy, even if this was disguised as 'early retirement' (Morris *et al.* 1994). The BRHS has also given us some insights into the effects of unemployment on cigarette smoking and alcohol consumption. Loss of employment did not seem to provoke an increase in smoking or drinking. This finding matches that of a study of 929 Scottish school-leavers (Peck and Plant 1986). However, the BRHS data did show that 6% more men who were destined to lose their jobs were smokers at the time of recruitment to the study and 3.1% more were heavy drinkers. Like poverty and poor-quality housing, cigarette smoking and heavy drinking are health hazards that susceptible individuals seem to carry with them into unemployment rather than being risky behaviour they adopt in response to job loss. In fact, unemployment may force smokers to curtail their consumption and offset the risks of their habit (Lee *et al.* 1991).

Two large follow-up studies have examined the consequences for teenagers who cannot find work after leaving school (Banks and Jackson 1982; Donovan *et al.* 1986). Both show that in those who found work after leaving school there were improvements in measures of emotional stability, whereas those in their jobless peers deteriorated.

Factory-closure studies

Factory-closure studies have several design attributes which should make them the best type of research in resolving the unemployment and health conundrum (Morris and Cook 1991). They are longitudinal studies where the cohort and the cause of the unemployment are defined by a shared circumstance – a mass redundancy. It may be difficult, however, to glean any objective evidence of the subjects' health in the period before they lose their jobs.

The pioneering study of Fisher (1965) was largely qualitative, but those of Kasl and colleagues (Kasl *et al.* 1975; Kasl *et al.* 1968; Kasl and Cobb 1970) were able to detect significant clinical and biochemical changes in blue-collar factory workers made redundant in Michigan, USA. Scandinavian research teams also published useful data (Iversen and Klausen 1981; Westin *et al.* 1989). Jacobsen (1972) first detected the clinical significance of the threat of unemployment. He was able to demonstrate a peak of general practitioner consultations associated with a strong rumour, denied by the employer, of a forthcoming mass redundancy. The studies of Beale and Nethercott (1985) and of Mattiasson and public-health colleagues (1990) were also able to prove the central importance of threatened redundancy. Detectable signs of clinical trauma seem to begin at this point even if it precedes actual job loss by as much as two years (Beale and Nethercott 1988*a, b*). However, the proof that the causal mechanism is the strongest link between unemployment and ill health still eludes us: we still need the benefit of data from a substantial prospective study based on the demise of a major industry.

Conclusions

An editorial in a recent volume of the leading academic journal of British general practice included the following: 'While it would be perverse to suggest that unemployment could have a beneficial effect on health, the adverse effects of unemployment on health remain uncertain and the relationship between the two is unclear.' (Anon 1985). A decade later, and after a further trough and peak in persistently high levels of UK unemployment, research findings remain sparse and inconclusive. The fact that the raw data can be accommodated in such detail in a brief review such as this can only mean a dearth of evidence. Contrast this with the background to a new report from the Royal College of Physicians on smoking and the young, where the working party was able to draw on the conclusions of 423 research papers (Turner-Warwick 1992). Investigating the epidemiology of unemployment morbidity has been underexplored (Wagstaff 1986), but some commentators are prepared to interpret the little data we have as 'almost irrefutable' evidence that unemployment kills (Smith 1991). Others have been confident enough to calculate a UK mortality rate for unemployment (Scott-Samuel 1985) – 3000 excess male deaths per annum. This would be the equivalent of a Lockerbie disaster every six weeks.

The realization that each of the possible sequential experiences in the workplace (Fig. 6.3) might have a discrete effect on individual health should dictate future research design (Bartley 1994). That the phase of perceived insecurity even prior to formal warning of redundancy is likely to be especially important is reinforced by recent reports on civil servants and miners respectively (A very, personal communication; Ferrie *et al.* 1995). And once a man has been unemployed for an extended period and adapted to the circumstances, a new job may fail to restore his former vigour (Claussen *et al.* 1993). One cannot assume that progress through the employment market is circular, as Fig. 6.3 would imply.

It is easy to recite a litany of what we do not know about unemployment and health. Will unemployed men waiting to see their general practitioner be old, young, single, married, separated? Will they be abusing their partners or their children? Will they be adopting palliative behaviour involving drugs? Will they be in trouble with the police? Will they be provoked into antisocial behaviour? What is the significance of their symptoms? Is there an 'unemployment syndrome'? Our ignorance can only become more and more embarrassing unless we collect more information.

Unemployment and health: what should doctors do?

Although any link between sickness in a population and the availability of work is yet to be defined, the effects of such an influence would be unavoidable in general practice

Fig. 6.3 *The sequential experiences of the workplace*

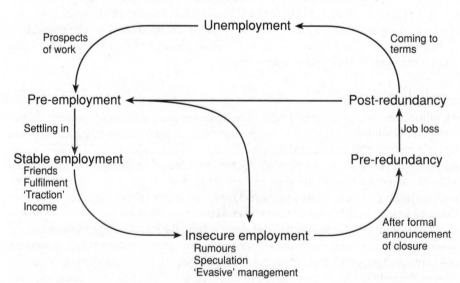

(Beale 1991; Smith 1992). At the same time it is ironic that the jobless and their immediate relatives will be counselled by the one individual in their community least likely to be made redundant – their family doctor. The most understandable response for a doctor consulted by a patient who has lost his job is by means of body language. Upturned palms, shrugged shoulders, and an apologetic tilt of the head says it all: unemployment is not a doctor's responsibility. But in many other, apparently hopeless, situations in medical practice we learn to resist such nihilism; we listen, we empathize, we 'do nothing skilfully' – the true art of the physician.

Doctors' attitudes have never been assessed properly but hearsay suggests that the profession is slowly learning to embrace the problems associated with, or exposed by, unemployment. We need to be more astute than merely inviting the unemployed patient to air his problems. The research evidence suggests that those merely threatened with redundancy are just as likely as the unemployed to appear in the GP's surgery more regularly than before (Beale and Nethercott 1985; Ferrie et al. 1995). We are all familiar with the 'tender spots' to prod when symptoms seem haphazard or inconsistent. We ask leading questions about fears, about finance, about relationships. For the middle-aged man who begins to consult repeatedly and who is reluctant to return to his job (Beale and Nethercott 1988c; Kristensen 1991), we must learn to tease out his perception of his job security. We also have a joint professional responsibility. If doctors with immediate clinical contact do not agitate about erosion of population health resulting from socio-economic disadvantage, who will? But politicians are unlikely to be convinced by case reports or other anecdotal evidence unless they want to be. The real sin of omission has been committed by the professional epidemiologists (Bartley 1992). Of all the original evidence on unemployment and health cited in this chapter and elsewhere, virtually none of it has been published by UK community physicians. This must be seen as a particular failure, for only in the British NHS – free at the point of clinical contact – does the abrupt change in financial circumstances associated with redundancy not affect the patient's ability to afford health care. It appears that the only attempt to conduct a study on unemployment and health of a scale and design that could have told us, with confidence, some of the mechanisms involved was conceived by members of two of the medical Royal Colleges, but was strangled at birth if not stillborn (Brown 1984, personal communication).

Directors of Public Health have become, in effect, the stockbrokers of the new market of health care. How many of them are convinced that unemployment in the communities for which they are purchasing health care is a factor dictating some of the demand is quite unknown. A study performed in 1986 (Harris and Smith 1987) showed that only 13% of UK health authorities were taking unemployment into account when allocating resources, and the latest preventive health catechism published by the Government – *The health of the nation: a strategy for health in England* (Anon 1992) – does not even mention unemployment.

The future of unemployment

Although history is reputed to repeat itself, jobs in the future are likely to be different to those we have now. Two probable trends are outstanding (Williams 1985): part-time and short-term jobs in the service sector will continue to increase; the number of stable and low-skilled jobs in the economy will fall as machines controlled by micro-processors replace human beings. Lifelong employment in one industrial niche will no longer be commonplace; the demand for gold watches will dwindle.

Changes in the nature of work will be in parallel with changes in the size of the work-force. We are just entering a period where the number of entrants into the UK workplace will diminish. At the same time we are finding that the demand for carers of the disabled and of the demented is rising exponentially. A less predictable factor is the influence the AIDS pandemic will have: the balance of nature may be at work.

However, the current general practice registrars are going to be senior partners before sociodemographic changes, alone, can 'cure' the present 'epidemic' of unemployment. The present generation of family doctors seem unsure of their role. Their academic mentors have organized no adequate research. The unemployed themselves do not voice specific demands other than for jobs. And the Government continues, as did Nelson, to peer down a telescope with a blind eye.

References

Anon. (1985). Job loss and the use of health services. *Journal of the Royal College of General Practitioners*, **35**, 507. (Editorial).

Anon. (1992). *The health of the nation: a strategy for health in England.* HMSO, London.

Arber, S. (1987). Social class, non-employment, and chronic illness: continuing the inequalities in health debate. *British Medical Journal*, **294**, 1069–73.

Archer, J. and Rhodes, V. (1987). Bereavement and reactions to job loss: a comparative review. *British Journal of Social Psychology*, **26**, 211–24.

Banks, M. and Jackson, P. (1982). Unemployment and risk of minor psychiatric disorder in young people: cross-sectional and longitudinal evidence. *Psychological Medicine*, **12**, 789–98.

Bartley, M. (1992). Authorities and partisans. The debate on unemployment and health. Edinburgh University Press, Edinburgh.

Bartley, M. (1994). Unemployment and ill health: understanding the relationship. *Journal of Epidemiology and Community Health*, **48**, 333–7.

Bartley, M. and Owen, C. (1996). Relation between socio-economic status, employment, and health during economic change, 1973–93. *British Medical Journal*, **313**, 445–9.

Beale, N. (1991). Dying to work. *Horizons*, **5**, 23–6.

Beale, N. and Nethercott, S. (1985). Job loss and family morbidity: a study of a factory closure. *Journal of the Royal College of General Practitioners*, **35**, 510–14.

Beale, N. and Nethercott, S. (1988a). The nature of unemployment morbidity. 1. Recognition. *Journal of the Royal College of General Practitioners*, **38**, 197–9.

Beale, N. and Nethercott, S. (1988b). The nature of unemployment morbidity. 2. Description. *Journal of the Royal College of General Practitioners*, **38**, 200–2.

Beale, N. and Nethercott, S. (1988c). Certificated sickness absence in industrial employees threatened with redundancy. *British Medical Journal*, **296**, 1508–10.

Beveridge, W. (1944). *Full employment in a free society*. George Allen and Unwin, London.

Brenner, M. H. (1971). Economic changes and heart-disease mortality. *American Journal of Public Health*, **61**, 606–11.

Brenner, M. H. (1979). Mortality and the national economy: a review and the experience of England and Wales, 1936–1976. *Lancet*, **ii**, 568–73.

Bunn, A. (1979). Ischaemic heart disease mortality and the business cycle in Australia. *American Journal of Public Health*, **69**, 772–81.

Claussen, B., Bjorndal, A., and Hjort, P. (1993). Health and re-employment in a two-year follow-up of long-term unemployed. *Journal of Epidemiology and Community Health*, **47**, 14–18.

Cole, J. (1995). *As it seemed to me*. Wedeinfeld & Nicholson, London.

Colledge, M. and Bartholomew, R. (1980). The long-term unemployed: some new evidence. *Employment Gazette*, **88**, 9–12.

Cook, D., Cummins, R., Bartley, M., and Shaper, G. (1982). Health of unemployed middle-aged men in Great Britain. *Lancet*, **i**, 1290–4.

Dean, M. (1993). Unemployment and health. *Lancet*, **341**, 230–1.

Donovan, A., Oddy, M., Pardoe, R., and Ades, A. (1986). Employment status and psychological well-being: a longitudinal study of 16-year-old school-leavers. *Journal of Child Psychology and Psychiatry*, **27**, 65–76.

Ennals, S. (1991). *Understanding benefits*. BMJ Publications, London.

Fagin, L. and Little, M. (1984). *The forsaken families*. Penguin, Harmondsworth.

Ferrie, J., Shipley, M., Marmot, M., Stansfield, S., and Davey-Smith, G. (1995). Health effects of anticipation of job change and non-employment: longitudinal data from the Whitehall II study. *British Medical Journal*, **311**, 1264–9.

Fisher, A. (1965). Psychiatric follow-up of long-term industrial employees subsequent to plant closure. *International Journal of Neuropsychiatry*, **11**, 267–4.

Forbes, J. and McGregor, A. (1984). Unemployment and mortality in post-war Scotland. *Journal of Health Economics*, **3**, 239–57.

Fox, A. and Goldblatt, P. (1982). *Longitudinal study: socio-demographic mortality differentials*. HMSO, London.

Franks, P., Adamson, C., Bulpitt, P., and Bulpitt, C. (1991). Stroke death and unemployment in London. *Journal of Epidemiology and Community Health*, **45**, 16–18.

Freud, S. (1930). *Civilisation and its discontents*. Hogarth Press, London.

Fryer, D. and Ullah, P. (1987). *Unemployed people*. Open University Press, Milton Keynes.

Fryer, D. and Warr, P. (1984). Unemployment and cognitive difficulties. *British Journal of Clinical Psychology*, **23**, 67–8.

Furness, J., Khan, M., and Pickens, P. (1985). Unemployment and parasuicide in Hartlepool, 1974–1983. *Health Trends*, **17**, 21–4.

Gallie, D., Marsh, C., and Vogler, C. (1994). *Social change and the experience of unemployment.* Oxford University Press, Oxford.

Greenwood, W. (1933). *Love on the dole.* Jonathon Cape, London. (Republished 1984, Penguin, Harmondsworth.)

Griffin, J. (1993). *The impact of unemployment on health.* Briefing Paper No. 29. Office of Health Economics, London.

Hansard, X. (1991). Lamont N. Parliamentary debates (Hansard) 6th series – Commons. Vol. **191**. 16/5/91.

Harris, C. and Smith, R. (1987). What are health authorities doing about unemployment and health? *British Medical Journal*, **294**, 1076–9.

Harrison, R. (1976). The demoralising experience of prolonged unemployment. *Employment Gazette*, **84**, 339–48.

Hawton, K. and Rose, N. (1986). Unemployment and attempted suicide among men in Oxford. *Health Trends*, **18**, 29–32.

Higgs, R. (1984). Life changes. *British Medical Journal*, **288**, 1556–7.

Hoggart, R. (1957). *The uses of literacy.* Penguin, Harmondsworth.

Howard, A. (1979). *The Crossman diaries.* Methuen, London.

Iversen, L., Andersen, O., Andersen, P., Christoffersen, K., and Keiding, N. (1987). Unemployment and mortality in Denmark 1970–1980. *British Medical Journal*, **295**, 879–84.

Iversen, L. and Klausen, H. (1981). Lukningen af Nordhavns-verflet. [The closing of Nordhavns shipyard.] Publication 13. Department of Social Medicine, University of Copenhagen, Copenhagen. [English summary pp. 199–207.]

Jackson, P., Stafford, E., Banks, M., and Warr, P. (1983). Unemployment and psychological distress in young people: the moderating role of employment commitment. *Journal of Applied Psychology*, **68**, 525–35.

Jackson, P. and Warr, P. (1984). Unemployment and psychological ill health: the moderating role of duration and age. *Psychological Medicine*, **14**, 605–14.

Jackson, P. and Warr, P. (1987). Mental health of unemployed men in different parts of England and Wales. *British Medical Journal*, **295**, 525.

Jacobsen, K. (1972). Afskedigelse of sygelighed. [Dismissal and morbidity.] *Ugeskr Laeger*, **134**, 352–4.

Jahoda, M. (1979). The impact of unemployment in the 1930s and the 1970s. *Bulletin of the British Psychological Society*, **32**, 309–14.

Jahoda, M. (1982). *Employment and unemployment. A social-psychological analysis.* Cambridge University Press, Cambridge.

Kasl, S. and Cobb, S. (1970). Blood pressure changes in men undergoing job loss: a preliminary report. *Psychosomatic Medicine*, **32**, 19–38.

Kasl, S., Cobb, S., and Brooks, G. (1968). Changes in serum uric acid and cholesterol levels in men undergoing job loss. *Journal of the American Medical Association*, **206**, 1500–7.

Kasl, S., Gore, S., and Cobb, S. (1975). The experience of losing a job: reported changes in health, symptoms and illness behaviour. *Psychosomatic Medicine*, **37**, 106–22.

Krahn, H., Lowe, G., and Tanner, J. (1985). The social-psychological impact of unemployment in Edmonton. *Canadian Journal of Public Health*, **76**, 88–92.

Kristensen, T. G. (1991). Sickness absence and work strain among Danish slaughterhouse workers: an analysis of absence from work regarded as coping behaviour. *Social Science and Medicine*, **32**, 15–27.

Lee, A., Crombie, I., Smith, W., and Tunstall-Pedoe, H. D. (1991). Cigarette smoking and employment status. *Social Science and Medicine*, **33**, 1309–12.

McMichael, A. (1976). Standardised mortality ratios and the 'healthy worker effect': scratching beneath the surface. *Journal of Occupational Medicine*, **18**, 165–8.

Marsden, D. (1982). *Workless*. Croom Helm, London.

Martikainen, P. T. (1990). Unemployment and mortality among Finnish men, 1981–5. *British Medical Journal*, **301**, 407–11.

Mattiasson, I., Lindegarde, F., Nilsson, J. A., and Theorell, T. (1990). Threat of unemployment and cardiovascular risk factors: longitudinal study of quality of sleep and serum cholesterol concentrations in men threatened with redundancy. *British Medical Journal*, **301**, 461–6.

Miles, I. (1983). *Adaptation to unemployment?* Occasional paper no. 20. University of Sussex, Science Policy Research Unit, Falmer, Brighton.

Morris, J. and Titmuss, R. (1944). Health and social change: a recent history of rheumatic heart disease. *Medical Officer*, **72**, 69–85.

Morris, J. K. and Cook, D. G. (1991). A critical review of the effect of factory closures on health. *British Journal of Industrial Medicine*, **48**, 1–8.

Morris, J. K., Cook, D. G., and Shaper, A. G. (1994). Loss of employment and mortality. *British Medical Journal*, **308**, 1135–9.

Moser, K. A., Fox, A. J., and Jones, D. R. (1984). Unemployment and mortality in the OPCS longitudinal study. *Lancet*, **ii**, 1324–9.

Moser, K. A. Goldblatt, P. O., Fox, A. J., and Jones, D. R. (1987). Unemployment and mortality: comparison of the 1971 and 1981 longitudinal study census samples. *British Medical Journal*, **294**, 86–90.

Moylan, S., Millar, J., and Davies, R. (1984). *For richer, for poorer. DHSS cohort study of unemployed men*. HMSO, London.

Murray-Parkes, C. (1972). Bereavement: studies of grief in adult life. Tavistock Publications, London.

Payne, R., Warr, P., and Hartley, J. (1984). Social class and psychological ill health during unemployment. *Sociology of Health and Illness*, **6**, 152–74.

Peck, D. and Plant, M. (1986). Unemployment and illegal drug use: concordant evidence from a prospective study and national trends. *British Medical Journal*, **293**, 929–32.

Platt, S. and Kreitman, N. (1984). Trends in parasuicide and unemployment among men in Edinburgh, 1968–1982. *British Medical Journal*, **289**, 1029–32.

Porter, A. M. D. (1989). Unemployment and ill health: is the question going away? *Family Practice*, **6**, 1–2.

Scott-Samuel, A. (1985). Does unemployment kill? *British Medical Journal*, **290**, 1905.

Seabrook, J. (1983). *Unemployment*. Granada, St Albans.

Sinfield, A. (1981). *What unemployment means*. Martin Robertson, Oxford.

Smith, R. (1987). *Unemployment and health. A disaster and a challenge*. Oxford Medical Publications, Oxford.

Smith, R. (1991). Unemployment: here we go again. *British Medical Journal*, **302**, 606–7. (Editorial).

Smith, R. (1992). 'Without work all life goes rotten'. *British Medical Journal*, **305**, 972. (Editorial).

Smith, R. (1993). Workfare and health. *British Medical Journal*, **306**, 474. (Editorial).

Taylor, D. (1990). *Creative counting*. Unemployment Unit Briefing, London.

Townsend, P. and Davidson, N. (1982). *Inequalities in health. The Black Report*. Penguin, Harmondsworth.

Turner-Warwick, M. (1992). *Smoking and the young*. Royal College of Physicians, London.

Ullah, P., Banks, M., and Warr, P. (1985). Social support, social pressures and psychological distress during unemployment. *Psychological Medicine*, **15**, 283–95.

Wagstaff, A. (1986). Unemployment and health: some pitfalls for the unwary. *Health Trends*, **18**, 79–81.

Warr, P. (1987). *Work, unemployment and mental health*. Oxford Science Publications, Oxford.

Westin, S., Schlesselman, J. J., and Korper, M. (1989). Long-term effects of a factory closure: unemployment and disability during ten years' follow-up. *Journal of Clinical Epidemiology*, **42**, 435–41.

Williams, S. (1985). *A job to live*. Penguin, Harmondsworth.

CHAPTER SEVEN

Male sexuality and its problems
Peter Barrett

> Sexual intercourse began
> In nineteen sixty-three
> Between the end of the Chatterley ban
> And the Beatles' first LP
> (Phillip Larkin, *Annus Mirabilis*)

Men are supposed to think about sex a lot and, if that is the case, purchases of this book may be made on the merits or otherwise of this chapter while the purchaser is perusing it in the bookshop. We think you will have made a good decision. Men often find it difficult to talk to GPs about their sexual problems, and GPs in turn fear that sexual counselling may take more time than is available. The author discusses normal and abnormal male sexual function, and uses case histories to illustrate specific approaches that GPs may find useful. He deals with both psychological and physical causes of sexual problems; the latter may well be underestimated and need to be considered. The chapter deals mostly with heterosexual problems as little seems to be known in the medical world about the sexual problems of homosexual men.

Normality

In 1959, two American sexologists first presented their papers to the New York Academy of Sciences in the course of a two-day 'Conference on the Vagina' (Masters and Johnson 1959). Dr William Masters and his research associate Mrs Virginia Johnson had been studying the physiology of normal human sexual response in a laboratory setting. They continued to produce a succession of papers on related subjects over the next six years. Their papers originally stimulated very little reaction from the medical establishment, rather surprisingly in view of their content, and it was not until 1966 when their book *Human sexual response* was published that popular interest was aroused (Masters and Johnson 1966).

Masters and Johnson made several hundred observations of the physiological changes that occur in the male and female sexual organs during sexual arousal, relying very heavily on couples volunteering for the rather intrusive sets of measurements that were required. It is not within the scope of this chapter to detail each experiment, but it is worth recording that, as a result of their measurements, four phases of sexual arousal were identified:

(1) excitement;
(2) plateau;
(3) orgasmic;
(4) resolution.

They pointed out that these phases did not occur as distinct separate entities, but ran into each other as sexual activity progressed.

Excitement

During this phase, the penis usually becomes fully erect. The exact mechanism by which engorgement occurs is still not fully understood, but intact nerves, anatomy, and circulation are essential for success (Lue and Tanagho 1987). As a result of a marked increase in the blood supply to the corpora cavernosa of the penis, it usually becomes engorged within a few seconds. The engorgement may be a response to physical stimulation or to an erotic sight or thought. A small penis can double in size but a large, resting penis will not increase in size nearly as much. There is in this a great source of consolation to those men who fear they are not as well-endowed as they would like.

The rigidity of the engorged penis is thought to be due to blood being trapped in the corpora cavernosa. The corpora are surrounded by a membrane called the tunica albuginea which contains a network of veins. As the penis expands these veins are compressed and cannot drain as much blood away as normal, resulting in a rigid penis.

Plateau

This is a continuation of the excitement phase and in the male produces a fully distended penis. There is a slight distension of the coronal ridge at the base of the glans of the penis and sometimes a change in colour of the glans itself to a purple hue. The testicles are often up to 50% bigger during this phase and due to the action of the cremasteric muscles are drawn up into the scrotum. This may be associated with a discharge of a little clear fluid from the urethra. Masters and Johnson (1966) described this as the 'point of no return' as it indicated that orgasm was imminent. During plateau, the rate of respiration increases and there is a rise in pulse rate and blood pressure. Tension of all muscles is increased.

Orgasm

Before orgasm, fluid containing millions of sperm has been collecting in the seminal vesicles and in the ampullae. As these organs contract, they eject their contents into the urethra where it is mixed with prostatic fluid produced by contractions of the prostate gland. The pleasurable feeling associated with orgasm is said to occur at this time. The second phase of ejaculation now occurs and involves rhythmic contractions of the urethral bulb and the penis. Semen can be ejected for a distance of up to two feet, though as men get older the contractions can become less intense. Voluntary muscles go into spasm. A man will sometimes get carpopedal spasm and may grasp his partner very firmly during this phase, though will often be unaware of this.

Resolution

The release of muscular tension throughout the body is occasioned by the completion of orgasm. The penis returns to its pre-engorged size in two stages. The rigidity disappears quite quickly but the penis may stay enlarged for some time. It can take up to half an hour for it to return to normal. Unlike the female, the male has a refractory period during which time he is unable to achieve another erection following orgasm. The timing of such a period is very variable. Masters and Johnson (1966) reported a young man who could achieve three orgasms in 10 minutes, measured under laboratory conditions, but it is much more common for this state to last for much longer and it tends to increase with age.

The above description of the normal physiology of male arousal is of interest and some-times a solace to men worried by their perceived lack of ability in this area, but the reverse is often true. The concentration on achieving a 'norm' can lead to excess pressure and consequent failure. Statistical analysis of the average number of times intercourse occurs, the length of time it lasts, the size of the penis, and the time taken before ejaculation happens is not relevant to most couples provided they are both happy with their own frequency and quality of lovemaking. Problems arise when one partner becomes or verbalizes for the first time their dissatisfaction with intercourse. It really does not matter whether couples make love once a year or twice a night if both are content, but as soon as one complains then both have a problem if they wish the relationship to continue. They might be convinced that their own level of sexual performance is perfectly normal and that it is their partner who needs help. When they seek help they will find that the doctor has his or her own sets of internal normal values. If not aware of the dangers, the doctor makes value judgements about the couple's problems, based not on the actual difficulties but on a comparison of their sexual activity with the doctor's own sense of normality. This can lead to a great deal of frustration for the doctor and the patient. It is essential that the doctor avoids any such comparison and listens to the nature of the complaint in an uncritical way. It does not matter whether the doctor feels that once a week is too much or too little. What does matter is whether each partner is happy with the level of sexual activity in their own relationship. Consider the patient who comes to the doctor to complain that her partner 'only' wants to make love twice a week. The doctor may well be faced with the other partner the following day complaining that his partner wants to make love 'as much as' twice a week. Who is right and who is wrong?

The fact that, 'on average', people make love 2.2 times a week is of little help to this couple. The fact that the doctor makes love once a week can influence his or her judgement and may interfere with the ability to deal with the complaints in an unbiased way. We all have our own concept of normality and I suspect that it is based not on physiological analysis but on our own internalized ideas about sex.

Sexual problems in men

For the sake of clarity, sexual problems in the male can best be divided into the following areas:

(1) problems of ejaculation;
(2) problems of erection;
(3) problems of libido;
(4) problems of sexual deviance.

Though the problems are distinct, there is often considerable overlap in the individual patient.

Problems of ejaculation

These fall into two groups:

(1) premature ejaculation;
(2) retarded or non-ejaculation.

Of these two groups, premature ejaculation is by far the most common. It is so common in younger or inexperienced males that it perhaps should be regarded as almost normal in this group. The great majority of men will not need to seek help about this provided they do not become convinced that they are suffering from a severe sexual abnormality. Their anxiety in these circumstances produces a marked worsening of the problem which is closely linked to the level of concern about their sexual adequacy.

Men are capable of reaching orgasm about two minutes from initial stimulation. This is a source of concern to women who, on average, need about eight minutes to reach their orgasm. Perhaps in the old days men were not so worried about fulfilling their partner's needs as they are today, and no doubt the relationships suffered because of that, but today there is an acceptance that mutual satisfaction is an important factor. Men therefore have to be able to control the timing of their ejaculation and this can cause problems on a mechanical level. Simple behaviourial techniques can be used for this group and their partners.

The 'squeeze' technique involves delaying ejaculation by firmly squeezing the penis between thumb and forefinger just behind the glans penis. The man and his partner are encouraged to face each other with legs across and outstretched. They masturbate until the man is on the point of ejaculation, at which time the penis is squeezed until the sensation of ejaculation disappears. The procedure is then repeated for a number of cycles, the partners deciding when to allow ejaculation to occur. Once this process has been practised for a few sessions over the course of a few weeks, the couple progress to the insertion of the penis into the vagina. It is important that they do not move too vigorously during this stage as the man needs to continue to feel in control of his ejaculation. If he feels the ejaculation coming then the penis is withdrawn and squeezed until the sensation goes, or if feeling confident they may just elect to freeze with the penis remaining inside the vagina until the feeling of ejaculation recedes. Gentle movement can then be resumed and the process repeated if necessary. The theory is that the man will gain confidence in his ability to control his erection, and in so doing relieves a lot of the attached anxiety, thus breaking the vicious circle.

Unfortunately, a large number of couples get into trouble with this method. There will be failure to realize that the ejaculation is about to occur and they will have to deal with the mess and disappointment that this produces. The penis may well go down and distress is caused when it does not immediately respond to further stimulation. This is a natural phenomenon of the refractory period of the penis and couples need to be reassured that the penis will respond again in time but cannot be rushed. With practise and patience on the part of the couple and the therapist, many uncomplicated cases of premature ejaculation respond. Whether this is merely as a result of the behavioural conditioning, or more to do with the effects of open discussion of a private problem between therapist and partners, is difficult to quantify.

Premature ejaculation may not simply be a problem of over-anxiety in an inexperienced man. It may reflect far deeper problems relating to the individual, his upbringing, emotions, and attitudes to women. The presentation of the problem may not occur until many years after the partnership began and can reflect a newly declared dissatisfaction on the part of the female. As mentioned above, no matter what the actual quality of intercourse, if both parties are happy then there is no need to interfere, but as soon as one complains then help to address the issues becomes necessary. This help is often required urgently, and long waiting-lists for psychosexual clinics only serve to drive the problem underground, cementing certain behavioural characteristics in the couple.

Mr A was aged 65 and had been married to his present wife for 35 years. He was referred to the psychosexual clinic with a diagnosis of 'impotence', but actually reported that he could get a perfectly good erection. The problem was that he could only last for a matter of three minutes inside his wife before he ejaculated and she had begun to complain. He appeared a very neatly dressed man who was articulate and puzzled by his problem. Up until four years ago he had considered that he performed well enough but then had noticed that he had started to come rather quickly. Trying to reassure this individual that his performance was actually normal would not have helped him. He needed help to understand the nature of his new difficulties. He had tried the squeeze technique but with little success. It had been too mechanical and he felt that it was not appropriate to continue. He started to discuss the background to the complaint. He lived with his wife in comfortable surroundings and over the past 10 years had looked after his mother-in-law who stayed with them. His wife had been keen to do alterations to the house so that she would hear her mother easily in case she got into difficulties at night. Her mother was very frail and needed a lot of help with her mobility. In an attempt to make it easy to care for her, he had knocked down a partition wall, and as a consequence there was no longer a door to their bedroom. He had thought that this would not matter as the children were off their hands and living away, but as the consultation progressed it became apparent that he felt very resentful about their lack of privacy. He was acutely aware of the noises that they made when they made love and always conscious of any possible interruption to their sexual activities. His wife did not see this as a problem. He had not wished to upset his wife as he loved her dearly, but had expressed his anxieties and anger by getting sex over and done with as quickly as possible. This was interpreted to him and he was able to express his feelings freely during the consultation, vowing to rebuild the door and wall as soon as he could!

Mr B was aged thirty and had been married for six years. He worked as a senior manager in a company and professionally was doing very well. His wife was also in senior management and both were very busy people. He had suffered from premature ejaculation for years but he and his wife had thought that it would go away in time. This had not happened and they had been referred to 'Relate' for behaviour therapy. They had both found this too mechanical, particularly his wife, and they abandoned the sessions after a few weeks. He had come from a very close family but when he was aged 13 his father died from a coronary thrombosis. His mother could not come to terms with this loss and committed suicide a couple of years later. He told the therapist this story without any trace of emotion. He appeared flat and over-controlled emotionally. This was fed back to him and he agreed that he always tried to keep in tight control of all his feelings. He could not face the thought of losing control. He had learnt as a teenager to avoid all emotional expression as this was too painful. He had not cried when his parents died, denying his grief. Those around him at the time colluded with his need to avoid emotion as this was also too painful for them to bear. Now he was faced with a wife who wanted him to express his emotions in lovemaking. All he could do was to get his feelings out of the way as soon as possible, and this had shown itself in his premature ejaculation. He made good use of the interpretations, and when he returned four weeks later, had achieved good intercourse.

Erectile problems

Various studies have indicated that erectile problems can affect up to 10% of the adult male population and 25–50% of men in their seventh and eighth decades (Jeffcoate 1991). Yet there is an apparent reluctance to present these difficulties to a doctor. Perhaps it is a reflection of the external nature of the male genitals and the fact that the problem cannot be covered up during intercourse that leads men to cover up in other ways. If given the right opportunity and the correct surroundings then men will be far more likely to discuss their sexual problem. Even when impotence is a known complication of a particular condition, such as diabetes, it is rarely discussed by the clinic doctors. Even if the subject is raised there will be denial of any difficulty by many men.

The causation of erectile dysfunction is, for convenience, divided into physical and emotional. Trying to distinguish between the two is important (Jeffcoate 1991; Slob *et al.* 1990), and there is often an overlap between the emotional and physical state. A man who cannot get an erection is going to have some feelings about this, and probably deeper feelings than if he were merely to suffer from bronchitis. Various tests to identify a physical problem have been devised and range from simple examination and blood tests to complex blood-flow monitoring and radiology (Gilbert *et al.* 1991). It is important to try to identify the cause of the impotence, but this should not blind the doctor to the fact that the patient's feelings will also be affected. A few years ago, many doctors would have said that impotence was all in the mind and merely reassured the patient that he would get better in time if he did not worry about it. However, it is now known that at least 50% of impotence has a physical cause, and this may be an underestimate.

Physical causes of impotence

There are several recognized physical causes for impotence. The most common are as follows:

(1) diabetes;
(2) circulatory disorders;
(3) surgery involving the pelvic area;

 (4) disease of the erectile tissue of the penis;
 (5) hormonal abnormalities;
 (6) side-effects of medication;
 (7) neurological disorders;
 (8) chronic physical disease;
 (9) trauma;
(10) alcohol and drug misuse.

1. *Diabetes.* Diabetes is a well-recognized cause of impotence, though the exact per-
    centage of diabetic patients affected is not certain (McCulloch *et al.* 1980) When
    men attend a diabetic clinic, most of the emphasis is understandably focused on
    maintaining good control of the diabetes. The clinics are busy and the thought of
    opening up a discussion of the patient's sexual life can be daunting, so questions are
    not asked. The patients are usually too embarrassed to mention such a private prob-
    lem in the often exposed environment of an out-patient setting. If the subject is
    raised then there follows an often mechanical consultation which leaves both doctor
    and patient dissatisfied. Impotence in a diabetic patient may be due to the effects of
    the diabetes on the nerve supply or blood supply to the penis. The history is one of a
    gradual decline in erectile ability, which affects not only attempts at lovemaking but
    produces a lack of morning and nocturnal erections. Masturbation results in no
    improvement and in these circumstances mechanical methods of treatment have to
    be considered, but only if the patient feels that it is an important part of his relation-
    ship. The need for the doctor to be active and to find an answer to the patient's prob-
    lem has to be guarded against. Just because the doctor feels that penetrative sex is an
    important part of his life does not mean that the patient feels the same. The wishes
    of the patient have to be respected and time given to allow a proper examination of
    the patient's needs. It is possible that many patients suffering from diabetes blame
    their impotence on this disease when other emotional causes are likely. It is far eas-
    ier to have a physical illness to blame than have to face the thought of looking at
    one's emotions and relationships. The history of the impotence is an important
    clue. If the onset of the impotence is sudden, if the patient can masturbate satisfac-
    torily, and if the morning or nocturnal erections are still present then the cause is
    likely to be emotional rather than physical. If one asks the patient outright 'Do you
    masturbate?', the likely response is going to be 'No', as no one readily admits to this
    activity. If, on the other hand, one asks 'Do you still get an erection when you mas-
    turbate?', then a much more honest answer is likely as the assumption has been
    made and the patient saved embarrassment. Trying to help a diabetic patient suffer-
    ing from impotence needs an awareness and readiness to discuss the problem. It
    needs quiet and private surroundings for the consultation to take place. Both emo-
    tional and physical aspects of the difficulty have to be looked at and the patient
    allowed to decide for himself the best method of treatment.

2. *Circulatory disorders.* In order for the penis to become erect there has to be an intact
    blood supply to the erectile tissue of the penis. If there is significant narrowing of
    the blood vessels due to atheroma then the penis cannot engorge, and although

ejaculation can still take place, penetrative sex is not possible. The other component involves the veins. If the veins drain the blood away from the penis too quickly then the penis cannot maintain any rigidity. The penis may become initially erect but after a few seconds rapidly decreases in size, much to the frustration of both partners. Attempts have been made to reduce this venous leak by sophisticated methods of radiographic imaging, identifying the venous culprit and then surgery to tie the vein off. Although the initial results of this technique looked promising, there was a worrying return to the preoperative state in the majority of men within a few months. Occasionally, there is an isolated narrowing of the arteries supplying the penis which may be amenable to surgery, but this is rare. The effects of smoking on potency have not been fully investigated but there may be a connection related to the general problems of smoking on the circulation.

3. *Surgery to the pelvic area.* As the engorgement of the penis depends on a sympathetic and parasympathetic nerves plus an intact blood supply, any surgery to the pelvic area affecting these could result in impotence. Surgeons are well aware of the complications of such surgery and warn the patient about the possibility of such a problem. When a patient has had surgery with such a warning, the anxiety to prove himself intact is enormous. This anxiety may result in impotence in its own right and can be very difficult to sort out. Probably the most common operation is prostatectomy, and although this operation does not result in impotence it often results in retrograde ejaculation. This can be devastating for some men who pride themselves on their ability to have a forceful ejaculation. The absence of such an ejaculation leads them to experience complete impotence, often linked to extreme anger, mainly directed at the medical profession.

4. *Disease of the erectile tissue.* The penis needs adequate erectile tissue to expand, and anything which interferes with the integrity of this tissue will result in varying degrees of impotence. The most common disease affecting this area is Peyronie's disease. This is a fibrous thickening and contraction of the fascia around the corpora, and as the penis expands the fibrotic area remains contracted, thus pulling the shaft of the penis to one side. This can lead to quite dramatic bends of the penis, rendering penetrative sex out of the question. If the bend is significant a surgical procedure is performed to remove the scarred area. This normally results in a little shortening of the overall length of the penis, and in a small number of cases can, in itself, produce impotence. If the bend is bad then there is no alternative to the operation. If the bend is minimal then it may be worth waiting a few months before embarking on a surgical solution.

5. *Hormonal abnormalities.* Many men assume that the reason they are impotent is due to lack of 'hormones'. It is true that a lack of testosterone may produce impotence, but it is much more likely to result in a loss of libido. It is rare to identify a low testosterone level but it is always worth arranging a blood test for testosterone and follicle-stimulating hormone (FSH) and luteinizing hormone (LH) in case this is so. Injections of testosterones (e.g. Sustanon) given intramuscularly at monthly

intervals in these circumstances can rapidly produce an improvement both in libido and erectile performance. For the majority of men the levels are normal, and then they and the doctor have to start the difficult process of looking at other causes. There has been a fashion for the 'male menopause' and treatments with testosterone, whether or not the levels are normal. There is, according to the endocrinologists, no rationale in this method of treatment and they discourage it. Anecdotal reports of wonderful improvements in male sexual performance abound but there is little scientific evidence to support it. It is very important to establish that the prostate is normal. Giving large doses of male hormone to a man with a hormone-dependent tumour will not endear the doctor to the medical defence organizations.

6. *Side effects of medication.* One of the most common problems is the underestimated effect of medication on male sexuality (Bateman 1980; British Medical Journal 1979). The prescription of drugs which lower the blood pressure is a major cause of impotence. The older thiazide diuretics are prone to give rise to iatrogenic impotence, and it may be a feature of many others. If faced with a man who has become impotent, it is worth trying to get him off all medication if possible. If this is not practicable then a change to one of the more modern hypotensives may well be worthwhile. Other medication affecting sexuality includes the phenothiazines, antidepressants, sedatives, and some H2 antagonists such as cimetidine (though this drug is more likely to reduce libido). It is always difficult to sort out whether it is the tablets or the emotions that are to blame for the problem. The doctor often has to take a pragmatic approach to treatment as costly and time-consuming investigations have yet to prove their worth.

7. *Neurological disorders.* An intact nervous system is essential for an erection to occur. Both sympathetic and parasympathetic systems are involved, and damage to either penile supply will preclude an erection. Spinal injuries, infections involving the spinal cord, cord compression, and demyelination, as found in multiple sclerosis, can all produce impotence. Treatment will usually take the form of mechanical aids or injections and these methods will be described later in this chapter.

Any man affected by such a physical problem will have some feelings about it. Doctors cannot ignore the emotional component to any physical illness, particularly when it affects sexual function. Men need to be able to express their emotional distress about their illness. Unfortunately, some doctors are likely to be so distressed by the patient's complaints that they try to retreat into the safety of the traditional medical model, asking questions and assuming control of the consultation. This has the effect of denying the patient the chance to say what they really want and reduces the consultation to a series of questions and answers. These questions and answers are more to do with what the doctor wants to know rather than what the patient wants to say. The doctor is, by this manoeuvre, protected from the feelings of the impotent man and the feeling that he might be impotent to help. Despite recent changes, medical training still largely produces doctors who are knowledgeable, active, and able to help. It is still less good at enabling doctors to cope with their patients' emotions, to listen without being directive, and to accept their own inabilities to produce a 'cure'. Active listening and interpretation of what seems to be happening between the doctor and the patient can be the major source of change in the patient. What happens in the consultation is often a reflection of what happens in the man's life outside the surgery.

8. *Chronic physical disease.* The effects of a chronic illness are far-reaching. To expect a man to perform well sexually when feeling debilitated is clearly unreasonable, but may reflect a need in their partner to defend against the illness and to try and create the illusion that all is well. The man may have a similar defensive system and will focus on his sexual dysfunction at the expense of his other disabilities. An empathetic ear, not denying his sexual distress but moving towards his physical problems, may be needed both for the patient and his partner. Our own expectations of sexual fulfilment may get in the way. If we assume that penetrative intercourse is the only method of sexual expression for a couple then we are guilty of denying them the chance for other forms of sexual happiness at a time of their lives when any such expression is of vital importance.

Mr and Mrs C had been married for 30 years and had a stable marriage with two grown-up children. After the children had left home, Mr C noticed a swelling on his penis. He attended the urological clinic, a biopsy was taken, and the diagnosis of carcinoma made. He was advised to have an amputation of the penis as a matter of urgency. There was no other alternative and the operation went ahead. He and his wife realized that they would not be able to make love again. The surgeon at the follow-up clinic opened up the subject of their sexual relations. They admitted that they were very distressed about the results of the operation and an appointment was made for the psychosexual clinic, with a somewhat apologetic letter of referral. The doctor listened to their distress. They had never had a satisfactory sexual relationship and the operation had merely exposed their pre-existing problems. He worked in a job where it paid to be obsessional and to keep all the emotions under control. He had never been able to share his feelings with his wife, who had been left feeling unloved and out in the cold. As the consultation progressed it became clear that his need to control his feelings was, in reality, based on a fear of failure. He had wanted to open up about these feelings on many occasions but somehow had never been able to do so before the operation. The fact that he was no longer in a position to attempt intercourse had freed him from the fear of failure and allowed him, for the first time in his life, to express these emotions to his wife. She was no longer excluded from his inner thoughts. She was able to express her anger at their previous situation and her guilt at feeling angry with a man who was ill. After two consultations they were able to move on to other means of giving each other sexual satisfaction. He felt able to give his wife pleasure by stimulating her and bringing her to orgasm. He felt potent in a way that he had never experienced before and, although mourning the loss of his penis, was happy with his new-found abilities.

9. *Trauma.* There are obvious problems with local trauma to the genital area but, as noted above, the effects of such trauma need careful evaluation. Any accident involving the nervous supply or the arterial supply to the penis will result in impotence. If the penis remains intact, plastic operations using implants can be performed or injections of vasoactive substances can be given. These mechanical treatments will be described later in this chapter. The doctor may feel unable to help

in any other way, but an ability to stay with the man's distress about such a loss is essential, as treating the physical side of the problem is only half the story.

10. *Alcohol misuse.* The fact that alcohol 'increases the desire but takes away the performance' has long been recognized. In the short term it is no more than a passing nuisance, but if the abuse of alcohol becomes chronic then a mixture of physical and emotional effects are noted. The liver's responsibility for metabolizing sex hormones is disrupted and the libido is reduced. The integrity of the blood supply to the penis is altered and the central nervous system depressed. An erection may be partly successful but be short-lived. The sense of failure will increase the man's anxiety and his need to escape into more alcohol. The man's need to use alcohol to avoid emotional difficulties has to be addressed and this is by no means an easy option for doctor or patient. The use of alcohol to avoid sex may be a problem for many couples. The traditional 'friday night out' and the inevitable argument when he returns home drunk successfully avoids any chance of lovemaking. It also protects him from having to attempt intercourse and his associated fear of failure. It is not the man who is failing but the alcohol that makes him fail. This option is much more acceptable to many men and explains their resistance to attempts at under-standing their behaviour.

Sex and the wheelchair

Until the recent introduction of injectable vasoactive substances, many men confined to wheelchairs had to resign themselves to a celibate future. Their lack of ability to express themselves emotionally in penetrative intercourse merely adding to their sense of impotence in other areas of their lives. For many, this situation has now changed, and a positive approach to their sexuality can be encouraged.

> A couple in their mid-fifties were referred to the psychosexual clinic. They were both confined to wheelchairs and had met in a local nursing home. They had both been married before but their marriages had not survived the traumas of wheelchair existence. They had developed a close, loving relationship and the staff of the home were as cooperative as they could be in facilitating their relationship. Unfortunately, he could not gain an erection. After some discussion, the use of papaverine injections was proposed, and as he had full dexterity he found them easy to inject into his penile shaft. The resulting erection enabled them to enhance their sexual relationship in a way that up until then had been impossible. They did have some initial difficulties in establishing an adequate level of privacy in their nursing-home room but their resilience and sense of humour overcame the nursing staff's embarrassment.

Investigations of physical causes

There have been many attempts to distinguish between physical and emotional impotence (Jeffcoate 1991). The man's history can be helpful. If the impotence came on gradually over a period of months, if there is no erection at all under any circumstances (including masturbation), and if there are no morning erections, then the cause is likely to be organic. If, in the absence of physical trauma, the impotence is of sudden onset, if the man can occasionally obtain an erection, and if morning erections are still present, then the cause is more likely to be emotional. The presence of physical disease, as mentioned above, can be causal but should not be assumed to be the reason for impotence without exploring the man's emotional state. It is much easier to blame physical illness, for both doctor and patient, than to open the emotional can of worms.

Blood tests can be helpful and measurement of serum testosterone, prolactin, and FSH are probably useful, though rarely abnormal. Urine testing for the presence of glucose and the assessment of liver function is also worthwhile if indicated clinically. Low serum testosterone should not be assumed to be the cause of impotence if found. The range of normal values of testosterone is large and many men function perfectly well on low normal values. If loss of libido is a major feature then giving supplementary male hormone may improve the symptoms. Doctors should be careful to assess prostatic function before giving extra male hormone in an effort to exclude neoplastic change which could be markedly worsened by its administration.

The assessment of penile blood flow has absorbed many workers and sophisticated techniques have been employed (Gilbert *et al.* 1991). At this stage it is not certain how these findings in practice will affect the treatment of the impotent man.

Emotional causes of impotence

All the above physical causes will have their emotional components, and the doctor will need to be ready to deal with both aspects of the man's distress. In the past, it was common for doctors to attribute almost all impotence to emotional causes. Understandably, men became frustrated with this approach and were reluctant to return to their doctor for help. It is now recognized that at least half the men presenting with impotence have physical reasons for their complaint and, just as with any other complaint, an attempt at diagnosis should be made. The need to look at the physical should not preclude looking at the emotional aspects of the illness, nor vice versa. There needs to be a parallel approach.

Common emotions involved in sexual difficulties can be broadly grouped under four headings:

(1) fear;
(2) anger;
(3) sadness;
(4) guilt.

1. *Fear.* Fear of failure, fear of loss of control, and, perversely, fear of success are common themes. Fear of failure leads some men to put themselves under enormous pressure to succeed. Any hint of an erection that is perceived as not being 'good enough' or an ejaculation that is not delayed long enough leads to a downward spiral of anxiety and failure. Simple reassurance is often regarded as being all that is needed to solve the problem but the doctor has to ask himself 'Who is being reassured?' Is it the patient or really the doctor who gains from the reassurance? Can reassurance actually conceal the doctor's true feelings? A doctor faced with a patient reattending for a minor sexual difficulty may send the patient away with repeated reassurance that 'all is well' and 'not to worry about it'. Could the doctor in fact be saying to the patient 'Look, I know that there is nothing wrong with you. Stop believing as you do and start believing as I do and I will feel much happier'. It is important that the reason for the patient's continued attendances at the doctor's are

studied. In this way, the real problems lying behind the patient's difficulties might be addressed.

Mr D was a fresh-faced student of 20, dressed in normal student attire, with long, greasy hair and a thin, worried look on his face that did not fit in with the casual student image. He had been referred to the sexual problem clinic with a full letter from his GP. The letter said that he could not achieve an erection that would stand up long enough to allow intercourse, and with each failure the problem got worse, to the extent that he now avoided any attempts at sexual contact with his girlfriend. He arrived early for his appointment and as soon as he was seated he spurted out his story, itself almost like a premature ejaculation. He was extremely anxious and the story was studded with anxious pleas for reassurance that he would get better and quickly.

He had attempted intercourse on several occasions and, although he could achieve a good erection with his trousers on, as soon as the time came for removing his clothes and inserting his penis the erection failed him. He could masturbate easily but if his girlfriend was present then the penis did not erect. The doctor was careful not to fall into the trap of thoughtless reassurance. Instead, the patient's anxiety about failure was studied. His parents were from a professional background and had high hopes for their only son. He was pressured into exam courses that he was not really interested in and, as a consequence, failed academically. He had then taken up an arts course at a polytechnic college and, although very gifted, had always managed to flunk the exams. He knew his parents were disappointed in him and he had a very low opinion of his own attributes. He was so anxious to please and yet convinced of his own inadequacy. This produced a huge conflict for him when attempting to make love. Then his private parts were exposed and had to meet a woman's approval. His feelings of inadequacy produced a tremendous need for reassurance, and yet he was unable to accept this reassurance when offered as it did not fit in with his own set of personal beliefs. No wonder his own doctor and girlfriend and parents had become so exasperated with him. His attendance at the clinic allowed him to explore these feelings and conflicts with a resolution of his impotence.

2. *Anger.* Unexpressed anger is a frequent cause of sexual dysfunction. The patient is often unaware of his own feelings and they only show themselves during intercourse at times when 'raw emotions' are allowed and expected.

The study of the doctor/patient relationship in seminars by Michael Balint (1964) and later Tom Main (1982) helped doctors understand the hidden agendas that patients bring to the surgery.

A man in his early sixties came to the doctor's surgery as a temporary-resident patient late on a Friday evening. The doctor was tired and wanted to go home. It had been a hard week. Agreeing to see the patient somewhat reluctantly, there was a loud knock on the door, and before the doctor could say 'come in', the door burst open. In strode a man of military bearing, dressed smartly in a three-piece suit. He said 'Good evening, Doctor', and before sitting down moved the stethoscope and blood pressure machine from the edge of the doctor's desk so that he could rest his elbow on the doctor's table. The doctor was aware that he already felt angry with this controlling and intrusive patient. Before the doctor could speak, the patient went on to say that he had a sore throat and would need some antibiotics. If the doctor would be kind enough to issue a suitable prescription he would be on his way. The doctor was not going to take this lying down. He asked to look in this man's throat 'to see if he really did need any medication'. Unfortunately (for the doctor), this patient did have a severe infection and antibiotics were justified. The patient then stormed on to say that there was one other small matter of a private nature and would the doctor refer him to a consultant for further help. When the doctor asked what the nature of the problem might be, the patient told him that he would rather not go into details and a simple letter of referral to a physician would suffice. This was turning into a real battle between the doctor and the patient. It was at this time that the doctor wondered what was going on. Why did this man need to be so controlling and where was all the anger coming from? He calmly said that if he was to be of help then he would have to know a little about the problem. The patient sighed and mumbled that he had been having trouble with getting an erection for a few months. The doctor suggested an examination, and to the resentful words 'If you insist', the man slowly got undressed. As he started to remove his clothing, his manner changed from a blustering colonel to a very worried and rather shy man. He admitted that his erections had gone since the preceding Christmas. He had been married for 20 years, but on returning home one day had found his wife gone and a brief note on the mantelpiece. He could not understand why she had gone (though the doctor had some ideas) but he resolved that it was not going to affect his life. He had a number of successful 'one night stands' but had then met 'a wonderful woman'. She was the best thing that had ever happened to him and, at first, sex had been good. He used to give her presents of cash each Christmas but this year she had wanted a fur coat. This turned out to be much more expensive than the cash presents. The doctor enquired whether he had any feelings about this. There then followed a brief pause, followed by an explosion of anger about how you can never satisfy women and how they always want more than you can give. This seemed to be well-reflected in his sexual performance of late. In his anger and frustration he had literally 'downed tools'. As he dressed he regained some of his former composure and control. He said 'I did not realize how angry I was until now. I think I will have to have it out with her'. The patient left the doctor with some anxieties about what he would do but he returned the next week saying that his throat was much better and that he no longer needed a referral 'about that other business'.

It was the study of the patient's reaction in the surgery and the doctor's response that allowed this consultation to progress. If the doctor had merely retaliated then nothing would have been resolved. The examination of this man played a key role. It was noted that as he removed his clothes so some of his defences were removed as well. Examination of his genitalia, his private parts, allowed the patient to open up in other ways about his private feelings. The doctor must be aware of the emotions attached to examination, especially examination of the genitalia. It is no use staring fixedly at the testicles and ignoring what is happening to the person attached to them. Does the patient look interested? Are they fearful? Have they got their eyes shut? Are their fists clenched? All these actions can provide insights to the presenting problem.

3. *Sadness.* The loss of a partner after many years of marriage leaves many men sad and lonely. Attempts to start new relationships often result in sexual failure and this adds to the sense of isolation. The exposure of genitalia and feelings that were previously shared only in the comfort of a long-lasting and mutually trusting relationship is often too much for men to bear, and yet some feel a need to perform and satisfy a new partner in the same way as they did when young. This may just be an attempt to ensure that they will not be left again, but will result in a great deal of pressure. There

may be a hidden agenda designed to fail and in this way let the man off the hook of having to perform sexually with a new partner.

Mr E was referred to the sexual-problem clinic with a history of being unable to sustain an erection with his new partner. He arrived on time and calmly told the doctor of his sexual difficulty. He could not understand why he had this problem as he had never had any difficulties when married. He had been married for 40 years and was devastated when his wife died. He lost weight, did not go out, and neglected himself. Luckily, an old friend of theirs had visited and she had encouraged him to put his life back together. She got him to go to the local social club and involved him in charity work. He said, 'without her I would have committed suicide'. He felt terribly grateful to her and their relationship became close. She wanted to live with him and he wanted to please her in any way he could, but every time he tried to make love his erection failed. He told the doctor this story in a very resigned way and kept saying 'I don't suppose you can do anything to help'. The doctor was taken in by the sadness of the story and there followed a long series of rather sterile consultations, interspersed with attempts using injections to produce erections to ease this man's problem. It eventually became clear to the doctor that no matter what methods were used, all were doomed to fail. This man did not want anything to succeed. Because he felt grateful to his new partner he felt he ought to please her, but he could not bring himself to commit himself to any other woman. He had demonstrated his apparent willingness to get something done, to show his partner that he cared, but underneath all this was his need to remain true to his wife and her memory. The relief on the patient's face when the doctor admitted defeat was a clear indication of his real wishes.

4. *Guilt.* The sense of guilt that some men feel about their sexual needs interferes with their sexual performance, but it can be extremely difficult to establish the root of their problems. Because they perceive their sexual longings as perverted, dirty, or shameful, they keep their needs well hidden. It is essential that a non-judgemental approach is taken and the patient allowed to express their secrets in a completely confidential atmosphere. Fear of homosexuality, of transvestism, masturbation, and fetishism are common.

Although the origin of the patient's problem may be obviously emotional, some men cannot deal with their emotions until they know that something can be done on a practical level. It is as if the emotional defences have to be manned until they feel safe enough to lower them, and the only way for them to feel this safe is to know that there is a practical solution. The use of papaverine, or, more recently, prostaglandin E1 injections has helped a great deal to achieve this. They are powerful, vasoactive substances, and if given directly by injection into the corpora of the penis, usually result in an erection lasting anything from half an hour to four hours. It does not work if there is significant damage to the vasculature supplying the penis. Up to 50% of men will not be able to face the thought of injecting themselves with papaverine but about 65% of men will gain an erection sufficient for penetrative intercourse (Gilbert and Gingell 1991). The sense of relief that can be achieved using papaverine allows the emotional dimension of the problem to be studied. If the problem is 'purely' physical, this may not play much part in the consultation. There is a danger that by just giving papaverine the doctor will assume that the problem is solved. If you only give an injection you only get an erection and the problems lying behind the original complaint may not be studied (Barrett 1990).

The vacuum method of obtaining an erection has found favour in some clinics. A tube is placed over the penis, forming a seal with the skin of the pubis. A small hand pump attached to the tube creates a vacuum around the shaft of the penis, causing blood to flow into the penis. Once the penis is engorged with blood, a small rubber ring is placed around the base of the penile shaft, the vacuum is released, and the tube removed. The ring holds the blood in the penis until intercourse is over, whereupon it is removed and the penis deflates. Many patients have found this an acceptable way of gaining an erection but many find it too mechanical. Only 27% of patients were willing to use these devices long term (Gilbert and Gingell 1992). Unfortunately, it is not generally available via the NHS and patients have to purchase it.

Whatever method is employed on the mechanical front, the patient's feelings about the situation have to be studied and his reactions to these mechanical treatments explored. It can offer valuable insights into otherwise hidden areas of their difficulties.

Libido

The use of the word libido can be a cause of confusion in describing a man's sexual difficulties. A patient will be referred with a diagnosis of impotence when, in fact, a loss of libido is the real problem. The wish or drive to make love is affected by hormonal activity as well as emotional factors. If a man complains of a loss of interest in making love, it is important to establish whether it is an actual absence of sexual feeling or merely described as this in order to avoid difficulties in making love. Fantasies or sexual dreams offer a clue as to whether there is a true absence of sexual feeling. A simple blood test measuring testosterone level may provide an answer but the doctor must not jump to conclusions if the testosterone is marginally low. Some men function perfectly well on very low male hormone levels and there is a wide range of normal values. If there is doubt, a therapeutic trial of male hormone injections can be used, but it is important to exclude prostatic cancer before commencing such treatment.

True loss of libido is relatively rare and, on close enquiry, most overt complaints of loss of libido hide a wish to avoid intercourse because of problems such as fear of failure. Sensitive consultation is needed to uncover the real problems.

Excess alcohol causing liver damage can result in a true secondary loss of libido and, if suspected, liver function tests should be performed and advice given (perhaps one of the rare cases when directive advice is appropriate).

Homosexuality

Homosexuality is not in itself a problem for most of the community, but fears of homosexuality and uncertainties about sexual preference can cause difficulties for some individuals. The nature of many homosexual relationships is still transitory and leads to problems in expressing deeper sexual feelings. Fear of discovery for many homosexual men makes brief promiscuous encounters the norm. The facility to share the ongoing intimacy of a long-term relationship in these circumstances is denied and expression of other relationship needs frustrated. A caring, accepting, and non-judgemental approach of the doctor to the patient is important in allowing the patient to express their fears and needs.

Sexual deviance

The highly charged emotions that surround sexual deviance make it difficult for the doctor to offer help. Our own ideas of right and wrong get in the way of non-judgemental consultation. Whether or not we can separate ourselves from the nature of the difficulty affects our ability to help a patient who might be in considerable distress. A convicted paedophile does not deserve sympathy, but if they genuinely have asked for help then the doctor has an ethical duty towards patients, recognized for general practitioners in the NHS under their terms of service as an obligation to provide 'all necessary and appropriate medical care'. The patient who is terrified of their feelings of paedophilia needs considerable help to explore the feelings and their origin. Often, they reflect an inability to face up to the challenge of an adult sexual relationship. Intense fears of inferiority lead to an absolute avoidance of adult intercourse and fantasies (or sadly the reality) of sexual relations with children. The treatment of convicted sexual offenders is not within the scope of most doctors nor this chapter.

Other sexual deviance may include fetishism or bondage. Some men have a great fear of women and particularly the vagina. The ability to get close to women without having to approach the vagina seems to be at the root of most fetishes. Foot fetishists manage to keep the furthest away from the vagina with the possible exception of voyeurs with telephoto lenses. If helped to understand the nature of their fears, many men can be helped to a more natural way of sexual expression.

Bondage reflects feelings about control and relates to either a need to be out of control and be bound, or a need to be in total control and bind the partner. The bondage does not necessarily lead to sexual problems, but if it becomes a replacement for a normal sexual experience then help may be required. Unfortunately, it is not usually the man who seeks such help. As with problems of other simple fetishes, such as requiring the partner to wear certain clothing, there is a danger that the sexual expression will relate to the object rather than the person behind the activity. The woman will feel used and uninvolved in the sexual relationship. The man sees little wrong in what for him has always been an almost masturbatory experience, just using his partner as a convenient clothes horse. If he wants help then his fears of women can be explored, but he will often be brought along to the doctor by his partner 'for help'. In this case, he will have little interest in getting better and counselling is likely to prove fruitless.

In this chapter, normal male sexuality and difficulties with ejaculation, erection, libido, and sexual expression have been studied. The constraints of such an overview have, of necessity, meant that the coverage is somewhat superficial, but a reading list is appended for those wishing to further develop their knowledge in this interesting field.

References

Balint, M. (1964). *The doctor, his patient and the illness.* Pitman, London.

Barrett, P. J. (1990). Papaverine: heresy or progress? *Journal of the Institute of Psychosexual Medicine,* **1**, 6–8.

Bateman, D. N. (1980). Drugs and sexual function. *Adverse Drug Reaction Bulletin*, **85**, 308–11.

Brecher, E. and Brecher, E. (1967). *An analysis of human sexual response.* Andre Deutsch, Manchester.

British Medical Journal (1979). Drugs and male sexual function. *British Medical Journal*, **ii**, 883–4.

Gilbert, H. W., Desai K. M., and Gingell, J. C. (1991). Non-invasive assessment of arteriogenic impotence: a comparative study. *British Journal of Urology*, **67**, 512–16.

Gilbert, H. W. and Gingell, J. C. (1991). The results of an intracorporeal papaverine clinic. *Journal of sex and marital therapy*, **6**, 49–56.

Gilbert, H. W. and Gingell, J. C. (1992). Vacuum constriction devices – a second-line conservative treatment for impotence. *British Journal of Urology*, **70**, 81–3.

Jeffcoate, W. J. (1991). The investigation of impotence. *British Journal of Urology*, **68**, 449–53.

Lue, T. F. and Tanagho, E. A. (1987). Physiology of erection and pharmacological management of impotence. *Journal of Urology*, **137**, 829–36.

McCulloch, D. K., Campbell, I. W., Wu, F. C., *et al.* (1980). The prevalence of diabetic impotence. *Diabetologia*, **18**, 279–83.

Main, T. F. (1982). Training for the acquisition of knowledge or the development of skill. In *Practice of psychosexual medicine* (ed. K. Draper), pp. 7–18. John Libby, London.

Masters, W. and Johnson, V. (1959). The sexual response cycle of the human female. *Annals of New York Academy of Sciences*, **83**, 301–17.

Masters, W. and Johnson, V. (1966). Human sexual response. Little, Brown, & Co., Boston.

Slob, A. K., Blom, J. H. M., and van der Werff ten Bosch, J. J. (1990). Erection problems in medical practice, differential diagnosis with relatively simple method. *Journal of Urology*, **143**, 46–50.

Further reading

Freedman, G. R. (1983). *Sexual medicine.* Churchill Livingstone, Edinburgh.

Skrine, R. L. (1987). *Psychosexual training and the doctor/patient relationship.* Montana Press, Glasgow.

Tunnadine, P. (1983). *The making of love.* Jonathan Cape, London.

Address for further advice

The Institute of Psychosexual Medicine,
11 Chandos Street,
London W1M 9DE.

CHAPTER EIGHT

Men and alcohol

Simon Smail and Stephen Rollnick

Alcohol is widely used in society but the heaviest users are young men. It is a great social lubricant that is associated with fun, enjoyment, and good life. It has a darker side which is often hidden from the general practitioner, particularly as adult males are absent from the doctor's consulting room anyway. We wanted this chapter to examine the transition from social lubricant to problem alcohol user. We also wanted to investigate the role of the GP in detecting and managing alcohol problems. Just asking about alcohol will pick up 50% of problem drinkers. Some are ready to change and a brief commonsense intervention is described which both informs the drinker about safe limits and may provide the motivation for reduction. The authors recognize that alcohol is a touchy subject and their approach is both shrewd and sensitive.

Alcohol has been used as a socially acceptable drug since the early days of human civilization. There has always been some concern about its use and there have been varied attempts to control or reduce the consumption of alcohol over the years. In the eighteenth century, the Royal College of Physicians sent a petition to Parliament, drawing attention to the 'fatal effect of the frequent use of several sorts of distilled spiritous liquors upon the great numbers of both sexes, rendering them diseased, not fit for business, poor, a burthen to themselves and neighbours, and too often the cause of weak, feeble, and distempered children' (Royal College of Psychiatrists 1986). The response by the government was to introduce controls on the sale of alcohol, the licensing of premises, and a reduction in the hours during which alcohol could be sold. In most Western countries there are a variety of laws controlling the sale and consumption of alcohol; in the 1920s its sale was banned completely in America during the era of prohibition. The recent trend in the United Kingdom has been towards a gradual relaxation of licensing laws, and an attempt by public bodies to encourage 'sensible drinking' by appealing to a sense of personal responsibility (Kendall 1987), a policy which has not been without its critics.

Alcohol consumption

In historical terms, alcohol consumption today in the United Kingdom is probably some-what less than in previous centuries (Royal College of Psychiatrists 1986). At the end of the seventeenth century, it is reported that beer consumption reached a peak level of 2.3 pints per head of population per day.

Nowadays, consumption is usually measured in 'standard units' of alcohol per week. A standard unit is taken as around 8.5 grams of absolute alcohol, which is contained in half a pint of beer (bitter or a beer of equivalent strength), a small glass of wine, or a bar measure of spirits (one-sixth of a gill is the standard measure used in England and Wales; one-fifth of a gill in Scotland). Figures published in government surveys which rely on self-report data suggest that overall intake for men has been fairly constant from 1984 to 1994, whilst it has risen slightly amongst women (OPCS 1995). Such surveys do, how-ever, consistently underreport overall consumption when compared with Customs and Excise statistics. The Customs data suggest that overall consumption is over nine litres of pure alcohol per adult per year. In 1993, 6.1% of total household expenditure was spent on alcohol (Social Trends 1995). Self-reported consumption figures show that 27% of men and 13% of women in 1994 were drinking over the recommended safe limits (Fig. 8.1).

The heaviest consumers of alcohol are young men. Men in the age group 18–24 consume on average around 20 standard drinks per week; consumption rates decline into later life (Fig. 8.2). The General Household Survey of 1990 undertook a detailed survey to characterize the consumption of alcohol in Great Britain at that time (OPCS 1992). The figures illustrate the range of consumption in the different age groups. In the 18–24 age group, 94% were drinkers and 36% were drinking more than 22 units per week, defined as a 'hazardous' level by the Royal College of Physicians (RCP 1987).

There is little doubt that experimentation with alcohol begins at an early age. The Health Promotion Authority for Wales has collaborated in an international comparison of drinking behaviour amongst teenagers (HPAW 1990a). The data show that even by the age of 11, more than 80% of boys and girls had already tasted alcohol. In 1988, 32% of boys between the ages of 13 and 16 were drinking at least weekly, and 23% of girls. Children in this age group were also asked if they had ever been drunk: 25% of boys and 17% of girls admitted to being drunk more than four times. These figures were higher than those obtained in any of eight other European countries.

Crude consumption statistics, however, mask an enormous variation in actual levels of intake by individuals. Of particular concern amongst men is the habit of binge drinking. The authors of a survey from Wales (HPAW 1990b) defined binge drinking as drinking half the recommended weekly intake on one occasion, i.e. 10 or more units for men and seven or more for women. Two-thirds of male drinkers and one-third of female drinkers reported binge drinking at least occasionally, with 28% of men and 8% of women reportedly doing so weekly. Age and social class differences were found, with higher proportions of younger and manual social groups reporting weekly binge drinking.

Fig. 8.1 *Alcohol consumption by sex, 1984–1994, persons aged 18 and over, Great Britain. Weekly consumption figures (OPCS 1992)*

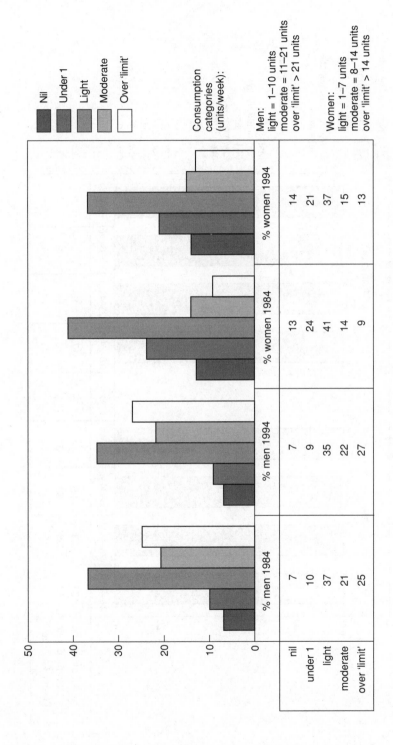

Consumption categories (units/week):

Men:
light = 1–10 units
moderate = 11–21 units
over 'limit' > 21 units

Women:
light = 1–7 units
moderate = 8–14 units
over 'limit' > 14 units

	% men 1984	% men 1994	% women 1984	% women 1994
nil	7	7	13	14
under 1	10	9	24	21
light	37	35	41	37
moderate	21	22	14	15
over 'limit'	25	27	9	13

Legend: Nil, Under 1, Light, Moderate, Over 'limit'

Fig. 8.2 *Alcohol consumption by age, 1990, men and women, Great Britain. Consumption per week (OPCS 1992)*

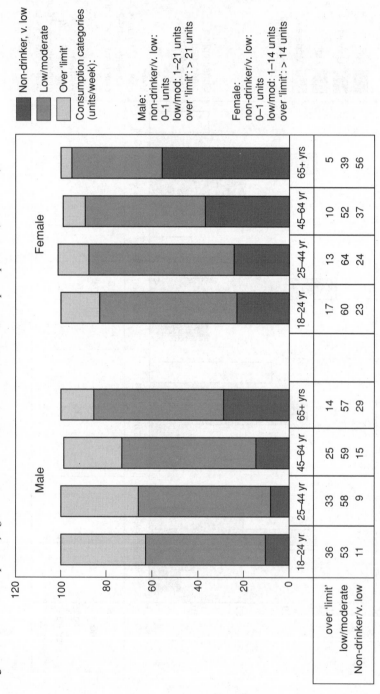

The social uses of alcohol

The pharmacological effects of a small amount of alcohol are well-documented, and include not only an anxiolytic effect but also some euphoria. There seems little doubt that many people deliberately use alcohol as an anxiolytic, and its use as a 'social lubricant' probably serves a useful purpose in improving the social discourse of society (Orford 1985).

Certain occupational groups are more at risk of hazardous or dangerous drinking. Those who work in the drinks industry top the list, closely followed by seamen, fishermen, financial agents, and, not far from the top, medical practitioners (Plant 1981). Many authors cite stress as a trigger factor, and in individual cases it is often possible to relate the onset of heavier drinking to a specific episode or stressful event, such as redundancy.

There are, however, some disincentives to drinking. Lack of time, the disapproval of family and friends, and a cultural milieu which disapproves of drinking or drunkenness may all be relevant factors. The cost of alcohol is also a key feature in determining overall consumption levels (Grant *et al.* 1982). There is an inverse relationship between the real price of alcoholic beverages, and the level of consumption per head, and most indices of alcohol-related harm. Between 1949 and 1979, the real price of alcohol dropped by about 50%; over the same period, alcohol consumption almost doubled.

Physical harm from alcohol

Almost every system in the body can be damaged as a result of excessive alcohol consumption (Table 8.1). The evidence for these associations has been well-reviewed elsewhere (Paton 1988; Royal College of General Practitioners 1986; Royal College of Physicians 1987; Royal College of Psychiatrists 1986).

Official figures for deaths from alcohol relate only to chronic liver disease and cirrhosis, alcoholic psychosis, alcohol dependence syndrome, toxic effects of alcohol, and accidental poisoning by alcohol. These statistics show a doubling in alcohol-related deaths from 1950 to the early 1990s. However, these official statistics are thought to under-report deaths from alcohol at least fivefold. They fail to include many accidental deaths that occur as a result of acute alcohol intoxication, and also do not include those deaths in which alcohol played a significant part, even though the immediate cause of death was something other than one of the more obvious alcohol-associated causes.

In order to establish a clearer estimate of the effects of alcohol on mortality, Kristenson and Hood (1984) carried out a prospective study of 10 000 middle-aged men in Malmo, Sweden who were recruited and initially screened with an intensive health-screening examination. A careful analysis of the subsequent deaths during the following 3.5 to 8 years showed that 32% were related to alcohol, and no less than 39% of those who died had a history of excessive alcohol consumption. Moreover, the death rates were six to seven times higher in those men whose gamma-glutamyl transferase levels were in the upper quintile (suggesting existing liver damage) at initial screening compared to those with GGT levels in the lowest quintile.

One of the most significant studies carried out into the effects of alcohol consumption on mortality in the UK was that of Marmot *et al.* (1981) who conducted a longitudinal survey

Table 8.1 *Potential physical hazards from alcohol (Paton 1988)*

Nervous system

Acute intoxication – loss of social inhibitions, slurring of speech, reduced intellectual performance, accidents, coma, death

Blackouts, loss of memory for events

Withdrawal symptoms

Wernicke's encephalopathy

Korsakoff's syndrome

Cerebellar deterioration

Head injury, subdural, extradural haematoma

Peripheral neuropathy

Liver

Symptomless enlargement

Fatty infiltration

Alcoholic hepatitis

Cirrhosis

Gastrointestinal symptoms

Oesophageal acid reflux

Cancer of oesophagus

Gastritis

Aggravation and impaired healing of peptic ulcers

Nutrition

Malnutrition

Obesity

Cardiovascular, respiratory

Arrhythmias, hypertension

Pneumonia from inhalation of vomit

Rib fractures

Endocrine

Increased production of cortisol, leading to obesity, increased facial hair, hypertension

Fall in blood glucose, sometimes leading to coma

Diabetes

Reproductive system

Loss of libido, reduced fertility

Fetal alcohol syndrome – small babies with developmental defects

Skin

Acne

Rhinophyma

of Whitehall civil servants. They reported a 'J-shaped' relationship between alcohol consumption and mortality. At zero consumption, the mortality rate was found to be higher than with modest levels of consumption, suggesting a slight beneficial effect from a small intake of alcohol. However, overall mortality rose when consumption reached 34 grams of alcohol a day (around four standard drinks). Much of this variation was a result of an increase in cardiovascular mortality. Men drinking more than 30 units a week had twice the mortality at 10-year follow-up than men who were drinking between one and eight units. The existence of the J-shaped or U-shaped relationship between mortality and alcohol consumption has been confirmed by other investigators, and possible mechanisms for the protective effects of alcohol have been discussed (Kannel and Ellison 1996).

Tofler (1985) conducted a very elegant prospective study of 'men about town' in Perth, Australia, and also reviewed other long-term follow-up studies. He concluded that the heart muscle of the social drinker can be damaged by more than 30 units a week, as evidenced by T-wave changes and left-axis deviation. Myocardial function deteriorates with consumption levels above 80 units a week. There is a linear relationship between consumption of alcohol and both systolic and diastolic blood pressure. At about 60 units per week a threshold is reached, after which the slope of the relationship increases.

In general practice, one of the early presenting physical features of excessive alcohol intake is likely to be gastrointestinal symptoms. Problem drinkers suffer an increased incidence of reflux oesophagitis, gastritis, diarrhoea, and diverticulitis. Of more significance is the increased incidence of pancreatitis, and carcinoma of the pancreas and the oesophagus.

Studies in the United Kingdom, in Sweden, and in America all suggest that around a fifth of medical admissions to hospital are a direct result of alcohol misuse, and possibly around a third of male admissions to casualty departments are alcohol-related (Paton 1988).

Alcohol-related morbidity in general practice has not been so thoroughly studied as that in hospital practice, although those surveys which have been published suggest a high prevalence of problems associated with alcohol consumption. Within a general practice population, at any one time around 10% of adult men will be drinking dangerously (more than 50 units per week).

In an urban practice in Cardiff, we sent a questionnaire to a sample of 1201 men between 17 and 70 years of age; 692 (58%) were returned (Rollnick *et al.* 1988). Sixty-one per cent of the respondents were drinking between 1–15 units per week, 11% between 16–30 units, 15% between 30–50 units, and 13% were drinking more than 50 units a week. However, when an audit of the notes of 38 of these problem drinkers was carried out, only eight were known to the practice as problem drinkers. Compared to a comparison group of social drinkers, problem drinkers consulted significantly more often, and were more likely to complain about gastrointestinal problems, headaches, and dizzy spells than controls (Table 8.2). Spouses of problem drinkers were also more likely to consult than spouses of the control group, with a significant excess of sleep disturbance symptoms, accidental injury, and gastrointestinal symptoms (Table 8.3) (Muir 1988).

Given the national prevalence figures for dangerous drinking levels, similar findings are likely in most practices. The level of morbidity and indeed mortality from problem drinking in any practice is therefore likely to be considerable; even though the morbidity is recognized, it may not be ascribed to problem drinking.

Table 8.2 *General practice morbidity over four years for 38 male 'excessive drinkers' compared with age-matched control population. Urban Cardiff practice (Muir 1988)*

Problem	Excessive drinkers (n = 38)	Controls (n = 38)
Gastrointestinal	14*	8*
Sleep problem	0	1
Irritable bowel	0	1
Accidental injury	13*	9*
Heart/circulation	1	0
Nutrition/endocrine	1	0
Genito-urinary	10	13
Musculoskeletal	11	8
Respiratory	8	7
Amnesia	1	0
Haematemesis and malaena	1	0
DTs	1	0
Headache/dizzy spells	10*	0*

* *t-test significant at p < 0.05*

Acute intoxication

One of the earliest effects of intoxication is loss of judgement. Even though small doses of alcohol are pharmacologically depressant, there is a paradoxical effect in some people who feel stimulated or disinhibited by alcohol. This, undoubtedly, is one of the factors in the association of alcohol with aggressive behaviour. With higher doses, there is slurred speech, impairment of coordination, thinking, and memory, and ultimately drowsiness and respiratory depression. Death can result from respiratory arrest or inhalation of vomit.

There is considerable circumstantial evidence that alcohol intoxication is associated with violence (Lancet 1990). UK studies have shown that alcohol intoxication is involved in 60% of parasuicides, 54% of fire fatalities, 50% of homicides, 42% of patients admitted to hospital with serious head injuries, 30% of deaths through drowning, and 30% of all domestic accidents (Taylor 1981). Some of the studies, in which those involved in violence have been screened for alcohol usage, have been criticized because many of them lack control populations. However, case–control studies do show that in the case of young men involved in urban violence, the consumption of more than eight units of

Table 8.3 *General practice morbidity over four years for 25 spouses/female partners of excessive drinkers compared with morbidity of spouses/partners of controls. Urban Cardiff practice (Muir 1988)*

Problem	Spouses of excessive drinkers (n = 25)	Spouses of controls (n = 25)
Gastrointestinal	15*	3*
Sleep problem	6*	1*
Accidental injury	7*	2*
Nutrition/endocrine	1	1
Genito-urinary	17	17
Musculoskeletal	12*	5*
Respiratory	1*	6*
Headache/dizzy spells	6	8
Smoking	8*	2*
Medication		
Antidepressants	1	2
Sleeping pills	3	0
Tranquillizers	7*	3*
Painkillers	3	1

* *t-test significant at p < 0.05*

alcohol was significantly associated with involvement in violence (Shepherd *et al.* 1990). Binge drinking, which is known to be a significant problem amongst British men, is therefore apparently associated with violent outcomes. Furthermore, alcohol consumption by young males increases the likelihood that the behaviour of others will be perceived as threatening or challenging (Pihl 1983); this phenomenon could contribute to a cycle of violence.

Many types of crime are associated with alcohol. Studies suggest that around half of all those in prison have alcohol problems (McMurran and Baldwin 1989). The highest rates of alcohol abuse are found in recidivists, especially those who are imprisoned for recurrent short periods.

There is now abundant evidence to demonstrate the link between drinking and road accidents. A survey conducted by the Grand Rapids police force (Borkenstein *et al.* 1964) demonstrated that the risk of an accident doubled when the driver's blood alcohol level reached 80 mg per 100 ml, and at 150 mg the risk was increased tenfold. Other studies have shown that there is a gradient of risk across the agegroups. Younger and less experienced drivers are far more at risk of an accident at low blood alcohol levels than older and more experienced drivers (Dunbar *et al.* 1985).

Family harm

Apart from harming themselves, those with alcohol problems also harm their families. Many families fall apart under the strain of an alcoholic parent. A third of all problem drinkers say that marital discord is one of their problems, and 40% of cases brought before family courts in the USA feature 'alcoholism' in some way. In a survey of 100 cases of wife-battering in Britain, the husband was 'frequently drunk' in 52 of the cases (Paton 1988).

The harm to children in a family with an alcoholic parent is of especial concern in general practice. Rydelius (1981) carried out a longitudinal study in Sweden in which 229 children from 141 families where there was an alcoholic father were followed up for a number of years. The outcome for these children was compared to the outcome of a control group of children recruited from families where there was no parental drinking problem. The study found that children of alcoholic fathers run the risk of becoming socially maladjusted themselves when they reach adulthood; the problems involved in this maladjustment included alcoholism. The children also continued to show excessively frequent ill health, with somatically oriented symptoms during adult life, and an increased frequency of mental illness. The results in respect of sons showed that they were more severely affected in the long term than were the daughters of alcoholic fathers. Other studies have similarly demonstrated eventual mental ill health or antisocial behaviour in the children of alcoholics. Children in families with an alcoholic father may be the victims of violence or incest, and are more prone to suffer from anorexia and hysterical symptoms.

The prospective studies quoted above found that children of alcoholics are more likely to develop alcoholism themselves, and it is clear that alcoholism does tend to run in families. However, twin studies and adoption studies have shown that in one-third of cases the development of alcoholism is genetically linked, and in the other two-thirds there are cultural or environmental influences which appear to determine alcoholism (Murray and Murray 1991).

Problem drinkers

There have been many varied usages of the terms 'alcoholism', 'problem drinker', etc. over the years, and it is false to imply that there is any one definition of 'alcoholism' which can apply to all circumstances. As has been discussed earlier, there are a whole range of physical, psychological, and social problems resulting from excessive drinking. It is perhaps more useful to consider drinking problems under two headings: 'alcohol-related problems' and the 'alcohol-dependence syndrome'. People may suffer from alcohol-related problems even if they are modest social drinkers but occasional binge drinkers. At the other end of the spectrum, dependent drinkers demonstrate the features of dependency common to dependency syndromes seen with other drugs of addiction (Edwards and Gross 1976). The dependence syndrome is described in an empirical fashion. It is useful to identify common features of the syndrome although individual symptoms and behaviours may vary; dependence levels can vary on a continuum from mild to severe. Significant features of the syndrome include an increased tolerance to alcohol, repeated withdrawal symptoms, a subjective awareness of the compulsion to take the drug, relief or avoidance of withdrawal symptoms, and reinstatement after a period of abstinence. However, the pattern of addictive behaviour varies with time. Heather and Robertson (1983) suggest that addictive behaviour can best be explained in terms of social-learning theory. The phenomenon of dependence is mediated through a learning process. The behaviours may change as different sets of learning conditions operate.

Several studies have been conducted which have followed the career of addictive drinkers. Vaillant and Milofsky (1982) followed up 110 male problem drinkers identified from within the general population and found that these men moved between different drinking styles at different times. Eighteen men had ultimately achieved asymptomatic drinking for two years or more. However, 21 men whom they described as 'securely abstinent' with a mean of 10 years' abstinence were nevertheless amongst those initially with the highest dependency ratings, suggesting that men with addictive behaviour can nevertheless achieve secure abstinence.

Another 10-year follow-up study (Taylor et al. 1985) found that around 25% of drinkers continued as 'troubled' drinkers, 12% became abstinent, whilst the remainder moved between these two categories and occasionally into 'social' drinking.

Studies of the occurrence of physical and psychological harm have demonstrated time and again that there is a clear relationship between consumption and the likelihood of the onset of damage, for example cirrhosis, hypertension, gastrointestinal problems, alcoholic brain damage, etc. The Royal Colleges of Physicians, Psychiatrists, and General Practitioners (Marmot 1995; RCGP 1986; RCPhys 1987; RCPsych 1986) have produced recommendations for 'sensible' drinking levels which have been widely adopted in the UK. The consensus medical view is that 'safe limits' are up to 21 units per week for men and up to 14 units per week for women. At such levels, most individuals are unlikely to come to any harm provided the total amount is not drunk in one or two bouts and that there are occasional drink-free days. 'Moderate' levels of consumption are defined as 20–50 units per week for men, and 15–35 units for women. High (or dangerous) levels are 51 or more units per week for men, and 36 or more for women.

An element of controversy was introduced into the discussion of sensible levels of alcohol consumption when the Department of Health issued new advice to the public at the end of 1995 (DoH 1995). The Government stated that 'regular consumption of between two and three units per day by women of all ages will not accrue any significant health risk' and went on to suggest that the ceiling for men could be three or four units per day. The report carefully avoided the use of the word 'limits' and proposed the term 'benchmark' be used. It also recommended that older people who did not drink might consider the possible health benefits of drinking. However, a number of influential medical bodies rapidly repudiated the advice given by the Government committee – which was composed 'exclusively of civil servants with no scientific experts from outside the civil service' (Edwards 1996). The advice of the Royal Colleges of Physicians, Psychiatrists, and General Practitioners and of the BMA remains in line with previous recommendations (Marmot 1995).

Attitudes to alcohol consumption

The 'sensible-drinking' levels have been publicized in many health education campaigns and publications, such as *That's the limit* (Health Education Council 1984); professionals, including doctors and nurses, have been advised to remind their patients of the safe limits for alcohol consumption. A number of surveys have endeavoured to find out if the public are aware of the concept of 'safe levels' of consumption. A question was included in the General Household Survey of 1990 asking drinkers about their own self-image of themselves as drinkers. No less than 16% of men who were drinking hazardously or dangerously thought they were drinking either 'a little' or 'hardly at all', suggesting a low level of insight, and possible difficulties in reaching such men with educational campaigns. Welsh data (Health Promotion Authority for Wales 1989) show that only a third of the population could correctly identify the appropriate measure of beer or wine as a unit of alcohol. Twenty-two per cent thought that a pint of beer was the equivalent of a unit. Generally, the majority of those questioned in the survey could correctly identify the safe limits for alcohol consumption, or underestimated the limits. However, a higher proportion of younger men overestimated the limits.

Detection of the problem drinker

Problem drinkers are frequently undetected in general practice. Not all of them, it should be remembered, are currently experiencing a medical problem connected to their drinking. Absenteeism from work and/or domestic difficulties are often the more pressing problems. It is therefore not surprising that they are sometimes difficult to detect. Both clinical experience and the findings of research point to the combined use of a number of detection methods. To begin with, attention will be given to the often valuable information which can be gleaned from talking to and observing the patient himself. Detection is not purely a technical matter but often one of engaging patients in dialogue about their drinking. Raising the subject of drinking in a sensitive and constructive manner is often the key to effective detection. It is important to remember that one is not merely looking for the severely alcohol-dependent patient, and that patients can be placed on a continuum, albeit a little crudely, from those without major problems at the one end to those with severe alcohol dependence at the other.

It is undoubtedly good practice to take a routine alcohol-consumption history whenever an adult screening interview is conducted. However, the accuracy of a straightforward alcohol history is not high. A simple history based on questions such as 'How much do you drink?' only has a sensitivity of 50% in detecting problem drinkers. Clues may be provided by the presentation of symptoms which could be alcohol-related, but the most accurate assessments of alcohol consumption, for practical purposes, are achieved by the use of a questionnaire.

The Michigan Alcohol Screening Test (MAST questionnaire) is well-validated and has a sensitivity of above 85%. However, in its full version, it is too long to be used routinely in primary care settings. The CAGE questionnaire is the most popular for use in general practice (Ewing 1984) and has a sensitivity of between 60 and 85%; it is certainly more accurate than a simple clinical history, and extremely quick to use:

1. Have you ever felt you should *Cut* down your drinking?
2. Have people *Annoyed* you by criticizing your drinking?
3. Have you ever felt bad or *Guilty* about your drinking?
4. Have you ever had a drink first thing in the morning to steady your nerves or get rid of a hangover? *(Eye-opener.)*

Biological markers for excess alcohol intake have some value as screening tools, although they have poorer sensitivity than a well-constructed questionnaire (Hays and Spickard 1987). No single biological screening test is as sensitive as the CAGE questionnaire. Elevation of hepatic enzymes and mean corpuscular volume do occur with excessive alcohol consumption, but these are not particularly sensitive screening tests for problem drinkers. Estimation of the liver enzyme gamma-glutamyl transferase is more sensitive than other biochemical tests (around 60%), but a false positive result may be found in 15–50% of tests since the blood level of this enzyme may be raised with diabetes, heart or kidney disease, and some medications such as anticonvulsants and steroid hormones.

A careful clinical history and the routine use of the CAGE questionnaire or the brief MAST questionnaire (Pokorny *et al.* 1972) are therefore more rewarding than undertaking routine blood tests in screening for problem drinkers. Blood tests do, however, have a place in monitoring the progress of drinkers who have been advised to moderate their intake of alcohol.

Evidence for the effectiveness of brief intervention

Following identification of a patient who appears to be drinking heavily – perhaps at the level of 'heavy social drinking' – it is reasonable to consider a brief intervention as an initial therapeutic response. During the 1980s, a large number of studies were conducted in medical settings, mostly among male heavy drinkers, using the rationale provided by secondary prevention (Babor and Grant 1992; Bien and Miller 1993). Within a controlled-trial format, heavy drinkers identified with a screening questionnaire were given brief advice about the need to reduce consumption. Among the conclusions to emerge from this research, which included studies in general practice (Anderson and Scott 1992; Wallace *et al.* 1988), were that brief advice led to significant reductions in consumption and alcohol-related problems. Although the proportion of heavy drinkers who changed was relatively small, a longer, more intensive intervention did not appear to improve the success rate. One way of interpreting these findings is to conclude that, even though the potency of brief advice is relatively weak, the benefits to public health of widespread GP intervention would be considerable (Kahan *et al.* 1995). A review of six studies of 'brief interventions' suggested that between five and 10 minutes of advice could lead to reductions of alcohol consumption of around 25–35% at follow-up six months or one year later (Anderson 1993). Furthermore, current evidence suggests that brief interventions are as effective as more expensive specialist interventions (Nuffield Institute 1993).

Another approach has been to explore the development of potentially more effective interventions which take into account the readiness to change of the individual (Rollnick *et al.* 1992; Rollnick and Morgan 1995). However this issue is resolved, it is quite clear that many male heavy drinkers do not appear to want help or advice; often, the doctor will be confronting the norms of a heavy-drinking subculture. Therefore, the following section on the conduct of brief intervention will pay some attention to how to negotiate this terrain in an effective and respectful manner.

The conduct of brief intervention

The general practice studies cited above started with the important question: what can GPs do in the course of routine consultations to encourage heavy drinkers to reduce consumption? The amount of training they received was minimal, and they were simply encouraged to 'give advice' to the drinkers. That these studies emerged with positive results is most encouraging since more recent developments offer the possibility of improving effectiveness rates even further.

Once the doctor has satisfactorily raised the subject of drinking, the content of brief advice for encouraging moderate drinking is fairly straightforward, involving a discussion of safe and harmful levels of consumption and of different methods for reducing consumption (Anderson and Scott 1992). One of the obvious limitations of simple advice-giving, experienced by many who were involved in conducting outcome studies, is that some of the recipients are not ready to change. The resulting dialogue can sometimes descend into disagreement. Among the new developments in this field has been the realization that motivation is not an all-or-none phenomenon; neither is it static. It can and does change, and the doctor can enhance it. Working with the less ready patients could be worthwhile; with a 'motivational nudge' provided by the doctor, drinkers might be able to go ahead and reduce consumption with little or no further assistance. These observations have given rise to the use of the 'stages of change' model (Prochaska and DiClemente 1986). In general practice, the most well-developed example of such an approach is the 'DRAMS' scheme ('Drinking Reasonably and Moderately with Self-Control') in Scotland (Heather *et al.* 1987). For drinkers who are not ready to change (called 'precontemplation stage'), the doctor simply provides information. For those who are uncertain about change ('contemplation stage'), the doctor provides an additional input which helps the drinker examine the pros and cons of drinking. Those who are ready to change ('action stage') receive concrete information and guidance about cutting down.

This approach will clearly help doctors structure their approach to heavy drinking and other behaviour-change problems. Many drinkers will be at the stage of 'readiness to change', but the challenge is to find ways of dealing with those who are less ready to stop drinking in the context of a brief consultation. This involves understanding their perceptions of the pros and cons of their behaviour. To succeed with this will mean paying attention to the social context in which drinking occurs. Negotiation, it has been suggested, might be the best term to describe this kind of consultation (Rollnick *et al.* 1993).

Managing the problem drinker

The problem drinker is harder to manage because their problems (personal, social, and medical) are more severe. One of the key issues here is the role of referral for specialist help. However this is resolved, the importance of continuing care from the GP is crucial since the patient inevitably ends up back in consulting room. It is not possible to general-ize about how to resolve the referral issue because local specialist services will vary, as will the attitudes and practices of GPs. Nevertheless, it is true to say that the last 15–20 years has seen an increased realization that the GP can do a reasonable amount to help the more severely disabled drinker.

If continuing care is crucial, then rapport with the patient is the first priority. From the specialist field has come the realization that a confrontational approach to problem drinkers only enhances their resistance and denial of the problem (Rollnick and Morgan 1995). A general practitioner therefore has to find the right balance between being under-standing on the one hand, and being firm about the need to do something about the prob-lem. Most reports of successful work with these patients in general practice find that the GP has taken a long-term view of the outcome, built a good rapport with the patient, and steadily 'chipped away' at the problem over a period of time. The problem drinker, like their less troubled, heavy-drinking counterparts, are not always ready to change. Fluctu-ating motivation is part of the problem itself. It is better to raise the subject of drinking in a non-confrontational way ('How do you feel about your drinking at the moment?') than by asking threatening questions like 'Don't you think it's time you stopped drinking?' Again, an examination of the pros and cons of drinking can often enhance motivation and readiness to change.

For the drinker who is ready to do something about the problem, how to withdraw from alcohol is often a terrifying prospect, something that has been avoided by repeated drinking to relieve withdrawal symptoms. Detoxification is dealt with in different ways in different areas. The current trend is to avoid in-patient admission to a specialist setting, unless there is a history of withdrawal fits. Home detoxification programmes are being developed fairly widely, in which a specialist nurse visits the patient at home to supervise closely the administration of a decreasing dose of supportive medication, such as diazepam. A dose of 20 mg of diazepam four times a day may be required, reducing daily and ending after seven days. Often, lower doses may be sufficient. Continued support from the general practitioner is often crucial to the success of this approach.

The general practitioner must also help the patient to make a judgement about whether additional counselling is needed from a specialist centre. If so, counselling is usually avail-able from a local, community-based, alcohol advisory service or community alcohol team. Some metropolitan centres also have NHS-based in-patient units run under the supervision of consultant psychiatrists. For longer-term care, some centres have hostels which operate in the voluntary sector. Whatever decision the patient comes to about spe-cialist help, the importance of maintaining contact throughout this period cannot be overemphasized. Many a drinker has returned to destructive drinking during or after a period of specialist counselling. Brief but regular contact with the GP can do a lot to pre-vent this. It should be recalled that the small amount of research on specialist versus gen-eral practitioner care points strongly to the efficacy of support in the primary care setting.

Conclusion

The challenge provided by male problem drinking is not just a clinical one. Because drinking is so much part of the social fabric of our culture and subcultures, general practitioners cannot avoid the social context by simply treating the problem as a clinical one. Helping a problem drinker to consider change means engaging in a frank dialogue about a sometimes touchy subject. A non-confrontational approach, based on a good rapport and supported by a clear understanding of the effects of heavy drinking, will produce better results than simply telling the patients that they should do something about the problem.

References

Anderson, P. (1993). Effectiveness of general practice interventions for patients with harmful alcohol consumption. *British Journal of General Practice*, **43**, 374, 386–9.

Anderson, P. and Scott, E. (1992). The effect of general practitioners' advice to heavy-drinking men. *British Journal of Addiction*, **87**, 891–900.

Babor, T. and Grant, M. (1992). *Project on identification and management of alcohol-related problems. Report on Phase II. A randomized clinical trial of brief intervention in primary health care.* World Health Organization, Geneva, Switzerland.

Bien, T. and Miller, W. (1993). Brief interventions for alcohol problems: a review. *Addiction*, **88**(3), 315–36.

Borkenstein, R. F., Crowther, R. P., Shumate, W. B., *et al.* (1964). *The role of the drinking driver in traffic accidents.* Department of Police Administration, Indiana University, Bloomingham.

Department of Health Inter-Departmental Working Group (1995). *Sensible drinking.* DoH, London.

Dunbar, J., Ogston, S. A., and Ritchie, A. (1985). Are problem drinkers dangerous drivers? An investigation of arrest for drinking and driving, serum y-glutamyltranspeptidase activities, blood alcohol concentrations, and road traffic accidents: the Tayside safe driving project. *British Medical Journal*, **290**, 827–30.

Edwards, G. (1996). *Sensible drinking.* British Medical Journal, **312**, 1. (Editorial).

Edwards, G. and Gross, M. M. (1976). Alcohol dependence: provisional description of a clinical syndrome. *British Medical Journal*, **1**, 1058–61.

Ewing, J. A. (1984). Detecting alcoholism: the CAGE questionnaire. *Journal of the American Medical Association*, **252**, 1905–7.

Grant, M., Plant, M., and Williams, A. (1982). *Economics and alcohol.* Croom Helm, London.

Hays, J. T. and Spickard, W. A. (1987). Alcoholism: early diagnosis and intervention. *Journal of General and Internal Medicine*, **2**:420–7.

Health Education Council (1984). *That's the limit.* HEC, London.

Health Promotion Authority for Wales (1989). *Drinking in Wales, 1988. Briefing Report 1.* HPAW, Cardiff.

Health Promotion Authority for Wales (1990a). *Health in Wales, 1990.* HPAW, Cardiff.

Health Promotion Authority for Wales (1990b). *Binge drinking in Wales. Briefing Report 2.* HPAW, Cardiff.

Heather, N., Campion, P., Neville, R., and MacCabe, D. (1987). Evaluation of a controlled-drinking minimal intervention for problem drinkers in general practice (the DRAMS scheme). *Journal of the Royal College of General Practitioners*, **37**, 358–63.

Heather N. and Robertson, I. (1983). *Controlled drinking*. Methuen, London.

Kahan M., Wilson L., and Becker, L. (1995). Effectiveness of physician-based interventions with problem drinkers – a review. *Canadian Medical Association Journal*, **152**(6), 851–9.

Kannel W. B. and Ellison R. C. (1996). Alcohol and coronary heart disease – the evidence for a protective effect. *Clinica Chimica Acta*, **246**, 1–2, 59–76.

Kendall, R. E. (1987). Drinking sensibly. *British Journal of Addiction*, **82**, 1279–88.

Kristenson, H. and Hood, B. (1984). The impact of alcohol on health in the general population: a review with particular reference to experience in Malmo. *British Journal of Addiction*, **79**, 139–45.

Lancet (1990). Alcohol and violence. *Lancet*, **336**, 1223–4. (Editorial).

McMurran, M. and Baldwin, S. (1989). Services for prisoners with alcohol-related problems: a study of UK prisons. *British Journal of Addiction*, **84**, 1053–8.

Marmot, M. G. (1995). *Alcohol and the heart in perspective: sensible limits reaffirmed*. Royal Colleges of Physicians, Psychiatrists, and General Practitioners, London.

Marmot, M. G., Rose, G., Shirley, M. J., and Thomas, B. (1981). Alcohol and mortality: a J-shaped curve. *Lancet*, **1**, 580–2.

Muir, H. (1998). *Problem drinkers and their problems*. B.Sc. dissertation. University of Wales, Cardiff.

Murray, A. and Murray, R. M. (1991). The role of genetic predisposition in alcoholism. In *Addiction behaviour* (ed. I. B. Glass). Tavistock/Routledge, London.

Nuffield Institute for Health, University of Leeds (1993). *Brief interventions and alcohol use*. Effective Health Care Bulletin No. 7, University of Leeds.

Office of Population Censuses and Surveys (1992). *General Household Survey 1990*. HMSO, London.

Office of Population Censuses and Surveys (1995). *Living in Britain. Preliminary results from the 1994 General Household Survey*. HMSO, London.

Orford, J. (1985). *Excessive appetites: a psychological view of addiction*. John Wiley, Chichester.

Paton, A. (ed.) (1988). *ABC of alcohol* (2nd edn). BMJ Publications, London.

Pihl, R. O. (1983). Alcohol and aggression: a psychological perspective. In *Alcohol, drug abuse and aggression* (ed. E. Gottheil, K. A. Druley, T. E. Skolada, and H. M. Waxman). Charles Thomas, Springfield.

Plant, M. A. (1981). Risk factors in employment. In *Alcohol problems in employment* (ed. B. D. Hore and M. A. Plant). Croom Helm, London.

Pokorny, A. D., Miller B. A., and Kaplan, H. B. (1972). The brief MAST: a shortened version of the Michigan Alcohol Screening Test. *American Journal of Psychiatry*, **129**, 342–5.

Prochaska, J. and DiClemente, C. (1986). Towards a comprehensive model of change. In *Treating addictive behaviours: processes of change* (ed. W. R. Miller and N. Heather). Plenum, New York.

Rollnick, S., Davies, R. G. W., and Smail, S. A. (1988). Preliminary report of WHO alcohol early intervention data, Llanedeyrn Health Centre. Personal communication.

Rollnick, S., Heather, N., and Bell, A. (1992). Negotiating behaviour change in medical settings: the development of brief motivational interviewing. *Journal of Mental Health*, **1**, 25–39.

Rollnick, S., Kinnersley, P., and Stott, N. C. H. (1993). Methods of helping patients with behaviour change. *British Medical Journal*, **307**, 188–90.

Rollnick, S. and Morgan, M. (1995). Motivational interviewing: increasing readiness to change. In *Psychotherapy and substance abuse: a practitioner's handbook* (ed. A. Washton). Guildford, New York.

Royal College of General Practitioners (1986). *Alcohol – a balanced view*. RCGP, London.

Royal College of Physicians (1987). *A great and growing evil: the medical consequences of alcohol abuse*. Tavistock Publications, London.

Royal College of Psychiatrists (1986). *Alcohol, our favourite drug*. Tavistock Publications, London.

Rydelius, P. A. (1981). Children of alcoholic fathers. *Acta Paediatrica Scandinavica*, Suppl. 286.

Shepherd, J. P., Robinson, L., and Levers, B. G. H. (1990). The roots of urban violence. *Injury*, **21**, 139–41.

Social Trends, No. 25 (1995). HMSO, London.

Taylor, C., Brown, D., Duckitt, A., Edwards, G., Oppenheimer, E., and Sheehan, M. (1985). Patterns of outcome: drinking histories over 10 years among a group of alcoholics. *British Journal of Addiction*, **80**, 45–50.

Taylor, D. (1981). *Alcohol: reducing the harm*. Office of Health Economics, London.

Tofler, O. B. (1985). *The Heart of the social drinker*. Lloyd-Luke, London.

Vaillant, G. E. and Milofsky, E. S. (1982). The etiology of alcoholism: a prospective viewpoint. *American Psychologist*, **37**(5), 491–503.

Wallace, P., Cutler, S., and Haines, A. (1988). Randomised controlled trial of general practitioner intervention in patients with excessive alcohol consumption. *British Medical Journal*, **297**, 663–8.

Sources of advice about alcohol problems

Alcoholics Anonymous,
PO Box 1,
Stonebow House,
Stonebow,
York Y01 2NJ.

Tel: 01904 644026.
(London area helpline number: 0171 352 3001, from 10.00 a.m. to 10.00 p.m. See under 'Alcohol' in local phone book for nearest branch.)

Alcohol Concern,
Waterbridge House,

32–36 Loman Street,
London SE1 0EE.

Tel: 0171 928 7377; fax: 0171 928 4644.

Medical Council on Alcoholism,
3 St. Andrews Place,
London NW1 4LB.

Tel: 0171 487 4445; fax: 0171 935 4479.

PART III

Clinical problems

CHAPTER NINE

Reproductive health: family planning and infertility

Richard Anderson

For many years, problems of fertility and contraception have been the preserve of women, and vasectomy the only point at which men became involved. However, there has been a considerable change in the recent past. Condoms have become much more widely promoted, fuelled by messages about HIV infection, and research continues for a reversible form of male contraception. Efforts are similarly being made to deal with male subfertility which makes a contribution in up to 30% of subfertile couples, and there has been a flurry of interest in the recent reports of falling sperm counts. This chapter presents the current state of the art: often enough knowledge to understand what is going on without always being able to remedy it, and a clear understanding of spermatogenesis without, as yet, a usable form of reversible contraception. Nevertheless, there are still some yawning gaps: for example, what is the psychological effect of infertility among men and how do they cope?

Introduction

Men and women have always wanted control over their fertility. In nations in which the demographic transition has not been achieved, uncontrolled population growth threatens both economic development as well as individual health and prosperity. Europe and North America have passed through this to achieve population stability.

Modern family planning depends on the availability of contraceptive methods, but the methods currently available place the major burden on the female. Thus, combined and progestogen-only pills, intrauterine contraceptive devices, diaphragms, implants, injectables, and now the female condom contrast with withdrawal or condoms for men. As comparatively recently as the 1960s, male methods were the most widely used, only overtaken by female methods in the late 1970s with the rapid increase in availability of hormonal methods. Despite this, there is increasing demand that men share the responsibility of contraception, fuelled by health scares about the combined pill. Condoms and vasectomy currently provide contraception for approximately 35% of couples in England and Wales (Oddens *et al.* 1994), demonstrating the size of the potential market for male methods of contraception. The recent emergence of the human immunodeficiency virus (HIV) has given a great boost to condom use, and young women starting on the contraceptive pill are routinely advised by some family planning clinics to use condoms in addition. The readiness of men to use new methods is supported by opinion polls: in 1991, 56% of German men were willing to accept a hormonal male contraceptive compared to 14% in 1977 (Nieschlag *et al.* 1992). Our own experience has been that it has become progressively easier to recruit couples to trials of hormonal male contraception, and although problems with the oral contraceptive pill is given most commonly as the reason for involvement in a male contraceptive trial, 33% of couples cited interest in the development of a hormonal male method as their prime motivation. We have recently carried out a survey of the attitudes of 450 men to contraception in general and proposed hormonal male methods in particular. This demonstrated the high level of dissatisfaction with current methods, with, for example, 61% claiming that condoms reduced sexual satisfaction. 88% of the sample wanted a reversible male method, and 66% either 'definitely' or 'probably' would use a male pill. This contrasts with only 17% who might consider a vasectomy at some point in the future. While 32% would use an injectable male contraceptive, nearly half thought such a method should be developed and 77% thought a male pill should be developed.

Increased interest in male contraception is paralleled by increased awareness of male infertility, which affects approximately 5% of men of reproductive age and is as common a cause of failure of a couple to conceive as female infertility. Advances in our knowledge of the process of spermatogenesis have led to advances in our understanding of the causes of male infertility and, to a limited extent, treatment modalities, although the therapeutic options remain very limited.

This chapter aims to discuss recent developments and future prospects for male contraception, and to provide a rational framework for the investigation and diagnosis of male infertility. An outline of the process of spermatogenesis and its regulation is also given to provide a foundation for the subsequent discussion.

Spermatogenesis and its control

The process

Spermatogenesis takes place in the seminiferous tubules, tightly packed coiled tubules arranged in lobules which drain at both ends into the rete testis, which in turn drains via several efferent ducts into the head of the epididymis. This is again a highly coiled tube, passing from the superior aspect of the testis inferiorly along the posterolateral surface of the testis to the tail of the epididymis, where it joins the vas deferens.

The seminiferous tubules are lined with Sertoli cells and germ cells and surrounded by peritubular myoid cells (Fig. 9.1). Spermatogonia, adjacent to the basement membrane of the seminiferous tubule, divide constantly by mitosis, followed by the two meiotic reduction divisions to produce haploid spermatids. The spermatids subsequently mature, with development of the characteristics essential for transport through the female

Fig. 9.1 *Human testis, epididymis, and vas deferens, with progressive enlargements to show anatomical and functional relationships with Leydig cells, Sertoli cells, and germ cells. Tight junctional complexes serve to divide the seminiferous epithelium into adluminal and basement compartments, and bidirectional secretion of some Sertoli cell products. T, testosterone; LH, luteinizing hormone; FSH, follicle stimulating hormone.*

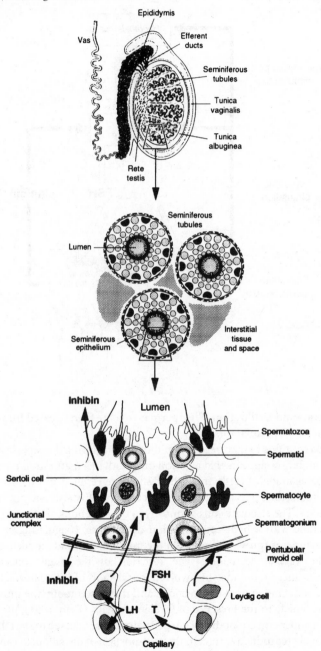

Fig. 9.2 *Representation of functional relationship in the hypothalamic–pituitary–testicular axis. Pulsatile secretion of gonadotrophin releasing hormone (GnRH) into hypophyseal portal blood stimulates pulsatile secretion of luteinizing hormone (LH) and follicle stimulating hormone (FSH). Secretion of testosterone (T) and inhibin by the testis results in negative feedback control at both the hypothalamus and pituitary, in addition to the effects of testosterone within the testis.*

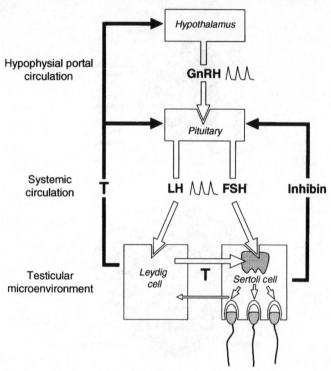

reproductive tract and fertilization. The spermatozoa are then released from the Sertoli cells in the process of spermiation.

Spermatozoa continue to mature in the epididymis, acquiring the capacity for motility and fertilization. It now appears that a period of epididymal maturation is not essential, as spermatozoa aspirated directly from the testis have resulted in pregnancies (Silber 1989). Spermatozoa then pass along the vas deferens by peristalsis and are stored in the ampulla of the vas. The ejaculate consists mostly of the secretions of the seminal vesicles, which are alkaline with a high concentration of fructose, coagulating enzymes, and prostaglandins. Fructose provides energy for the spermatozoa, and the alkalinity neutralizes the acidic vaginal secretions. The function of the huge concentration of prostaglandins is unclear, but may be involved in transport of spermatozoa through the female tract by inducing uterine contractions and may also modify the immunological response of the female to the presence of foreign antigens (Kelly 1991), preventing the development of antisperm antibodies. The spermatozoa are released to start their journey through the female reproductive tract to the mid-portion of the fallopian tube, the usual site of fertilization. By that stage, of the approximately 50 000 000 spermatozoa contained in the ejaculate, only 200 or so remain.

Control

The classical concept is that the pituitary glycoproteins luteinizing hormone (LH) and follicle stimulating hormone (FSH) stimulate Leydig cell steroidogenesis and Sertoli cell/seminiferous tubule function respectively. Despite the complexities of intratesticular control of spermatogenesis, LH and FSH are required for the initiation of spermatogenesis at puberty and its maintenance thereafter. The intratesticular concentration of testosterone is approximately 50 times that in peripheral blood, apparently far in excess of that required to saturate the androgen receptors present. It appears that this high concentration of testosterone, together with FSH, is required for the maintenance of quantitatively normal spermatogenesis. Testosterone diffuses into the bloodstream directly (into the testicular veins) and via testicular lymphatics, where it is mostly (60%) bound to sex hormone-binding globulin (SHBG) with high affinity, and to albumin (38%) with low affinity. Only approximately 2% is therefore free in solution, but that bound to albumin is freely available to the tissues and that bound to SHBG may also be specifically taken up in some organs.

The secretion of LH and FSH by the anterior pituitary is predominantly under the control of gonadotrophin-releasing hormone (GnRH), secreted into the hypothalamo-pituitary portal capillaries. Pulses of LH are secreted every 140 minutes and reflect pulses of GnRH secretion. Pulse frequency is reduced by testosterone in a classical negative feedback mechanism, and testosterone also acts on the pituitary to reduce the amount of LH secreted per pulse of GnRH. Testosterone also regulates FSH secretion in combination with the glycoprotein inhibin. Inhibin is a Sertoli cell product, and although its precise contribution to the control of FSH secretion is debated, it is now clear that the elevated FSH levels seen with seminiferous tubule damage are related to reduced inhibin secretion.

Male contraception

The condom

The use of condoms has come full circle since their description in the 16th century as protection against syphilis with the current promotion of use of a hormonal method in addition to a condom (Bromham and Cartmill 1993). This century has seen their development from linen and animal intestine via vulcanized rubber to latex, and to the multi-coloured, multi-flavoured varieties available today. Polyurethane condoms are also under development (Rosenberg et al. 1996). Condoms are currently used by 20% of couples as contraception in the UK and by approximately 40 million couples worldwide. They are particularly popular in Japan where they are used by 50% of couples.

Two of the major issues relating to condom use are their reliability and the degree of protection against infection. The efficacy of condoms as contraceptives varies greatly between populations, Pearl Indices (number of pregnancies if used by 100 women for one year) of between 2 and 12 being found (Vessey et al. 1988). Reasons for failure include inconsistent use and problems such as breakage and slippage. Barrier methods are especially unforgiving of inconsistent use, and user-related problems outweigh manufacturing defects. Breakage or slippage have been reported to occur in as many as 12% of acts of intercourse and are more common in the young and inexperienced (Sparrow and Lavill 1994). Others have found a wide range of breakage rates, between 0.6 and 2% and up to 12% (Cates and Stone 1992; Rinehart 1990), but these may be reduced by the use of additional, water-based lubrication (Gabbay and Gibbs 1996). Breakage rates also vary widely between countries, and while there is a good correlation between 'expected' breakage rates on the basis of laboratory testing and actual rates, in one study the best predictor of breakage rate was age of the condom (Steiner *et al.* 1992).

Other problems are caused by the expectations of the 'one size fits all' approach. While unrolled condoms can expand greatly, this is not possible when they are rolled up, as when being put on, and condom failure is significantly higher in the 19% of men who report that condoms are too tight (Tovey and Bonell 1993). The two major UK manufacturers also supply narrower condoms, 48 mm and 49 mm flat width. The EC has recently issued a new standard of condom manufacture, allowing condoms between 44 and 56 mm flat width, with harmonization of manufacturing and testing procedures across Europe (Carnall 1996).

Attitudes to condoms continue to be negative in a large proportion of the population, being regarded as messy and inconvenient, reducing sexual pleasure, and carrying connotations of infidelity (Choi *et al.* 1994; Oddens *et al.* 1994; Stewart *et al.* 1991).

The practice of condom usage as protection against infection combined with use of another method as primary contraception has been mentioned above, and is widely promoted. Individuals will differ with regard to their priorities, and these priorities will change over time, within and between relationships. Studies that have attempted to investigate dual usage have suggested that consistent use of condoms is lower the more effective a contraceptive the primary method is (Polaneczky *et al.* 1994): this may reflect the greater immediacy of the threat of pregnancy and the problems inherent with coitally-dependent methods. The hope that promotion of such double use is the answer to the problem of combining protection against both pregnancy and infection is thus naive. This also demonstrates on an individual level the importance of assessment of the needs and attitudes of the couple, and at a public health level the requirement for more acceptable and effective barrier methods.

Vasectomy

Vasectomy is increasingly popular as a method of contraception, and is now used by more couples in the UK than female sterilization (Oddens *et al.* 1994). The reasons for this include its ease, being performed as an out-patient under local anaesthesia, infrequency of complications, and low failure rate as well as reflecting a change in attitude in the population.

As with female sterilization, counselling of the couple is of the greatest importance in reducing the incidence of regret, which is estimated to be 3%. Women who have made a positive decision to have no children are less likely to regret sterilization than those who have had several by their mid-twenties (Leader *et al.* 1983), and the same is likely to be true of men. Points which may be covered during counselling include reasons for requesting the procedure, the ages of the couple and their children, past reproductive history, general health of the man, as well as a description of the procedure and postoperative course.

Particular attention should be paid to previous local anaesthesia, the presence of hernias, varicocele, and previous scrotal surgery which may necessitate more extensive surgery to allow confident identification of the vasa: such problems may indicate the need for general anaesthesia. A checklist is useful to ensure that all areas have been covered. The couple should be made aware of the possibility of failure of the method, estimated to be between 0 and 2.2% (Liskin *et al.* 1983), due to failure to await the confirmation of azoospermia and late recanalization. Azoospermia (the complete absence of spermatozoa from the ejaculate) is routinely confirmed by analysis of two ejaculates 12 and 16 weeks post-operatively, which will allow identification of those patients in whom the surgical technique was incorrect. Motile sperm are absent from the semen after 10 ejaculates in 35% of men, but this can take up to 50 ejaculations to occur in others (Sivanesarantham 1990). It is thus essential that sexual activity is resumed after only a brief period of abstinence of approximately one week. This is to allow sufficient healing of the cut ends of the vas deferens, to prevent 'blow out' by the forceful peristalsis which occurs during ejaculation. Earlier testing has been recommended recently, with the absence of motile spermatozoa in the ejaculate after four weeks being found to be as reliable as complete azoospermia (Edwards 1993). Further testing was required only if there were motile spermatozoa present, and this regime was found to be independent of the number of postvasectomy ejaculations. This testing regime has, however, yet to gain widespread acceptance, despite the inconvenience to the couple of waiting longer than necessary and the expense of additional semen analyses.

Late recanalization probably occurs more frequently than has been recognised. Cases of proven paternity (by DNA analysis) in the presence of azoospermia have been reported (O'Brien *et al.* 1995), and a survey of 1000 men one year after successful vasectomy demonstrated the presence of spermatozoa in six, although only intermittently and at very low density (Smith *et al.* 1994).

Complications include haematoma formation, granulomas (either from suture material or spermatozoa), infection, and the development of antisperm antibodies. In a recent retrospective study of men four years after vasectomy, significant early complications were reported by only 3.5% of patients, but as many as 33% complained of chronic pain, although only three of these 56 men regretted the operation as a result (McMahon *et al.* 1992). This may be sufficient to require further surgery, for example epididymectomy, which has been reported to give good results in only 50% of cases (Chen and Ball 1991). Other surveys have found less worrying results, finding chronic pain in only one in 200 men (Denniston and Kuehl 1995).

The possibility that vasectomy may cause an increase in the incidence of prostatic and testicular carcinoma has attracted considerable attention both scientifically and in the media. Large studies in the UK and US (involving over 600 men with testicular carcinoma) found no increase in cancer risk if the vasectomy had been carried out over 20 years before (Giovannucci *et al.* 1992), and the Oxford linkage project study, comparing 13 246 men after vasectomy with 22 196 controls, suggested a reduced risk of testicular carcinoma (Nienhuis *et al.* 1992). With regard to prostatic carcinoma, two large US studies have suggested an association between vasectomy and prostatic carcinoma, particularly after a delay of 20 years or more, with a relative risk of 1.6 (Giovannucci *et al.* 1993*a*; Giovannucci *et al.* 1993*b*). Some doubt about the validity of these studies arises from the selection of subjects from a population with a high and rising incidence of prostatic cancer. Both the World Health Organization and the US National Institute of Health have issued statements discussing these points (Farley *et al.* 1993; Healy 1993), and concluded that there is no reason to change current practice. The increase in atherosclerosis seen in monkeys after vasectomy appears not to be of relevance in man.

Reversal

The use of microsurgical techniques for reversal of vasectomy has led to a considerable increase in the success rate. After vasovasostomy, up to 90% of men show sperm in the ejaculate and pregnancy rates of up to 80% have been reported (Silber 1989). However, this appears to depend on the time interval between vasectomy and reversal as well as operation technique. Sophisticated techniques have been developed to deal with the processes believed to impede successful reversal operations, and good pregnancy rates have been reported (Silber 1989). The appropriateness of diverting scarce NHS funds to such procedures may be questioned, but the development of such microsurgical techniques are also of relevance to the treatment of obstructive causes of azoospermia in the context of infertility.

An alternate approach is the development of a vasectomy technique which is designed to be reversible, and several techniques have been introduced (Hargreave 1992). The 'no scalpel' technique, popular in Thailand, Indonesia, and parts of China, is quicker and associated with fewer complications, but is not easier to reverse. The World Health Organization has been sponsoring clinical trials of chemical occlusion of the vas, and in China more than 300 000 occlusions have been performed using a carboxylic acid-cyanoacrylate glue. An inert polyurethane elastomer plug can also be injected into the vas, and a recent report has suggested that fertility was restored in all 130 subjects who had the plug removed after 3–5 years (Zhao *et al.* 1992). Questions remain, however, as to the completeness of azoospermia in all men, whether azoospermia is the result of simple blockage or whether fibrosis is important, and the development of long-term secondary effects on the testis and epididymis. As most requests for reversal are within 5–10 years of vasectomy, such effects may be of little practical relevance from that perspective, although the concerns regarding prostatic and testicular cancer discussed above remain valid.

Withdrawal

In the National Survey of Sexual Attitudes and Lifestyles (Wellings *et al.* 1994), 6.8% of men reported having relied on withdrawal as a method of contraception in the past year compared with 12.8% relying on vasectomy and 4.9% on an intrauterine contraceptive device. The use of this method was evenly spread over all socio-economic classes, but was more frequently used in the younger age groups.

Future prospects

The clearest gap in male methods of contraception is the lack of availability of a hormonal method: this is reflected by the use of the phrase 'the male pill' whenever the subject is mentioned in the media. This area of research has a clear physiological basis in our understanding of the gonadotrophin-dependent nature of spermatogenesis, and is the area closest to becoming a reality. Other areas of research include chemical and thermal interference with testicular and epididymal function, but many avenues thus far explored have been hampered by problems of toxicity.

Hormonal methods

Hormonal methods of contraception in the male have been investigated for over 50 years, following the demonstration that administration of testosterone (as the propionate ester) to normal men caused a reversible reduction in spermatogenesis without affecting libido or potency (McCullagh and McGurl 1939). This has subsequently been confirmed and enlarged upon in many other studies using a variety of testosterone derivatives, alone or in combination with progestogens; but the goal of complete suppression of spermatogenesis to provide the required degree of contraceptive efficacy with the maintenance of libido, without side effects, and in an acceptable method of delivery, remains elusive.

In one study where testosterone was used alone, plasma levels of gonadotrophins became undetectable in all men, but only 65% became azoospermic within six months of testosterone treatment. Only one pregnancy was reported in a total of 1486 months of contraceptive exposure, giving a Pearl Index of 0.8. Side-effects largely reflected the supra-physiological dose of testosterone, and included acne, hypertension, and polycythaemia (World Health Organization Task Force for the Regulation of Male Fertility 1990). Incomplete suppression of spermatogenesis has been a consistent finding in all studies of hormonal male contraception, whether using androgens alone or in combination with progestogens or GnRH analogues, with azoospermia being achieved in 50–70% of men in most studies.

The degree of contraceptive protection resulting from incomplete suppression of spermatogenesis has been the object of a second WHO study (World Health Organization Task Force on Methods for the Regulation of Male Fertility 1996). In this study, all men whose sperm count fell below 3×10^6/ml were then required to use the testosterone injections as their only form of contraception for one year. Ninety-eight per cent of 357 men who entered the trial were successfully suppressed to below this level, and the overall pregnancy rate was only 1.4 per 100 woman years, comparable to the combined contraceptive pill. Following discontinuation of the testosterone injections, sperm density recovered to normal in all men.

Progestogens also inhibit gonadotrophin secretion in men, with subsequent suppression of spermatogenesis. There is also suppression of testicular testosterone synthesis and secretion, and replacement androgen therapy is therefore required for the maintenance of libido and potency in particular. Levonorgestrel with testosterone replacement caused profound suppression of spermatogenesis in a recent study (Bebb *et al.* 1996), with azoospermia achieved in 12 out of 18 men and sperm density of less than 3 million/ml in the remaining men. The recent advances in progestogen preparations, such as the Nor-plant device (Roussell) which slowly releases progestogen from a subcutaneous implant over several years and which is easily removable, provide a new impetus for an androgen–progestogen preparation in men. Such a device potentially avoids the high plasma concentrations of testosterone caused by conventional administration methods, while producing long-lasting effects.

It therefore appears that inhibition of gonadotrophin secretion by progestogen or GnRH analogue with replacement testosterone administration results in azoospermia in the majority of men, and the use of these agents rather than androgen alone avoids or reduces the incidence of side-effects related to the supraphysiological doses of androgen required when used alone (Pavlou *et al.* 1991). This will also have the advantage of reducing the risks associated with high doses of testosterone, which include adverse changes in lipid profile and possible stimulation of prostatic growth. The use of GnRH antagonists may result in a greater rate of azoospermia with presumably increased contraceptive efficacy, but this has yet to be established in a large trial. A hormonal method of male contraception for widespread use therefore remains elusive for the present, although the most recent results outlined above provide some grounds for continuing optimism that such a method is a realistic possibility.

Non-hormonal methods

A logical approach to the development of non-hormonal methods of male contraception requires an adequate understanding of the relevant physiology and biochemistry of specific processes in sperm maturation in the testis or epididymis. This is not the case at present, and a serendipitous approach has generally been used in the past. The best known non-hormonal agent is gossypol, an extract of cotton-seed oil. The recognition that gossypol resulted in severe suppression of spermatogenesis led to large-scale clinical studies in China, in which it was 99% effective in producing azoospermia or severe oligozoospermia (Qian and Wang 1984). Unfortunately, recovery is slow, in 10% the effect is irreversible, and there were other serious side-effects.

Extracts of *Tripterygium wilfordii* Hook.f., a vine used in Chinese herbal medicine for a wide variety of complaints, may have more promise. Systematic experiment in rats revealed a marked effect on sperm motility, with less of an effect on density, which was reversible without apparent toxicity (Qian *et al.* 1986*b*). Similar effects were noted in a small group of men (Qian *et al.* 1986*a*), and subsequently a systematic approach to fractionated extracts has been undertaken, identifying six compounds with antifertility action. Much needs to be done to investigate the toxicity of these compounds, but this work demonstrates the potential value of a systematic approach.

While a specific epididymal action is very attractive as it avoids interference with the endocrine function of the testis, lack of understanding of epididymal function has limited this approach. Several compounds with epididymal effects have been investigated, including α-chlorohydrin and the 6-chloro-6-deoxysugars. Both groups of compounds act by inhibition of spermatozoal glucose metabolism, but their clinical use is again limited by toxicity.

Scrotal warming reduces spermatogenesis in experimental animals, and this approach has also been used in humans using a modified athletic support worn either continuously or only during the day (Mieusset and Bujan 1994; Shafik 1992). In these studies, 37 couples used this as a contraceptive for a total of 311 months, with only one pregnancy to a man who did not use the support consistently.

Conclusion

Male methods make a substantial contribution to overall contraceptive use, despite the major deficiencies of existing methods. Two-thirds of couples who took part in a recent

WHO contraceptive efficacy trial in Edinburgh gave 'inability to find a contraceptive method with which they were happy' as the main reason for taking part, despite the experimental and uncertain contraception offered. The remaining third gave 'the desire to see new male methods becoming available' as their main reason for participating. It is clear that there is considerable hidden demand for safe and effective male methods, hormonal or chemical, but the current involvement of the pharmaceutical industry is minimal. Nevertheless, the developments discussed above show the range of approaches being investigated, and, particularly with epididymal methods, illustrate the importance of increasing our basic knowledge of male reproductive function.

Male infertility

Infertility affects approximately one in seven couples in the UK, and a male factor can be identified in at least 30% of these, often in combination with a female factor (Hull *et al.* 1985). The science of andrology lags far behind our understanding of the female reproductive processes, and the therapeutic options are correspondingly limited. The conception rate without assisted reproductive techniques remains poor. Much, however, can be done to help the infertile, or, more usually, subfertile male, both in terms of information about the diagnosis and reassurance about implications for the general health of the patient, as male fertility is not clearly distinguished from 'virility' in the minds of many. Thus an accurate diagnosis allows directed counselling based upon a realistic estimate of the couple's likelihood of spontaneous conception, with consideration given as to when assisted conception would, and would not, be appropriate.

There is now good evidence that there has been a dramatic decline in sperm density over the last 50 years (Carlson *et al.* 1992). There has also been a twofold increase in the incidence of testicular maldescent and a threefold increase in the incidence of testicular carcinoma over the same time period. Antenatal exposure of male fetuses to oestrogens has been proposed to be a possible link between these observations (Sharpe and Skakkebaek 1993).

The basic investigation of male fertility is the semen analysis, and many clinicians involved in infertility work, both as GPs and in hospital clinics, will request a semen analysis without seeing the patient himself, and indeed may never do so if the semen analysis is reported as normal. This approach is not without pragmatic value, but it perpetuates the inequality of the burden of childlessness between men and women both socially and clinically. In our practice, both partners are routinely seen together, which as well as reinforcing the idea that infertility is a problem for the two partners as a couple, greatly increases communication and the potential for effective counselling.

Investigation

Semen analysis has been the benchmark investigation for over 60 years, but cut-off values between normal and abnormal remain controversial. In view of the substantial variation in semen quality, at least two or three analyses should be performed. The World Health Organization has published guidelines (World Health Organization 1992) which include the following standards:

volume > 2 ml
sperm density $> 20 \times 10^6$/ml

motility	$> 50\%$ with forward progression or $> 25\%$ with rapid linear progression
morphology	$> 30\%$ normal
viability	$> 75\%$ live
white blood cells	$< 1 \times 10^6$/ml.

None of these parameters individually gives good discrimination in terms of likelihood of pregnancy, but the 20×10^6/ml density has been in clinical use for many years and serves the purpose of highlighting those men requiring further study: thus in those men with a sperm density of $< 20 \times 10^6$/ml, sperm morphology and motility should be critically evaluated. A density of 5×10^6/ml is also a useful clinical guide, as below this density fertilization *in vitro* is unlikely, and donor insemination or more advanced assisted reproductive technology may be appropriate.

Antisperm antibodies can be detected by the immunobead or mixed agglutination reaction, and sperm–cervical mucus interaction can be investigated using the postcoital or *in vitro* penetration tests. These tests are very poorly standardized, and their diagnostic and therapeutic relevance are questioned. Newer tests include assessment of acrosome function, sperm-zona binding, and the production of reactive oxygen radicals, but these tests are very labour-intensive and remain largely of research importance at present (Aitken 1995). A simple test with good correlation with fertilizing ability is greatly needed.

Endocrine evaluation is used to identify the uncommon but treatable case of hypogonadotrophic hypogonadism. The FSH level is also used to distinguish obstructive azoospermia, with normal FSH, from azoospermia resulting from testicular damage, with high FSH. Chromosomal studies are of value in patients with azoospermia, particularly if the testicular volumes are low and the FSH high. Testicular biopsy can be used to assess the degree of spermatogenesis in the presence of obstruction, but is rarely required.

The causes of male infertility can be divided into pre-testicular, testicular, and post-testicular, resulting in disorders of spermatogenesis, sperm autoimmunity, genital tract obstruction, and coital disorders (Table 9.1).

Idiopathic infertility

In approximately 50% of men the aetiology of spermatogenic dysfunction is unknown, and descriptive terms are used for classification. Terms include azoo- and oligozoospermia (zero or low sperm density), asthenozoospermia (reduced motility of spermatozoa), and teratozoospermia (high proportion of morphologically abnormal spermatozoa). These terms may be combined, e.g. asthenoteratozoospermia. There is electron microscopy evidence of defects in the microtubules of the sperm tail in some cases of asthenozoospermia, and such structural abnormalities arising during spermatogenesis are unlikely to be correctable. Similar defects may be present in cilia in other body systems, particularly the respiratory system, and there may be a history of chronic respiratory infections. This is most evident in the immotile cilia syndrome, and more minor defects may not have clinical effects elsewhere in the body.

The degree of maturational development of spermatozoa is thought to be reflected in

Table 9.1 *Causes of male infertility. This table is not intended to be exhaustive, but to illustrate the possible aetiological categories. Idiopathic oligozoospermia/asthenoteratozoospermia accounts for approximately 60% of male infertility.*

Pre-testicular (with underandrogenization)	General pituitary (Panhypopituitarism) Specific hypothalamo-pituitary (Kallmann's syndrome) General endocrine (haemochromatosis, Cushing's syndrome)
Testicular (some with underandrogenization)	Idiopathic hypospermatogenesis Varicocele Maldescent Chromosomal (Kleinfelter's syndrome) Viral orchitis
	Drugs (sulphasalazine, alcohol, alkylating agents) Toxins Autoimmunity Androgen resistance (androgen receptor defects) Systemic disease (including febrile illnesses) Radiation
Post-testicular (no underandrogenisation)	Obstruction (post-infective) Malformation (cystic fibrosis) Coital (impotence, retrograde ejaculation)

the morphological appearance, with abnormal spermatozoa showing lower fertilizing potential. The morphological characteristics of an individual spermatozoon may be the best indicator of function, and correlate with movement characteristics associated with the ability to undergo the acrosome reaction, essential for egg penetration. The isolation of a population of spermatozoa with good motility and morphology is an important part of sperm preparation for assisted conception programmes.

Specific causes

Varicocele

The role of varicocele in the aetiology of male infertility remains controversial, as does the benefit of treatment. Venous blood from the testis drains into the pampiniform plexus, which is closely applied to the testicular artery, and forms the spermatic vein. This drains into the left renal vein, and into the inferior vena cava on the right. Reflux increases scrotal temperatures, and increased concentrations of adrenal metabolites or reduced removal of toxic substances may also contribute to the testicular damage. Varicoceles are more common on the left, and a varicocele is present in approximately 15% of young men. The presence of a varicocele therefore does not imply subfertility, and before recommending treatment other causes of infertility in both partners should be excluded. The current treatment of choice, where available, is transfemoral embolization under X-ray screening control, which has a lower risk of complications and recurrence. The results of trials carried out so far are inconsistent, with some suggesting an improvement in semen parameters and conception rates, and others showing none (Nilsson *et al.* 1979; Okuyama *et al.* 1988). A large, prospective, randomized trial has recently been performed by WHO (as yet unpublished), and demonstrated a benefit of treatment.

The issue of screening and treatment of adolescents for varicocele is currently attracting considerable debate. It is estimated that the risk of varicocele to cause subfertility is around 12–15%, i.e. threefold higher than in the general male population (Comhaire 1989). Surgical treatment results in hydrocele in approximately 5% of cases, and persistence of the varicocele in 10–20%. Thus the risk of surgical treatment is greater than the potential benefit. However, transfemoral embolization has a much lower complication rate (under 1%), with a risk of recurrence of 2%, and may therefore offer a favourable risk–benefit ratio. This has been recently investigated in a study of 88 adolescents (Laven *et al.* 1992). Embolization of the left testicular vein resulted in an increase in size of both left and right testes in the treatment group after one year of follow-up (to the same size as a control group without varicocele) compared to no change in the non-treated group. Sperm concentration also increased in the treated group while there was no change in the untreated group. While this study suggests that early treatment may be of benefit, it is too early to say whether later testicular function and fertility will be improved, and, on the available evidence, treatment of adolescents cannot yet be recommended.

Genital infection

Infection may account for approximately 8% of male infertility. Orchitis is most commonly the result of mumps infection, and may be bilateral in 17%. If so, spermatogenesis may be impaired, temporarily or permanently, with testicular atrophy. Recovery may take many months. Unilateral orchitis does not appear to affect spermatogenesis significantly, but the incidence of infertility after mumps orchitis is unknown.

Other pathogenic organisms include the gonococcus, *Chlamydia trachomatis* and gram-negative enterococci, which cause acute infections with dysuria, epididymitis, pelvic pain, or pain on ejaculation, and large numbers of polymorphonuclear leucocytes in the ejaculate. These acute infections may cause structural damage with obstruction to the passage of spermatozoa and formation of antisperm antibodies, and may also involve the accessory glands (prostate and seminal vesicles) which may result in defective function. Tuberculosis and syphilis may also cause orchitis, but the significance of other organisms such as *Mycoplasma hominis* and *Ureaplasma urealyticum* is uncertain, as they may be commensals. Febrile illness may depress spermatogenesis for several weeks, but recovery is complete.

Maldescent

Cryptorchidism continues to be a common paediatric problem, with an incidence of up to 2% at one year of age. The pathophysiology of failure of descent of the testis is poorly understood, and indeed there are differing theories of normal descent, with both mechanical and endocrine factors contributing. Current hypotheses stress the importance of a functional hypothalamic–pituitary–testicular axis, and both androgen-dependent and independent developmental changes in the gubernaculum. There may be abnormalities of the testis or epididymis present, and there is a high incidence of inguinal hernia, but while there is a high incidence of histological abnormalities of structure in undescended testes, it is not clear whether it is the abnormality that causes the maldescent or vice versa. It is generally accepted that the lower temperature in the scrotum is required for spermatogenesis. Treatment is with either human chorionic gonadotrophin (particularly if the testis is prescrotal), or by orchidopexy. Orchidopexy should be performed as early as the diagnosis is made, and ideally, from the point of view of future fertility, by the age of two years (Hadziselimovic and Herzog, 1987). Even so, fertility may be preserved in only 50%. There is no evidence that operation after this age is of benefit in terms of fertility, although at younger ages surgery is associated with increased risk of complications, including secondary hypoplasia and obstruction of the vas deferens. Currently, in Britain, despite screening programmes only 39% of those undergoing orchidopexy are aged under six years (Kaul and Roberts 1992). Apart from the psychological benefit, the major purpose of orchidopexy at older ages is to enable clinical detection of testicular malignancies, of which 10% occur in men with a history of cryptorchidism (Mead 1992).

Chromosomal abnormalities

Chromosomal abnormalities are found in 2% of infertile men (Chandley 1979), the most common abnormality being Kleinfelter's syndrome (47, XXY). This affects one in 500 men, and results from the fusion of a XX ovum or XY sperm with a normal gamete. Clinically, they are usually tall and thin, with gynaecomastia and small but firm testes, and hormonal estimation may show plasma testosterone levels at or a little below the lower end of the normal range, with elevated plasma LH and FSH levels. Many cases remain undiagnosed even in adult life, as the only phenotypic abnormality may be the presence of small testes. The frequency of chromosome abnormality increases as the sperm density falls, being found in 15% of azoospermic men, of whom most have Kleinfelter's syndrome. A specific Y chromosome deletion has been characterized in some men with azoospermia (Chandley 1995), providing important information about the control of spermatogenesis. Other chromosome defects include reciprocal sex chromosome-autosomal translocations, other reciprocal or robertsonian autosomal translocations, or may rarely affect only the germ cell population. This is only detectable by testicular biopsy and is therefore largely of research interest.

Bilateral congenital absence of the vas deferens (CAVD) is found in approximately 25% of cases of obstructive azoospermia, and is found in almost all men with cystic fibrosis. It is now recognized that approximately 60% of otherwise healthy men with CAVD carry one of the several identified genetic mutations associated with cystic fibrosis (Patrizio *et al.* 1993), and screening for these mutations should be performed in such men.

Drugs and toxins

The rapidly dividing nature of the seminiferous epithelium makes it very sensitive to toxins, both environmental and iatrogenic. A huge range of chemicals to which we are exposed in normal life are testicular toxins, including chemicals in paints, plastics, and foods (Lucier *et al.* 1977). Such considerations are occasionally of value in the individual patient, and may become apparent on taking an occupational history. The commonest iatrogenic causes are chemotherapy or radiotherapy for Hodgkin's disease and other malignancies both before and after puberty, and the prescription of sulphasalazine for inflammatory bowel disease. Chemotherapy usually causes azoospermia within eight weeks, and the subsequent degree of restoration of fertility is dependent on the degree of destruction of germ cells. Improvement in germ-cell function can continue over many years. Various strategies have been tried to protect the seminiferous epithelium from cytotoxic drug damage, including down-regulation with LHRH analogues, but without consistent success (Morris and Shalet 1989). Furthermore, the urgency in starting chemotherapy in these conditions often allows for little more than cryopreservation of two or three ejaculates. The issue of future fertility is often a low priority at such a stressful time as diagnosis of these conditions, particularly when the patient is adolescent and has yet to consider starting a family, but close communication between family doctor, haematologist, and donor insemination clinic may allow the subject to be broached and semen storage organized. Young men considering starting a family who have been previously treated with chemotherapy may also request semen analysis to assess whether their fertility has been impaired. An abnormal semen analysis at that stage may warrant specialist referral for counselling, and reassurance as to the availability of donor insemination if appropriate. Sulphasalazine is the most common example of a drug which reversibly impairs spermatogenesis, and 70% of men may be affected (Giwercman and Skakkebaek 1986). If it is possible to convert the patient to maintenance on an alternative medication then fertility is often restored. Other drugs occasionally associated with impaired spermatogenesis include anticonvulsants, nitrofurantoin, steroids, and alcohol, tobacco, and cannabis.

Endocrine causes

While a variety of endocrine disorders may cause infertility as a secondary effect, for example Cushing's syndrome, one endocrine disorder that primarily affects spermatogenesis and is amenable to treatment is hypogonadotrophic hypogonadism. This condition has a wide clinical spectrum, varying from complete absence of gonadotrophins (Kallmann's syndrome when associated with anosmia) to states of partial deficiency, and there is therefore evidence of hypoandrogenism with low or absent gonadotrophins. Treatment consists of administration of gonadotrophins or of subcutaneous pulsatile administration of GnRH at 90-minute intervals and will induce the secondary male sexual characteristics if not already present. Such therapies may need to be continued for over a year to induce fertility and therefore require considerable patient dedication as well as staff backup and resources. Secondary hypogonadotrophism may result from pituitary damage from haemochromatosis, tumours, trauma, and irradiation, and may therefore coexist with other endocrine abnormalities. In these conditions, the seminiferous tubules are regressed, but will often have developed normally originally (if the patient was postpubertal at the time of damage) and will respond to gonadotrophin replacement.

Autoimmunity

Autoimmune infertility may result from the breaching of the blood-testis barrier with subsequent generation of antisperm antibodies, and such antibodies are found in 5–10% of infertile men. This may result from testicular infection, trauma, surgery (including vasectomy), or may be associated with a family history of autoimmune disease. The anti-sperm antibodies may be directed at a variety of sites on the spermatozoa, including the tail piece resulting in impaired motility, or the head interfering with fertilization. A major problem has been the development of laboratory tests which distinguish between specific antibodies which impair function (which are those of the IgA class) and those with no clinical relevance. Antisperm antibodies may also be found in the female partner, and may interfere with transit through the cervical mucus. Treatment with high dose corti-costeroids is controversial, as although such treatment may improve pregnancy rates (Hendry *et al.* 1990), the price in terms of the risk of significant side-effects, including peptic perforation and avascular necrosis of the femoral head, is high. *In vitro* fertilization offers a higher pregnancy rate without these risks.

Androgen receptor defects

Androgen receptor defects may be associated with oligozoospermia in an unknown pro-portion of men. This effect is at the least severe end of the spectrum of defects associated with androgen insensitivity, which varies from the complete form, testicular feminiza-tion, to mild undervirilization (Griffin 1992). This is a rapidly expanding area of research as the androgen receptor DNA has now been cloned.

Sperm transport defects

Genital tract obstruction secondary to infection has been discussed above. Other specific causes include congenital absence of the vas deferens or associated structures. This is almost always found in patients with cystic fibrosis as discussed above, or may be a result of *in utero* exposure to stilboestrol which causes a variety of other urogenital abnormal-ities in males as in females. Young's syndrome may cause obstruction as a result of the inspissation of secretions within the lumen, and be the result of similar pathology to that which causes the chronic pulmonary infections and bronchiectasis in these patients. A history of chronic respiratory disease may therefore be the clue to two different causes of genital tract obstruction. Diagnosis may be suggested clinically by the inability to feel a vas within the scrotum and supported by a semen volume of < 1 ml, which is acidic and non-coagulating being composed largely of prostatic fluid, with low levels of fructose from the seminal vesicles. The combination of azoospermia, normal testicular volumes, and a nor-mal plasma FSH level suggest the presence of obstruction. This may be surgically remedi-able, e.g. by epididymovasostomy to bypass a localized blockage. An alternate therapeutic manoeuvre is the aspiration of spermatozoa from the epididymis followed by *in vitro* fertilization.

Coital disorders

Infrequent sexual intercourse is an under-recognized cause of failure to conceive, and may be a result of one or other partner's job, e.g. travelling or shift-working. Sexual prob-lems may present in three ways: infertility causing psychosexual problems, psychosexual problems masquerading as infertility, or incidental findings of psychosexual problems in cases of infertility (Elstein 1975). The emotional stresses of infertility may be sufficient to cause frank impotence, or more often reduce desire as a reaction to the need for timed intercourse and the repeated failure to conceive (Berg and Wilson 1991). 'It's all too clinical' is a common complaint. Less frequently, there may be an organic cause, such as depression, alcohol abuse, spinal cord injury, diabetes mellitus, or the result of drug administration (β-blockers, psychotropic drugs). Endocrine causes will often also cause reduced libido, which may be the presenting complaint, and prolactin and testosterone levels should be checked. Bladder neck surgery may cause retrograde ejaculation, diagnosed by examination of post-ejaculatory urine sample. Viable spermatozoa may be recovered from the urine and used for intrauterine insemination or *in vitro* fertilization.

Treatment

As 50% of men have no identifiable aetiological factors associated with their infertility, a precise pathophysiological diagnosis cannot be made. This is frustrating for both patient and doctor, but a clear understanding of the principles discussed above will allow identification of those men where there is a specific diagnosis to be made. For all, the most important factor is an accurate assessment of the degree of subfertility, on which a discussion of the treatment possibilities can be based. A convenient framework involves division into three groups: untreatable sterility, potentially treatable subfertility, and untreatable subfertility or idiopathic hypospermatogenesis (Baker 1987). The group of untreatable sterility includes primary gonadal failure, with small testes, high plasma FSH levels, and azoospermia or extreme oligozoospermia, e.g. Kleinfelter's syndrome, the results of mumps orchitis, or post radiotherapy/chemotherapy. There is no prospect of any treatment to restore fertility and patients should be counselled regarding therapeutic donor insemination or adoption. The group of potentially treatable subfertility includes excessive smoking and alcohol consumption, drugs and other toxins, genital tract obstruction, varicocele, sperm autoantibody, gonadotrophin deficiency or other systemic endocrine disease, and coital disorders. Those with untreatable subfertility are the majority, with reduced sperm counts of defective spermatozoa from no identified aetiology. It is also important to remember that a normal semen analysis is no guarantee of the ability of the spermatozoa to fertilize oocytes.

Currently, the only proven method of increasing the chance of conception is *in vitro* fertilization (IVF), and there is variable availability of this in the NHS. The application of IVF to male infertility is based on the realization that relatively few spermatozoa (approximately 100 000) are sufficient for fertilization, and this number of active spermatozoa can be prepared from the ejaculate of most men with oligozoospermia. Fertilization and pregnancy rates in IVF for male factor infertility are lower than for other indications, with pregnancy rates of under 5%, compared to approximately 25% overall. This figure will, however, depend on the stringency of the local criteria for acceptance for IVF as well as the unit's expertise, and a high success rate may largely indicate that men with only mildly abnormal semen analyses are included. This is a rapidly expanding area, with improvements in sperm handing and preparation as well as micromanipulation techniques. Most centres are currently using intracytoplasmic sperm injection (ICSI), which involves injection of individual spermatozoa into an oocycte. This technique is rapidly replacing other methods of microassisted IVF for the treatment of severe oligospermia, and excellent pregnancy rates, often exceeding those of IVF with apparently normal gametes, have been reported (Palermo *et al.* 1993). Spermatozoa can be aspirated from the epididymis in obstructive azoospermia for use in ICSI, and pregnancies have also been reported following extraction of sperm cells from testicular biopsies. Such techniques, while providing the opportunity for successful treatment for almost all men, are rapidly pushing back the limits of technology, and concerns remain about the possibility of unexpected abnormalities. An excess of sex chromosome abnormalities has now been recognised. All children born as a result of such advanced technologies are at present being registered and followed up, and it is essential that couples are adequately informed about the still experimental nature of this treatment. A second hazard is that because the natural barriers of fertilisation have been bypassed, genetic causes of male infertility may be transmitted to male offspring. The success rates for IVF and its more advanced forms emphasize the fact that most couples with male factor infertility will not conceive as a result of this type of treatment, and this may not be in line with the couple's own perception of the likelihood of pregnancy. Other than in severe cases, frank discussion with the couple as to a best estimate of their spontaneous pregnancy rate is therefore of major importance in their management, together with maximizing this with general advice such as reduction in alcohol and tobacco consumption and the timing of intercourse. Referral for IVF is as a procedure of last resort when a suitable time period has elapsed. Much depends on the individual circumstances of the couple, and to make more definite recommendations may be at best misguided and at worse detrimental to the best interests of the couple. The role of the physician, after as accurate a diagnosis as possible has been made, will remain in counselling rather than treatment until much more is known about the basic pathophysiology of human spermatogenesis and its control.

References

Aitken, R. J. (1995). Male infertility: prognostic value of old and new tests. *Assisted Reproduction Reviews*, 5, 26–31.

Baker, H. W. G. (1987). Clinical evaluation and management of testicular disorders in the adult. In *The testis* (ed. H. Burger and D. de Kretser), p. 149. Raven Press, New York.

Bebb, R. A., Anawalt, B. D., Christensen, R. B., Paulsen, C. A., Bremner, W. J. and Matsumoto, A. M. (1996). Combined administration of levonorgestrel and testosterone induces more rapid and effective suppression of spermatogenesis than testosterone alone: a promising male contraceptive approach. *Journal of Clinical Endocrinology and Metabolism*, 81, 757–62.

Berg, B. J. and Wilson, J. F. (1991). Psychological functioning across stages of treatment for infertility. *Journal of Behavioural Medicine*, 14, 11–26.

Bromham, D. R. and Cartmill, R. S. V. (1993). Are current sources of contraceptive advice adequate to meet changes in contraceptive practice? A study of patients requesting termination of pregnancy. *British Journal of Family Planning*, 19, 179–83.

Carlson, E., Giwercman, A., Keiding, N., and Skakkebaek, N. E. (1992). Evidence for decreasing quality of semen during past 50 years. *British Medical Journal*, 305, 609–13.

Carnall, D. (1996). Condom trade barriers come down across Europe. *British Medical Journal*, 312, 597.

Cates, W. and Stone, K. M. (1992). Family planning, sexually transmitted diseases and contraceptive choice: a literature update – part 1. *Family Planning Perspectives*, 24, 75–84.

Chandley, A. C. (1979). The chromosomal basis of human infertility. *British Medical Bulletin*, **35**, 181–6.

Chandley, A. C. (1995). The genetic basis of male infertility. *Reproductive Medicine Reviews*, **4**, 1–8.

Chen, T. F. and Ball, R. Y. (1991). Epididymectomy for postvasectomy pain: a histological review. *British Journal of Urology*, **68**, 407–13.

Choi, K.-H., Rickman, R., and Catania, J. A. (1994). What heterosexual adults believe about condoms. *New England Journal of Medicine*, **331**, 406–7.

Comhaire, F. H. (1989). Vasculature of the testis: assessment and management of varicocele. In *The testis* (ed. H. Burger and D. de Kretser), p. 515. Raven Press, New York.

Denniston, G. C. and Kuehl, L. (1995). Open-ended vasectomy: approaching the ideal technique. *Journal of the American Board of Family Practitioners*, **7**, 285–7.

Edwards, I. S. (1993). Earlier testing after vasectomy, based on the absence of motile sperm. *Fertility and Sterility*, **59**, 431–6.

Elstein, M. (1975). Effect of infertility on psychosexual function. *British Medical Journal*, **3**, 296–9.

Farley, T. M. M., Meirik, O., Mehta, S., and Waites, G. M. H. (1993). The safety of vasectomy: recent concerns. *Bulletin of the World Health Organization*, **71**, 413–19.

Gabbay, M. and Gibbs, A. (1996). Does additional lubrication reduce condom failure? *Contraception*, **53**, 155–8.

Giovannucci, E., Ascherio, A., Rimm, E. B., Colditz, G. A., Stampfer, M. J. and Willett, W. C. (1993*a*). A prospective cohort study of vasectomy and prostate cancer in US men. *Journal of the American Medical Association*, **269**, 873–7.

Giovannucci, E., Tor, D., Tosteson, Sc. D., Speizer, F. E., Martin, P., Vessey, M. P., *et al.* (1992). A long-term study of mortality in men who have undergone vasectomy. *New England Journal of Medicine*, **326**, 1392–8.

Giovannucci, E., Tosteson, T. D., Speizer, F. E., Ascherio, A., Vessey, M. P. and Colditz, G. A. (1993*b*). A retrospective cohort study of vasectomy and prostate cancer in US men. *Journal of the American Medical Association*, **269**, 878–82.

Giwercman, A. and Skakkebaek, N. E. (1986). The effect of salicylazosulphapyridine (sulphasalazine) on male fertility. *International Journal of Andrology*, **9**, 38–52.

Griffin, J. E. (1992). Androgen resistance – the clinical and molecular spectrum. *New England Journal of Medicine*, **326**, 611–18.

Hadziselimovic, F. and Herzog, B. (1987). Cryptorchidism. *Paediatric Surgery International*, **2**, 132–40.

Hargreave, T. B. (1992). Towards reversible vasectomy. *International Journal of Andrology*, **15**, 455–9.

Healy, B. (1993). Does vasectomy cause prostate cancer? *Journal of the American Medical Association*, **269**, 2620.

Hendry, W. F., Hughes, L., and Scammell, G. (1990). Comparison of prednisolone and placebo in subfertile men with antibodies to spermatozoa. *Lancet*, **335**, 85–8.

Hull, M. G. R., Glazener, C. M. A., Kelly, N. J., Conway, D. I., Foster, P. A., Hunton, R. A., *et al.* (1985). Population study of causes, treatment, and outcome of infertility. *British Medical Journal*, **291**, 1693–7.

Kaul, S. A. and Roberts, D. P. W. (1992). Preschool screening for cryptorchidism. *British Medical Journal*, **305**, 181.

Kelly, R. W. (1991). Seminal plasma and immunosuppressive activity: the achilles heel of reproduction. *International Journal of Andrology*, **14**, 243–7.

Laven, J. S., Haans, L. C., Mali, W. P., te Velde, E. R., Wensing, C. J. and Eimers, J. M. (1992). Effects of varicocele treatment in adolescents: a randomised study. *Fertility and Sterility*, **58**, 756–62.

Leader, A., Galan, N., George, R., and Taylor, P. (1983). A comparison of definable traits in women requesting reversal of sterilization and women satisfied with sterilization. *American Journal of Obstetrics and Gynecology*, **154**, 198–202.

Liskin, L., Pike, J. M., and Quillin, F. (1983). Vasectomy: safe and simple. *Population Reports*, Series D, no 4.

Lucier, G. W., Lee, I. P., and Dixon, R. L. (1977). *The testis*, Vol. **IV**, p. 577. Academic Press, New York.

McCullagh, E. P. and McGurl, F. J. (1939). Further observations on the clinical use of testosterone propionate. *Journal of Urology*, **42**, 1265–7.

McMahon, A. J., Buckley, J., Taylor, A., Lloyd, S. N., Deane, R. F. and Kirk, D. (1992). Chronic testicular pain following vasectomy. *British Journal of Urology*, **69**, 188–91.

Mead, G. M. (1992). Testicular cancers and related neoplasms. *British Medical Journal*, **304**, 1426–9.

Mieusset, R. and Bujan, L. (1994). The potential of mild testicular heating as a safe, effective and reversible contraceptive method for men. *International Journal of Andrology*, **17**, 186–91.

Morris, I. D. and Shalet, S. M. (1989). Endocrine-mediated protection from cytotoxic-induced testicular damage. *Journal of Endocrinology*, **120**, 7–9.

Nienhuis, H., Goldacre, M., Seagroath, V., Gill, L., and Vessey, M. (1992). Incidence of disease after vasectomy: a record linkage retrospective study. *British Medical Journal*, **304**, 743–6.

Nieschlag, E., Behre, H. M., and Weinbauer, G. F. (1992). *Spermatogenesis–fertilization–contraception. Molecular, cellular and endocrine events in male reproduction* (ed. E. Nieschlag and U.-F. Habenicht), p. 477. Springer-Verlag, Berlin.

Nilsson, S., Edvinsson, A., and Nilsson, B. (1979). Improvement of semen and pregnancy rate after ligation and division of the internal spermatic vein: fact or fiction. *British Journal of Urology*, **51**, 591–6.

O'Brien, T. S., Cranston, D., Turner, E., MacKenzie, I. Z., and Guillebaud, J. (1995). Temporary reappearance of sperm 12 months after vasectomy clearance. *British Journal of Urology*, **76**, 371–2.

Oddens, B. J., Visser, A. Ph., Vemer, H. M., Everaerd, W. Th. A. M., and Lehart, Ph. (1994). Contraceptive use and attitudes in Great Britain. *Contraception*, **49**, 73–86.

Okuyama, A., Fujisue, H., and Matsui, T. (1988). Surgical repair of varicocele: effective treatment for subfertile men in a controlled study. *European Urology.*, **14**, 298–300.

Palermo, G., Joris, H., Derde, M. P., Camus, M., Devroey, P., and Van Steirtegham, A. C. (1993). Sperm characteristics and outcome of human assisted fertilization by subzonal insemination and intracytoplasmic sperm injection. *Fertility and Sterility*, **59**, 826–35.

Patrizio, P., Asch, R. H., Handelin, B., and Silber, S. J. (1993). Aetiology of congential absence of vas deferens; genetic study of three generations. *Human Reproduction*, **8**, 215–20.

Pavlou, S. N., Brewer, K., Farley, M. G., Lindner, J., Bastias, M. C., Rogers, B. J., *et al.* (1991). Combined administration of a gonadotropin-releasing hormone antagonist and testosterone in men induces reversible azoospermia without loss of libido. *Journal of Clinical Endocrinology and Metabolism*, **73**, 1360–9.

Polaneczky, M., Slap, G., Forke, C., Rappaport, A., and Sondheimer, S. (1994). The use of levonorgestrel implants (Norplant) for contraception in adolescent mothers. *New England Journal of Medicine*, **331**, 1201–6.

Qian, S. Z. and Wang, S. G. (1984). Gossypol: a potential antifertility agents for males. *Annual Review of Pharmacology and Toxicology*, **24**, 329–60.

Qian, S. Z., Zhong, C. Q., Xu, N., and Xu, Y. (1986*a*). Antifertility effect of *Tripterygium wilfordii* in men. *Advances in Contraception*, **2**, 253–4.

Qian, S. Z., Zhong, C. Q., and Xu, Y. (1986*b*). Effect of *Tripterygium wilfordii* on the fertility of rats. *Contraception*, **33**, 105–10.

Rinehart, W. (1990). Condoms – now more than ever. *Population Reports*, **H8**, 10–12.

Rosenberg, M. J., Waugh, M. S., Solomon, H. M., and Lyszkowski, A. D. L. (1996). The male polyurethane condom: a review of current knowledge. *Contraception*, **53**, 141–6.

Shafik, A. (1992). Contraceptive efficacy of polyester-induced azoospermia in normal men. *Contraception*, **45**, 439–51.

Sharpe, R. M. and Skakkebaek, N. E. (1993). Are oestrogens involved in falling sperm counts and disorders of the male reproductive tract? *Lancet*, **341**, 1392–5.

Silber, S. J. (1989). Results of microsurgical vasoepididymostomy: role of epididymis in sperm maturation. *Human Reproduction*, **4**, 298–303.

Sivanesarantham, V. (1990). Vasectomy – an assessment of various techniques and the immediate and long-term problems. *British Journal of Family Planning*, **16**, 97–100.

Smith, J. C., Cranston, D., O'Brien, T., Guillebaud, J., Hindmarsh, J., and Turner, A. G. (1994). Fatherhood without apparent spermatozoa after vasectomy. *Lancet*, **334**, 30.

Sparrow, M. J. and Lavill, K. (1994). Breakage and slippage of condoms in family planning clients. *Contraception*, **50**, 117–29.

Steiner, M., Foldesy, R., Cole, D., and Carter, E. (1992). Study to determine the correlation between condom breakage in human use and laboratory test results. *Contraception*, **46**, 279–88.

Stewart, D. L., DeForge, B. R., Hartmann, P., Kaminski, M., and Pecukonis, E. (1991). Attitudes towards condom use and AIDS among patients from an urban family practice center. *J.Nat.Med.Assoc.*, **83**, 772–6.

Tovey, S. J. and Bonell, C. P. (1993). Condoms: a wider range needed. *British Medical Journal*, **307**, 987.

Vessey, M. P., Villard-Mackintosh, I., McPherson, K., and Yeates, D. (1988). Factors affecting the use-effectiveness of the condom. *British Journal of Family Planning*, **40**, 43.

Wellings, K., Field, J., Johnson, A. M., and Wadsworth, J. (1994). *Sexual behaviour in Britain. The National Survey of Sexual Attitudes and Lifestyles.* Penguin Books, London.

World Health Organization (1992). *WHO laboratory manual for the examination of human semen and semen – cervical mucous penetration* (3rd edn). Cambridge University Press, Cambridge.

World Health Organization Task Force for the Regulation of Male Fertility (1990). Contraceptive efficacy of testosterone-induced azoospermia in normal men. *Lancet*, **336**, 955–9.

World Health Organization Task Force on Methods for the Regulation of Male Fertility (1996). Contraceptive efficacy of testosterone-induced azoospermia and oligozoospermia in normal men. *Fertility and Sterility*, **65**, 821–9.

Zhao, S. C., Lian, Y. H., Yu, R. C., and Zhang, S. P. (1992). Recovery of fertility after removal of polyurethane plugs from the human vas deferens, occluded for up to 5 years. *International Journal of Andrology*, **15**, 465–7.

CHAPTER TEN

Sexually transmitted diseases

George Kinghorn

Genito-urinary medicine (GUM) has become a more prominent specialty over the last 20 years, and general practitioners are more likely to work with genito-urinary physicians as our patients increasingly acquire sexually transmitted diseases (STDs). GPs have not traditionally been involved by patients who suspect a venereal origin to their symptoms. Our lack of expertise in the field has, in part, contributed to patients bypassing us. However, the changing epidemiology of STDs, the changing role of the GU clinics, and health education means that general practice will be increasingly involved in the management of the more chronic conditions. This chapter provides an introduction to the common STDs and their management.

Introduction

Gonorrhoea can be traced back almost further than any other disease, and *Leviticus*, **15**: 2–33, contains a description of the disease and the measures taken to prevent it. An epidemic of syphilis spread throughout Europe during the late fifteenth century. While there are conflicting theories as to its origin, most historians adhere to the notion that sailors returning with Columbus brought back the disease from the New World. Venereal syphilis, other sexually transmitted diseases, and their treatments continued to cause huge, premature loss of life and chronic illness during the next four centuries. Until the twentieth century, the treatment of venereal diseases was largely in the hands of surgeons, principally involving the management of complications such as strictures and fistulae. Most voluntary hospitals had limitations on admissions of those suffering from venereal diseases, and Poor Law institutions offered appalling treatment to sufferers. Whilst the upper classes could obtain private treatment, of uncertain value and usually at great expense, the really needy often had to resort to quacks or just fate.

In 1916, a Royal Commission on Venereal Diseases reviewed the prevalence and effects of venereal disease and its means of alleviation and prevention, and made recommendations of action to be taken. Amongst the then startling facts which emerged were the high mortality and morbidity rates of syphilis, which then affected no less than 10% of London's working-class males, and the role of gonococcal ophthalmia as the cause of 15% of infantile blindness. During the following year the hospital service for treating STDs was established. County Councils and Boroughs were instructed to organize clinics for the free and confidential treatment of persons suspected of suffering from venereal diseases. The clinics allowed for open patient access, without the necessity of general practitioner referral. The 1917 Venereal Diseases Act prohibited unqualified persons from treating these diseases and forbade advertising about their treatment other than by the local authorities. This service has now evolved into the specialty of genito-urinary medicine.

Genito-urinary medicine clinics

The major functions of GUM clinics are:
(1) the diagnosis and treatment of patients suffering from STDs;
(2) the control of STDs within the community;
(3) the prevention and treatment of AIDS/HIV infection.

Integration of clinics within the out-patient department and close liaison with allied disciplines have aided other efforts to de-stigmatize attendance. Patient awareness of STDs has been increased by health education.

Speed of diagnosis is vital to promote good control. GUM clinics provide immediate microscopy and have sophisticated laboratory support for diagnosis of genital infection by culture, antigen detection, and serological tests. The predominately out-patient approach permits diagnosis of early disease, the prevention of complications and transmission, and is very cost-effective.

Referral to GUM

Although urgent cases can always be seen the same day, most clinics now operate an appointments system in addition to the walk-in service, which may permit an appointment time tailored to the patient's needs. It is not the norm for a GP to receive letters from the clinic about patients who self-refer, unless the patient has given consent and/or has a condition(s) which requires continuing treatment.

Epidemiological aspects

Incidence

There has been a dramatic increase in the reported incidence of STDs during the past 25 years. The sexual revolution of the Sixties, facilitated by the wider availability of reliable contraception and changing sexual mores, was followed by a rising incidence of all STDs. This trend was augmented by the earlier sexual maturity amongst girls and earlier age of onset of sexual activity in both sexes. Changes in sexual behaviour now means that STDs are as common in women as men. In the UK, the importance of prostitutes as vectors of STD transmission has declined, although they remain of major importance in disease transmission in developing countries.

Other sociological changes which contribute to the increased incidence of STDs include urbanization, increased mobility amongst the young, and the greater ease of worldwide travel. The latter has also promoted the importation of unusual 'tropical' STDs and antibiotic-resistant infections. Despite the availability of effective treatment for most STDs during the past 40 years, their incidence has increased in many developed and developing countries alike.

Changing pattern

During the past decade, in the UK, the traditional bacterial venereal diseases have subsided whereas those infections caused by chlamydia, viruses, and other non-specific genital conditions have become more widespread. The reasons for this changing pattern are not fully understood but may, in part, reflect the effectiveness of control methods for bacterial infections contrasting with the difficulties encountered with diseases due to other micro-organisms. The changing pattern of STDs is mirrored by the changed aetiology of STD complications, such as epididymitis, pelvic inflammatory disease, and neonatal opthalmia, where chlamydial infections now far outnumber gonococcal infections.

At-risk groups

Young people who are starting out on their sexual careers remain at high risk of acquiring STDs. They are likely to be involved in, or exposed to, partner change, and are less likely to use condoms, especially when their judgement is further impaired by alcohol or drugs. Amongst males, STDs are more common in those living away from home, such as students and migrant workers, and those with a mobile occupation, such as lorry drivers, servicemen, and businessmen who travel abroad.

Homosexuals have been, until recently, particularly susceptible to infections such as syphilis and hepatitis B. Changed sexual behaviour, as a consequence of the HIV threat, dramatically reduced the incidence of all STDs amongst some older gay men. However, a relapse in unsafe sexual behaviour exposes them to risk of new infection. There has been far less of a change to safe sexual practices among heterosexuals. Sexual partner change, the rate of which is the single most important factor in determining risk for STDs, remains common in many groups of young people. STD risk is not necessarily related to social class, to educational attainment, nor to standards of personal hygiene.

STDs not infrequently occur in apparently stable relationships where neither partner admits infidelity. It is important to recognize that many STDs have long latent phases and that asymptomatic carriers may occur in either sex.

Routine assessment of male patients

History-taking

Genital health is of prime importance to the majority of men. Minor blemishes or symptoms appearing on the genitals, which would be ignored or trivialized if they occurred elsewhere, can be the cause of considerable anxiety. This anxiety, which is often associated with embarrassment and guilt if there has been recent, risky sexual exposure, may interfere with the taking of a rapid, comprehensive history.

Many patients prefer to seek the anonymity of the confidential environment provided by GUM clinics, rather than present to their GP. For those who do, the history should include details of the present complaint and the time sequence of symptom appearance. Knowledge of recent drug therapy and topical applications, both physician and self-administered, is essential as this may be causative of or mask the condition. The past medical history and current state of general health may be relevant although it is rarely necessary to pursue a full, formal symptomatic enquiry in young, fit men. In taking a sexual history, it is important that the GP feels comfortable with the choice of words and that these are tailored to the individual patient's cultural and educational background, and linguistic ability. Establishing the sexual orientation as well as the place, time, and type of recent sexual practices is routine in a genito-urinary clinic but is much more difficult in general practice. Such questions need to be introduced sensitively and reasons given for the line of history-taking. Sexual orientation is most easily ascertained by asking the patient if he has sex with men, women, or both. Open questions such as 'When did you last have intercourse?' and 'When did you last have intercourse with another partner?' are likely to elicit truthful answers. The place and time of last sexual contact may alert the clinician to an incubation period and to the possibilities of unusual or antibiotic-resistant infections acquired abroad. The type of sexual practices (oral, genital, and anorectal) will help define the extent of the physical examination and the sites from which specimens should be taken for microbiological investigators. The use of condoms with different partners should be enquired about.

Examination

If the GP has decided to refer, it is doubtful that an examination will add much to a good history. If the patient is reluctant to attend the clinic, an examination may help make his mind up. As a minimum, the entire genital region should be exposed; it may be necessary to perform a full physical examination. A thorough examination of the genitalia will include inspection of the skin of the entire anogenital area and of the pubic hair, palpation of the scrotal contents, and exposure of the glans penis, subpreputial sac, and urethral meatus in uncircumcised men. In the GU clinic, examination of the oropharynx is mandatory in men who admit to orogenital contact, and is also useful in others, for example to elicit mucosal lesions of Reiter's syndrome, syphilis, and HIV infection. Proctoscopy is performed in homosexuals who have had ano-receptive intercourse.

Principles of STD management

The drug treatment for STDs is often simple, but for each affected individual there are also psychological and social consequences which require additional management. If the patient is willing to involve his GP, this aspect of care becomes easier for the patient and the clinic.

STDs frequently occur together so that, for example, in patients presenting with genital warts or pediculosis pubis, screening for other infections is routine. Control of STDs demands that a precise diagnosis is reached before treatment is commenced, that follow-up is made to ensure that both clinical and microbiological cure is achieved, and that contact tracing is routinely carried out. Non-judgmental presentation of the facts about the methods of transmission, risks of reinfection, and the development of disease complications in untreated asymptomatic partners is most likely to promote patient cooperation with partner referral. Most men choose to inform their partners themselves; in only a small proportion of cases will home visits by a health adviser be necessary.

Health adviser functions

Health advisers are responsible for counselling patients and for conducting contact tracing. In many parts of the UK, health advisers are experienced nurses who have training both in hospitals and in the community. In GUM clinics, they are directly accountable to the consultant medical staff as this arrangement protects patient confidentiality.

The attendance of the partners of patients with genital tract infections can be sought by one of two methods. It is preferable to encourage the index patient to seek their partner's attendance – such patient referral is more cost-effective and is usually simple to achieve when education about their condition and means of preventing reinfection are explained to the index patient. A 'contact slip' which contains details of the clinic, the index patient's clinic number, and coded diagnosis is often provided to the index patient to be given to the partner. Occasionally, male partners will present with these to their general practitioner. Where the index patient requests assistance and gives sufficient information to allow identification of the consort(s), the health adviser may attempt to contact the sexual partners in the community. The health advisers have a role in contact tracing in those unusual situations where the general practitioner arranges treatment and follow-up in the community.

Urethral discharge

Presentation with a complaint of urethral discharge is very common in men. Although the symptom is often the result of sexually acquired infection, physiological causes also need to be considered.

Spermatorrhoea may present as a clear discharge in adolescents who have not had penetrative intercourse. Typically, the symptom occurs after sexual excitement, or after the passage of a bulky or constipated stool which causes pressure on the prostate gland. There is no accompanying dysuria or frequency. Simple reassurance and explanation is all that is required. Some men, particularly if they have a history of urethritis or who have had recent unsafe sex will milk their urethras and/or examine their urine for signs of discharge and threads. Overenthusiastic self-examination can cause overactivity of the paraurethral glands and the appearance of a clear mucus discharge. The mucus threads in the first passed urine specimen float, in contrast to the sinking of the threads and flocculations of purulent urethral exudate associated with urethritis.

Urethritis

Urethritis commonly presents as a discharge associated with dysuria and frequency. Diurnal frequency is common in urethritis. However, urgency, strangury, and nocturia are rarely present which helps to differentiate urethritis from cystitis associated with bacterial urinary tract infection (UTI).

Gonorrhoea

Gonorrhoea is caused by a gram-negative diplococcus which can usually be easily identified within pus cells on a stained smear, and is fragile, with special culture media and incubation requirements that are difficult to provide in general practice. Urethral swabs, which can be extremely uncomfortable for the patient, need to be placed into either Amies or Stuart's transport media and left at room temperature before being transported to the laboratory. Ideally, specimens of urethral exudate should be placed directly onto a suitable, selective culture medium and then immediately into a carbon dioxide incubator. Such facilities are rare outside GUM clinics, hence most patients with urethritis are best referred immediately to the clinic.

Clinical features

The incubation is characteristically short – usually 2–7 days – although in some men the recognition of symptoms is delayed for several weeks. About 10% of infections are asymptomatic at diagnosis, particularly those occurring in extragenital sites such as the rectum or oropharynx. Gonococcal urethritis is typically acute with the sudden appearance of a purulent urethral discharge and severe dysuria. If untreated, complications can occur. These may be local, such as involvement of paraurethral glands.

Treatment

During the past 15 years, beta-lactamase-producing strains of gonorrhoea, which are resistant to penicillin, have become more widespread throughout the world. Although such strains were initially imported from Africa and south-east Asia into the UK, there are endemic foci of these strains in various parts of the UK. These strains frequently also carry plasmids which confer resistance to multiple antibiotics. As a result, most clinics will use quinolone antibiotics, such as ciprofloxacin, in place of combined ampicillin and probenecid as first-line treatment. In complicated infections, continuous treatment is given for 7–14 days.

It is mandatory to investigate men with gonorrhoea for other sexually transmitted diseases – accompanying chlamydial infection will occur in at least one-third of patients and, if unrecognized, will cause persistent urethritis even after apparently successful treatment for gonorrhoea. Tests of cure for the gonococcus are usually carried out on two occasions in the two-week period following treatment. Both rectal and pharyngeal infections are more difficult to eradicate with single-dose treatment than are the corresponding urethral infections, and continuing treatment for five to seven days is often required.

Follow-up for up to three months to perform serological tests for syphilis is a time-honoured practice in GUM clinics. With the decline of syphilis in the UK, this is less often observed. However, the increasing risk of HIV, especially in sub-Saharan Africa and south-east Asia, requires that patients who may have been exposed to this risk should have follow-up serological testing for HIV infection.

Chlamydial infections and non-gonococcal urethritis

Non-gonococcal urethritis (NGU) is now four times more common than gonorrhoea. Its commonest cause is infection with *Chlamydia trachomatis* (35–50% cases), an unusual, intracellular bacterial pathogen which requires specialized cell culture for growth. The cause of other cases of NGU remains uncertain although genital mycoplasmas, including *Ureaplasma urealyticum*, cause some cases. *Trichomonas vaginalis* in men is often asymptomatic, may be associated with a balanoposthitis, and is occasionally found as a cause of urethritis in Afro-Caribbean men. Herpes simplex virus, especially in first episodes, often causes a terminal urethritis; urethritis may be the sole manifestation of recurrent disease. Sometimes, urethritis can occur as an extension of a bacterial cystitis, or as a result of trauma, foreign body, tumour, or stone in the urethra. Even when all of these causes have been excluded, some 25% of cases of urethritis remains unexplained. In men with recurrent or persistent urethritis, micro-organisms are less often detected on investigations, and many clinicians consider that the disease may have an immunological basis.

Clinical features

The incubation period of NGU tends to be longer than that of gonorrhoea, typically one to three weeks, and the symptoms are less acute. Up to 20% of affected men are symptomless or have minimal symptoms and signs. The onset or urethral irritation and dysuria is often gradual and urethral discharge is frequently only observed first thing in the morning or when voiding has been postponed for six or more hours. When examination is performed at such times, the discharge is mucopurulent and there may be signs of congestion and oedema of the terminal urethra.

The diagnosis requires that microscopy and culture of urethral specimens are performed to demonstrate the presence of pus cells and to exclude gonococcal infection. Macroscopic examination of the urine will show pus, as flocculations or threads which sink to the container base, in the first voided specimen in anterior urethritis; extension to the posterior urethra, which precedes the onset of ascending complications, may be manifest as the presence of pus in subsequent voided specimens. Chlamydial infection of the urethra is diagnosed by culture of endourethral specimens which require special antibiotic-containing transport media.

Treatment of choice are tetracyclines given for 7–14 days. Because of the risk of ascending complications like epidymitis and prostatitis, review is required, and it is necessary that partners are also investigated. In a minority, urethritis persists and longer courses of tetracyclines or erythromycins may be combined with metronidazole. Reiter's syndrome occurs in 1–2% of men with urethritis and is characterized by conjunctivitis, arthritis, and skin and mucous membrane manifestations. Referral to a genito-urinary physician is advised as the condition may become chronic and progressive.

Genital warts

Genital warts or condylomata acuminata are the commonest viral STD in the UK and are caused by human papilloma virus (HPV) types 6, 11, 18, and 31. Patients exhibiting warts are a subgroup of the total population affected, as most HPV infections are subclinical.

The incubation period varies from a few weeks to nine months or longer. They occur mainly on the penis, at sites of maximal trauma during intercourse, but can occur anywhere in the anogenital area, including inside the meatus. About 25% of patients presenting with warts will have other STDs.

Treatment is with podophyllin which is washed off four hours later. Trichloroacetic acid may be used in warts not responding to podophyllin. Liquid nitrogen, curettage, diathermy, and laser therapy are also used.

Other conditions, such as pediculosis pubis and scabies, commonly occur in the genital area and treatment is that in any other area of the body. What is different for the general practitioner is the association with other sexually transmitted diseases.

Genital ulcer disease

Syphilis is now a rare cause of genital ulceration in the UK but remains extremely common in developing countries. There has also been a resurgence of heterosexually acquired cases in the USA and large Soviet cities. The primary chancre of syphilis is typically a single, non-painful, indurated penile ulcer which appears three weeks after infection. Some cases of syphilis do not present until the secondary stage with a widespread, non-irritant skin rash which affects the palms and soles, together with a generalized lymphadenopathy. Early syphilis should also be suspected in cases of genital ulceration where there has been recent travel with sexual contact abroad. The differential diagnosis also includes other tropical causes of genital ulceration such as chancroid, donovanosis, and lymphogranuloma venereum.

The most common cause of genital ulceration in the British Isles is genital herpes, which can be caused by both type 1, usually transmitted by orogenital contact, and type 2 herpes simplex viruses. The incubation period is generally less than one week and vesicles precede the development of multiple, superficial, tender ulcers which are accompanied by inguinal lymphadenitis.

As a general rule, all cases of genital ulceration are best referred to GUM clinics for investigation, even if the patient suggests that the lesions are the result of trauma. GU physicians have found many chancres in so-called 'zip injuries'.

Further reading

Kinghorn, G. R. and Spencer, R. S. (1996). Sexually transmitted diseases. *Medicine*, sections 24.10, 24.11, 24.12. Medicine Publishing Company Ltd, Oxford.

This is a comprehensive, up-to-date, multi-author review of sexually transmitted diseases and related disorders in three sections. They contain practical advice on the clinical assessment of patients, and descriptions of the most important conditions and their management.

CHAPTER ELEVEN

HIV/AIDS

George Kinghorn, Richard Slack, and Gerard Bury

While HIV/AIDS has not reached the apocalyptic predictions of the mid-1980s, it is a disease that demands a wide range of knowledge and expertise, from screening to terminal care. Fortunately, many of the skills needed are already in the domain of medicine. A male patient with HIV will spend over 90% of his life in the community being looked after by his GP. Some patients do not disclose their HIV status to their GP because of fears about confidentiality and competence. As the illness progresses, its management becomes increasingly complex, like many of the chronic diseases we already manage. This complexity is reflected in the authorship of this chapter which includes a genito-urinary physician, an infectious disease specialist, and a GP. The authors have dealt with many aspects of HIV/AIDS, but such is the pace of progress in its treatment that they expect some of it will be out of date by the time the book is published.

Introduction

Outside the large conurbations, infection with the human immunodeficiency virus (HIV) and the clinical condition resulting from it, acquired immune deficiency syndrome (AIDS), are uncommon events in the UK. Most British general practitioners are unlikely to have looked after a case by the mid-1990s. On seeing a young adult with an acute febrile illness and enlarged lymph glands, the diagnosis of acute HIV infection is far from the mind; and the care of people with AIDS dying from unusual opportunist infections, malignancy, or neuronal damage is outside the experience of most British doctors in hospital or the community. How much should general practitioners know? In this chapter we will try to concentrate on the essentials, realizing that the literature is enormous and expanding more quickly than with any other medical condition. A shortened bibliography is appended, but the reader must realize that knowledge, especially about treatment, is changing rapidly. It is almost certain that some of what has been written here will have been superseded by the time the book is published.

More than any other disease, AIDS has transformed the relationship between doctor and patient. Both client-led treatment and client care are becoming more widely accepted, as a consequence of the initial recognition of the epidemic in an articulate, well-educated, politically active group in the USA. The early days of the AIDS story are well-known to most who read newspapers or glance at the television and are extensively described by Randy Shilts (1987). It is to be hoped that the second decade of the story will see equal advocacy for the poor and deprived, especially women and children, who make up the majority of newly infected cases outside the industrialized countries.

Mostly because of issues of confidentiality and stigma, patients have been seen almost exclusively in specialized settings, in particular in genito-urinary medicine (GUM) clinics. A survey in 1991 (Tolley *et al.* 1991) showed that 67% of people diagnosed as HIV positive by a London clinic were not known by their general practitioners to be infected. Even in those with advanced disease and an AIDS diagnosis, 33% had not discussed the condition with their registered practitioner. Because AIDS management has become a specialty, with scores of highly trained, full-time staff devoted to the illness, there has been a misguided notion that all the care could (or should) be managed by special units. This has, in turn, engendered the feeling in some patients that only specialists can deal with them. Some patients are seen regularly miles from their residence and lead a 'double' medical existence which results in confusion and potentially serious mistakes. This situation is slowly changing. Most GU physicians actively encourage the patient to inform his general practitioner so that a shared care plan can be developed. This is vital if antiviral or other potentially toxic medication is prescribed. In some parts of the UK, GPs are actively involved in shared care and an increasing amount of terminal care is being managed in the home by the primary health care team. This can only be achieved with the consent of all parties, especially that of the patient. Crucial to this agreement is trust in confidentiality within the practice and in the expertise available. Complete management of any patient in the community must involve the general practitioner and team and we need to explore ways of gaining the trust of HIV-positive individuals. One way this has been achieved, especially by gay men, is by using general practitioners known to be sympathetic. This has occurred mainly in the large cities where choice is much greater, but has further polarized the care of people with HIV.

Prevention

The epidemiology of HIV infection varies significantly throughout the British Isles. More than 80% of the 19 000 cases diagnosed in England and Wales between 1984 and 1994 were due to sexual transmission, mainly through homosexual intercourse. Worryingly, a review of incidence of HIV infection in homosexual men in London, between 1988 and 1994, showed a rate of about nine per 100 person years for men aged under 30 and about three per 100 person years for men aged over 30; these rates showed no evidence of falling over the seven-year period (Miller *et al.* 1995).

Advice from the GP about safer sex in either heterosexual or homosexual activity should be non-judgemental, honest, and easily understood. Options for safer sex range from monogamy, to use of protective materials, to avoidance of high-risk practices. Good, practical advice is available in leaflet form from a number of sources (Department of Health 1993).

In Scotland and Ireland, around half of all cases are due to use of contaminated needles and syringes during injecting drug use, with men being infected four times more often than women. While the rate of new infections due to injecting drug use has slowed in recent years, this may be due more to effective programmes of harm reduction than to a fall in the numbers who are using illicit drugs (Robertson 1994). While harm-reduction measures for injecting drug use, such as needle exchanges or methadone maintenance, are effective, the risk of sexual spread of HIV from infected drug users is high (Ronald *et al.* 1993).

Injecting drug users have usually sustained their habit by criminal activity and almost all have had contact with the police and judicial systems. Many started to inject heroin in their early teens and come from backgrounds of deprivation, hopelessness, and low self-esteem (Brettle *et al.* 1987; Bury and O'Kelly 1989).

Information, motivation, and non-judgemental support are all important in changing behaviour. Whether among homosexual men, injecting drug users, or among people who are not members of any high-risk group, the GP is in an important position to influence behaviour. Consultations about contraception, unwanted pregnancy, possible STDs, or new relationships are some of those which may present opportunities to offer simple, sensible advice about avoiding HIV.

HIV/AIDS as a men's issue

HIV/AIDS in England and Wales is predominately a disease of men. Even in eastern Scotland where intravenous drug use has contributed greatly to the extent of the epidemic, males greatly outnumber females in HIV statistics. From the start of HIV testing in 1984 to April 1993 there were over 17000 men known to be positive compared with 2468 women. AIDS diagnosis and deaths attributed to AIDS show similar disparities. In an 'average' general practice looking after a population of 10000, if cases were evenly distributed there would be three known HIV-positive patients, at least one of whom would have clinical illness if not an AIDS-defining condition. The ratio of seven men to every woman infected in the UK means that HIV is likely to be seen as a men's issue. Most of those infected with HIV were infected in the earlier 1980s. Where newly acquired infection has been found by examining sequential sera for change on positivity (seroconversion), those identified in the UK without exposure outside the country are largely men who have sexual relationships with men. Some of these are men who have reverted from 'safer sex' techniques to riskier behaviour – even though they know the risk. Some are young, gay men who were not sexually active at the height of the public education campaigns and may have missed the message.

The problems associated with health promotion and sexual behaviour have aroused much public discussion. The dilemma of overemphasizing heterosexual risk, at a time when UK statistics showed plainly that the epidemic was confined to certain groups with high-risk behaviour, has produced the predictable reaction among young heterosexuals that AIDS is not their problem. In spite of many national and local campaigns attempting to modify sexual behaviour, there is little evidence of adoption of 'safer sex' methods by UK youth. Should AIDS be an issue for men outside the traditional 'risk groups'? If so, what strategies should be adopted by practice staff to raise awareness among young, sexually active men who traditionally are rarely seen by GPs? One opportunity to reach this group is through travel advice. In a small study of a Nottingham general practice, 9% of 16–40 year-old men had new sexual encounters on holiday and only half used condoms (Gillies *et al.* 1992). Changing sexual behaviour in men has not been sustained even amongst some gay men who are fully aware of the consequences.

The infection

In spite of continuing fierce debate, the body of scientific information supports the idea that HIV causes AIDS. There may be co-factors which speed up the progress from initial infection to overwhelming immune depression. The first virus described by the French virologist Luc Montagnier and his team at the Institute Pasteur has now been named HIV-1 (human immunodeficiency virus 1), and many isolates of a genetically similar virus have been made throughout the world. HIV-2 is sufficiently different in its biochemical makeup, serological response, and natural history to be considered a separate virus. It is worth remembering that some of the standard HIV antibody tests do not give a positive response in HIV-2 infections and the laboratory may need to be warned if there is a likelihood of HIV-2. There are many related animal viruses infecting monkeys and cats, the study of which is assisting in understanding infection in humans and the development of vaccines.

There are three main routes of infection:

(1) sexual;
(2) blood-borne;
(3) materno–fetal.

All routes require viable virus, which in the complete form is surrounded by a fragile envelope, to reach and attach to specific receptors on susceptible cell surfaces. Free virus can be found in plasma and secretions in large numbers at the end stages of the disease ('full-blown' AIDS) and in the early primary infection, especially if it is clinically apparent (glandular fever-like). The long, latent period of asymptomatic HIV infection is generally less infectious, although it is important for people known to be carrying the virus and their partners to realize there is no 'safe period' (see risk factors below). This is because viral replication and infection of new cells is occurring continuously and, until recently, there was no easy way of determining the infectivity of an individual's secretion by viral load measurements outside specialized laboratories.

As with most infectious diseases, it is macrophages which are initially attached by the microbe and then the main target cell, in this case the T lymphocyte, is infected. The damage done by the virus is to continue infecting and depleting 'helper' T lymphocytes which carry the CD4 receptor. In common with many infections, intact skin and mucous membranes are impervious to attack, but traumatized or ulcerated surfaces are more likely to establish HIV infection. For example, work in East Africa has shown that men with genital ulcers (due to chancroid, syphilis, and herpes) were approximately 10 times more likely to acquire HIV infection. These conditions are made worse in uncircumcised men who are also likely to acquire infection without genital ulcers.

Testing for HIV infection

When a patient requests a test for HIV infection, a number of areas need to be covered. While the GP may be the ideal person to provide both pre- and post-test counselling, most GUM clinics have expert support available should it be needed.

Pre-test counselling

Why have a test? What risks has the patient been exposed to (unprotected sexual intercourse, injecting drug use, transfused blood products)? Occasionally, requests for HIV testing are based on inaccurate information about risks.

Who wants the result? Patients may request a test because a partner or parent is anxious for the information and has persuaded them to ask for the test. It does not mean the patient has made a considered decision or is ready to cope with the result.

Who will you tell? An important step in coming to terms with what a HIV test means is considering what might happen immediately after a positive result. A patient who would tell everyone or no one about their positive result probably does not yet have a realistic grasp of what is involved.

The nature of the test. It is essential that patients appreciate the difference between HIV infection and AIDS. A positive HIV test gives no information about the progress of the disease or its prognosis.

The implications of a test. Whatever the result, the possibility that a test has been carried out might be asked about by an insurer or prospective employer. A positive result will have serious effects on insurance, mortgage, job, or family life but will allow effective treatment now.

Procedures for follow-up. As it can take six weeks to three months for seroconversion after infection, further tests may be needed even if the first is negative. In the event of a positive result, further investigations and specialist assessment are needed.

Post-test counselling

Lifestyle changes. Whatever the result, anyone whose lifestyle has put him (or her) at risk should be counselled about ways to reduce that risk.

Support. Coming to terms with the diagnosis, deciding who to tell, and coping with the anger, guilt, and grief of a positive result all require non-judgemental and positive support. Many GPs are ideally placed to provide this support.

Medical assessment. Newly diagnosed patients should have specialist assessment of their immunological status to decide on the need for prophylaxis or other treatments.

Continuing care. The GP's role as a source of ongoing support, advice, and reassurance is invaluable. Other clinical roles during the asympomatic and symptomatic phases are discussed below.

Classification of HIV infection

The classification system for HIV disease provides a framework for the identification of the many pathological problems which constitute HIV disease. The most widely used system of classification is that of the Center for Disease Control (Table 11.1) (Center for Disease Control and Prevention 1992).

Management of minor illness

There is a long, asymptomatic phase of the illness during which most patients feel, and are, well. Not surprisingly, however, minor symptoms may be interpreted as the onset of something much more serious. Rapid and easy access to the general practitioner can be of great reassurance to patients when these symptoms – such as 'flu or gastrointestinal upsets – cause alarm.

The following is a list of illnesses which are common in patients with HIV and can be dealt with in general practice:
- oral thrush
- sinusitis
- respiratory tract infections
- seborrhoeic dermatitis
- molluscum contagiosum
- herpes simplex.

Anxiety, depression, or difficulty in coping may also be presented to the GP under the guise of minor physical ailments. All of these problems can be initially dealt with using standard therapeutic strategies. Failure to respond, deterioration, or diagnostic uncertainty are good reasons for prompt consultation with a specialist colleague. The possibility that this episode represents the first signs of opportunistic infection or other manifestation of immunodeficiency needs to be kept in mind.

Monitoring asymptomatic disease

HIV disease has assumed many of the characteristics of a chronic disease: 8–10 years after acquiring the infection, only about 50% of people will have developed AIDS (Hendriks *et al.* 1993). Even when an AIDS-defining illness occurs, many patients will survive for years. During the asymptomatic phase, most people are very well but may be understandably anxious about their health. The GP's main roles during the phase include:

(1) *support and reassurance for patients and their families;*

(2) *management of minor illnesses;*

(3) *health promotion.* This requires a special emphasis on safer sexual practices for all and harm-reduction measures such as needle exchange/opiate substitution for problem drug users (Advisory Council on the Misuse of Drugs 1988; Cravell and Hart 1990);

(4) *monitoring disease progression.* Regular physical examination and laboratory investigations can help to identify immunosuppression in an asymptomatic patient. At present, the most useful of these surrogate markers of disease progression is the CD4 (T cell) subset count (normally $> 800/\mu L$) (Phillips *et al.* 1994). Assays to assess viral load, by HIV RNA polymerase chain-reaction tests are now becoming more widely available. Elevated viral loads measured by this test have a clearer prognostic significance than older tests for the p24 (viral antigen). It is likely that viral load measurements will be increasingly used to guide clinicians as to the most appropriate time to initiate and change antiretroviral treatment regimes.

Table 11.1 *Classification of HIV (Center for Disease Control and Prevention 1992)*

I	*Acute HIV infection* Acute transient viral illness, within days to a week of infection. Difficult to distinguish and rarely recognized.
II	*Asymptomatic infection* This phase may last for up to eight years or more.
III	*Persistent generalized lymphadenopathy (PGL)* Lymph node enlargement lasting at least three months at two or more extra-inguinal sites; 10–15% with PGL progress to AIDS within 24–36 months.
IVa	*Chronic constitutional disease* Malaise, wasting, sweats, diarrhoea
IVb	*Neurological disease* Neuropathy, AIDS dementia complex
IVc1	*Opportunistic infections* – pneumocystis carinii pneumonia – cryptosporidiosis with diarrhoea > 1 month – candida: oesophagus, trachea, bronchi, lungs – cytomegalovirus (CMV): retina, colon, oesophagus – herpes simplex: oesophagus, lungs, bronchi – cerebral toxoplasmosis – atypical mycobacterial infection
IVc2	*HIV-related secondary infections* – oropharyngeal candidiasis – herpes zoster (involving several dermatomes) – tuberculosis – oral hairy leukoplakia
IVd	*Malignancies* – Kaposi's sarcoma – non-Hodgkin's lymphoma – primary intracerebral lymphoma
IVe	*Other HIV-related conditions* – HIV-related thrombocytopenia – seborrhoeic dermatitis

The following approach is suggested at around 12-week intervals, and a flowsheet can be created to monitor the results and kept in the patient's file or by the patient himself:

1. *Laboratory monitoring*:
   FBC
   platelets

CD4 count
HIV RNA polymerase chain reaction

2. *Clinical monitoring*:
   weight
   mucous membranes (e.g. for thrush or oral hairy leukoplakia)
   skin (e.g. for Kaposi's sarcoma)
   new symptoms
   lymphadenopathy

3. *Review of medication*

(5) *Early signs of serious illness.* The latent period between infection and the onset of symptoms of immune deficiency is highly variable. Progression rates are faster with certain infecting virus types, a large viral inoculum, the presence of pre-existing immune deficiency at the time of primary infection, and older patient age.

A variety of constitutional symptoms appear, their onset usually being associated with a decline in CD4 counts to less than $350/\mu L$. These include malaise, fever, night sweats, weight loss, and intermittent diarrhoea. Symptoms are usually intermittent in early symptomatic disease but become more constant with progressive immune deficiency. In association with symptoms, the immune deficiency causes the appearance of signs which particularly affect the skin, mouth, and lymph nodes. Common skin problems include extensive seborrhoeic eczema, folliculitis, pityriasis versicolor, fungal infections, and recurrent anogenital or orofacial herpes simplex. Herpes zoster is also very common – and its appearance in a young patient with an at-risk lifestyle should alert the clinician to HIV infection as a possible underlying cause.

Mouth problems are also very common. These include angular stomatitis, recurrent or persistent oral candidiasis, gingivitis with blunting of the interdental papillae, dental abscess, and recurrent aphthous ulceration. Oral hairy leukoplakia, which is caused by EBV infection and has an adverse prognostic significance, usually begins with warty-like white projections or parallel striae on the lateral margins of the tongue. Unlike candida plaques, the lesions cannot be removed by abrasion.

Lymphadenopathy may persist in patients with early symptomatic HIV infection. Haematological indices are frequently affected by HIV infection. Lymphopenia is extremely common. Thrombocytopenia is also relatively common and is caused by autoimmune phenomena, but it rarely causes severe bleeding. Similarly, unusual tumours such as Kaposi's sarcoma (KS) (which resemble small flat bruises) or non-Hodgkin's lymphomas may be easily missed without regular monitoring. Unlike the classical form of the disease, which is usually confined to the lower limbs of elderly patients, KS in AIDS is widespread, affects mucocutaneous surfaces and viscera, and often has an aggressive course. The lesions are macular at their onset but progress to raised, indurated, violaceous plaques. On the trunk, these tend to follow skin cleavage lines. They are also often visible on the face, the extremities such as the nose or penis, and the palate. Lymphoedema and pain may occur in long-standing lesions. If KS occurs alone in patients with high CD4 counts, then the outlook is better than for those presenting with other opportunistic infections. Treatment is by excision, radiotherapy, local or systemic cytotoxic drugs, or systemic interferon. In many cases, cosmetic treatment alone is required.

Serious opportunistic infections include tuberculosis, atypical mycobacterial infections, cytomegalovirus (CMV) retinitis, cerebral toxoplasmosis, or gastrointestinal cryptosporidiosis.

Certain other problems, such as HIV enteropathy or dementia, may be direct viral effects and are not necessarily mediated through opportunistic infections or tumours.

Close liaison with specialist colleagues, a high index of suspicion, and good clinical judgement are all essential in the early identification of serious but potentially treatable problems.

(6) *PCP prophylaxis.* Pneumocystis carinii pneumonia (PCP) has been one of the most common presenting problems in HIV disease and a serious cause of morbidity and mortality.

Once the CD4 count falls below 200/μL, PCP prophylaxis with oral cotrimoxazole 960 mg per day is highly effective in preventing what has become the commonest AIDS-defining illness in northern Europe. Sulphonamide sensitivity eruptions are common in AIDS patients. Nebulized pentamidine or dapsone/trimethoprim are alternative regimens for prophylaxis in those who are unable to take cotrimoxazole.

(7) *Help with complex drug regimes.* Patients who need treatment with antiretroviral drugs should be continuously monitored in collaboration with a specialist centre. This is a rapidly developing therapeutic area and combinations of two or more such drugs are now the norm. Patients often need help from the primary care team on managing complex drug regimes. Antiretrovirals, prophylactic drugs, and therapy for intercurrent problems can create complex regimes which can confuse and demoralize patients.

There are now three groups of antiretroviral drugs which can be prescribed, nucleoside reverse transcriptase inhibitors, protease inhibitors, and, most recently, the non-nucleoside reverse transcriptase inhibitors (NNRTI).

Drugs such as zidovudine, didanosine (ddl), and zalcitabine (ddC) are nucleoside analogues which inhibit reverse transcriptase, a viral enzyme essential for replication. Initial studies showed that use of zidovudine in AIDS patients increased survival duration. Subsequent studies in asymptomatic patients with less severe immune deficiency showed that zidovudine monotherapy did not influence mortality from AIDS (Concorde Coordinating Committee 1994). Subsequently, it has been shown that combinations of zidovudine with either ddl or ddC reduce disease progression and mortality from AIDS (Delta Coordinating Committee 1996). Because of this, and the rapid development of antiviral resistance by HIV, combination antiviral therapy has become the accepted norm.

Zidovudine treatment is associated with initial gastrointestinal effects, such as nausea and vomiting, headaches, myalgia, and insomnia. These tend to diminish with time. In late disease, toxicity may restrict zidovudine use. Myelosuppression causing macrocytic anaemia, which may necessitate repeated transfusion, leukopenia, and thrombocytopenia, occurs in 40% of treated AIDS patients but fewer than 5% of patients with early HIV infection.

Recent studies have shown a definite benefit of zidovudine therapy administered to pregnant women and to neonates in reducing materno–fetal transmission of HIV (Connor *et al.* 1994).

ddl and ddC have different toxicities and their major dose-limiting side-effects are peripheral neuropathy and pancreatitis. Lamivudine (3TC) is similar, is generally well-tolerated, and is often used as a replacement for these two drugs in combination with zidovudine. Stavudine (d4T) is another new drug in this class which can be used in combinations as a replacement for zidovudine.

The protease inhibitors are a recently introduced class of antiretroviral drugs. They are potent, but induce resistance rapidly unless they are part of combination therapy. There are three drugs of this class now available (saquinavir, ritonavir, and indinavir) which differ in their bioavailability after oral administration but have similar initial gastrointestinal side-effects and dose-limiting hepatotoxicity. They may also be associated with nephrolithiasis and a high fluid intake should be encouraged in treated patients.

The NNRTI drugs are the newest class of antiretroviral drugs. Delavirdine and neverapine have shown promise as adjuncts to other combination therapy. They appear to be potent and relatively free of side-effects but may interact with protease inhibitors, causing elevated levels leading to hepatotoxicity.

As a result of the rapid increase in the number of antiretroviral drugs, there is a multiplicity of possible combinations, and the potential for complex drug interactions. International trials are continuing to determine which combinations are most effective in reducing HIV replication, associated immunosuppression, and disease progression. A consensus is emerging that treatment initiated before symptomatic disease has developed will be beneficial in reducing long-term morbidity and mortality from HIV infection.

(8) *Liaison with specialist HIV services.* It is probably inevitable that the hospital emphasis should have been on specialist supervision of this condition rather than on its care in the community, as with any other chronic illness. Much, however, has been achieved in 'normalizing' care at the GP/specialist interface (Guthrie and Barton 1995; Mansfield and Singh 1993; Smith *et al.* 1993). Recent evidence has shown that by providing GPs with prompt discharge information, easy access to specialist advice, and up-to-date continuing education, hospital stays can be substantially reduced, and there can be a noticeable increase in contacts between patients and GPs (Smith *et al.* 1996). In addition, both patients and GPs felt that the standard of health care provided had improved.

Managing advanced disease

What is advanced disease?

In the CDC classification system, stage IV reflects the onset of symptomatic disease, which in most people represents advanced disease (see Table 11.1). However, it is not simple as not everyone with stage IV disease has AIDS. Some asymptomatic patients may have advanced disease or AIDS, perhaps because of immunodeficiency, a low CD4 count, or thrombocytopenia. Therefore, a patient may technically not fulfil the criteria for AIDS but be quite ill. Conversely, patients may have had an AIDS-defining illness but return to good health.

What is AIDS?

AIDS-defining illnesses include a wide number of problems; some examples are given in Table 11.2. All of these presume the patient's HIV status is positive or unknown.

Table 11.2 *Examples of AIDS-defining illnesses*

Problem	Description	Stage
AIDS encephalopathy	Severe cognitive or motor impairment	IVb
Wasting syndrome	Involuntary loss of more than 10% of baseline weight	IVa
Opportunistic infections	PCP, CMV, toxoplasmosis, etc.	IVc1
Malignancies	Kaposi's sarcoma	IVd
CD4 < 200 (Newly added in 1993 in USA)	Must be HIV positive	IVe

A staging system for AIDS based on the number and type of AIDS-defining diagnoses and CD4 count at the time of diagnosis of AIDS has recently been reported and may help to predict more easily the likely risk of death for individual patients (Morcroft *et al.* 1995).

How does AIDS present?

In a study of 436 patients with an AIDS-defining diagnosis at one London hospital between 1991 and 1993, 22% were diagnosed at the same time that they had a positive HIV test. Tuberculosis and PCP were common AIDS-defining diagnoses in this group but were rare among patients who had been diagnosed HIV positive some time before their AIDS-defining diagnosis. In the latter group, cryptosporidiosis, CMV infection, and wasting were common AIDS-defining diagnoses. Interestingly, patients who were HIV positive and presented late survived at least as long as their previously diagnosed counterparts, reflecting the benefits of medical intervention on disease progression after a diagnosis of AIDS (Poznansky *et al.* 1995).

Neurological manifestations

Cerebral toxoplasmosis is the commonest cause of acute neurological illness with fits, ataxia, altered level of consciousness, and focal signs. Often, there is a history of preceding headache for several days. Diagnosis is by computed tomography (CT) or magnetic resonance imaging (MRI) scan. First-choice treatment is with pyrimethamine and sulphadiazine.

Cryptococcal meningitis causes headache, nausea, and vomiting, and sometimes photophobia, although classical signs of meningitis are often absent. There are usually non-specific symptoms such as fever, malaise, and weight loss. Initial treatment is with IV amphotericin with or without flucytosine and subsequently with oral fluconazole which has to be continued in high dosage, 400 mg daily, indefinitely thereafter. Primary prevention of cryptococcal meningitis with fluconazole has been reported to be effective in patients with CD4 < 250/μL, and may become a routine part of the GP's role in management (Quagliarello *et al.* 1995).

Progressive multifocal leucoencephalopathy, which is caused by a papovarvirus infection, causes aphasia, blindness, ataxia, and hemiparesis. It is progressive until death.

Cytomegalovirus retinopathy is the commonest cause of impaired visual acuity in AIDS. The characteristic and florid 'cottage cheese and tomato ketchup' retinal changes result from perivascular exudates and haemorrhages. The condition is rapidly progressive and the associated retinal infarction may cause bilateral blindness. Treatment is with intravenous ganciclovir or foscarnet and needs to be continued indefinitely. Many patients on such treatment at home will be able to administer regular intravenous treatment to themselves via an indwelling IV catheter; others will need help from the primary care team.

HIV encephalopathy. Although there were initially fears that some HIV-infected patients would develop a dementing illness without other systemic illness, HIV encephalopathy is almost always a later preterminal AIDS manifestation. It begins with subtle cognitive changes with forgetfulness, impaired concentration, and deterioration in handwriting. Later, there are associated signs in the motor system with ataxia, weakness, and incontinence. Scans show dilated cerebral ventricles and cortical atrophy. Many patients are aware of their deteriorating cerebral function and this condition often causes them and their families great distress. Many elect for the replacement of active with palliative treatment at this stage, which is where the general practitioner and the specialist physician need to work closely with the community nursing team.

Gastrointestinal manifestations

Opportunistic infections may affect the whole of the GI tract and are directly or indirectly responsible for the progressive weight loss and wasting which is characteristic of AIDS.

Candida oesophagitis. This is becoming less common as a presenting symptom of early AIDS because systemically active antifungals, such as fluconazole and itraconazole, are given prophylactically after the onset of persistent oral candidiasis in patients with symptomatic HIV infection. It presents with retrosternal discomfort and dysphagia; diagnosis is confirmed by barium swallow or by endoscopy. Both CMV and herpes simplex virus can also cause oesophagitis.

Cryptosporidium is a common protozoal cause of persistent or torrential diarrhoea with colicky abdominal pain and electrolyte disturbance which can be diagnosed by finding acidfast cysts in the stools. Multiple specimens may be necessary to establish the diagnosis. It is difficult to eliminate but requires persistent symptomatic treatment.

Non-Hodgkin's lymphoma. These are usually high-grade B-cell lymphomas which often occur in extranodal sites. These include the central nervous system, bone marrow, and GI tract. Systemic symptoms such as fever and weight loss are frequent and the response to chemotherapy is generally poor. Mean survival after presentation is less than one year.

The deteriorating patient

Patients with advanced disease or severe immunodeficiency are at risk of sudden deterioration due to a range of special problems; some of these are listed in Table 11.3, together with one or two clinical characteristics with which the problem may present.

Table 11.3 *Presentations to be concerned about*

Characteristics	Possible problem
Fever, non-productive cough, dyspnoea, rapid or insidious deterioration	PCP
Dysphagia	Oesophageal candida
Fever, headache, meningism, seizures unusual	Cryptococcal meningitis
Focal neurological signs, confusion, lethargy, psychosis, ataxia	Cerebral toxoplasmosis
Plain visual deterioration, may be bilateral	CMV retinitis
Dehydration	Severe diarrhoea

Reasons for admission to hospital

Acute hospitalization should be urgently considered for patients with any of the following problems:

    progressive respiratory symptoms
    focal neurological signs
    progressive dementia or confusion
    severe dehydration
    unexplained fever
    unexplained, persistent headache
    persistent leg weakness
    depression
    inability to cope (either patients or carers)

Hard and fast rules about the need for hospitalization are very difficult to prescribe, so clinical judgement, common sense and early consultation with specialist colleagues remain the touchstones to what can be a difficult decision.

Terminal care

There is a great sense of waste in the death of a person with much to contribute to society. This loss to family and friends is often complicated by stigma, communication difficulties, and cover-up. In situations involving intravenous drug use, family members may have become alienated from the patient due to prolonged abuse, criminal activity, and hurt. In the final years or months it is possible for families to come to terms with their loss and to be reconciled and strengthened. Being able to accept a son or brother who has caused great pain to the family can be the most therapeutic thing that can happen to the family. Facilitating reconciliation is time-consuming and exhausting for the doctors and nurses involved. Many, of course, are not reconciled and such families will place demands on their GP in the longer term, often at key times like anniversaries and birthdays.

Family members often want to become involved in the care of the dying son or daughter and should be encouraged to do so – they will provide the very best care and attention and will treasure the opportunity to become close to someone from whom they may have thought themselves irreconcilably distanced.

With obvious deterioration, patients may want to make plans for their terminal care at home, in hospital, or in the hospice. The availability of HIV or hospice home-care teams provides excellent support to the primary care team in dealing with any problems that may arise. In general, the problems of pain relief, hydration, withdrawal of unnecessary medicines, and nursing care are familiar ones to any GP with experience of terminal care. Patients with opiate addictions generally find that less and less methadone or other opiate is needed to meet their needs.

Once reassured that the option of hospital or hospice is there should it be needed, family and friends usually opt to continue home care to the end and benefit greatly from the GP's support.

Family and partner management

Should the patient die in the community, it will often fall to the GP to complete the death certificate. Unless knowledge of the patient's condition is well-known to the immediate family, it is a kindness to omit writing this fact on the death certificate. It is still almost always possible to provide an accurate description of the cause(s) of death, which will allow the relatives to complete the necessary formalities, and to tick the box to indicate that further information will be available later. AIDS is not a notifiable disease in the UK although the hospital unit should provide information about the death to the Communicable Diseases Surveillance Centre at Colindale. The necessary form includes details of the patient's age, risk group, and clinical details, but identifiable personal information is not necessary.

Support groups

People with HIV/AIDS are in a similar position to others with a terminal illness. The need for support varies considerably between individuals and during the course of the infection. Nevertheless, anyone seeing a patient with HIV infection or AIDS regularly should determine what groups he has already contacted and if he needs more support outside partner, friends, family, and professionals. The early history of the epidemic indicated that insufficient attention was paid to this by physicians, especially in the US.

Homosexual men who declare their sexuality and identify themselves as gay are more likely to be in contact with a network of groups run by organizations within the gay community. Self-help groups are available in most large cities and contact may be made through the local genito-urinary medicine clinic or HIV/AIDS coordinator. Many of these organizations are listed in the National AIDS manual and some, such as Body Positive, are coordinated nationally (an abbreviated list is included in the appendix). Unfortunately, local voluntary groups vary greatly in composition and quality and several have had difficulties sustaining enthusiasm. Special Health Service funds have been available to assist voluntary AIDS organizations which have been run separately from other self-help and care groups. Because of the predominance of gay men with HIV, most local-run groups tend to serve their needs and have not been found suitable for those from different communities. This applies even to men who have sex with other men but for reasons of class, ethnicity, or individual preference do not find existing groups useful. Many patients in the early asymptomatic stage of HIV infection prefer not to associate with others with the disease and feel that positive groups remind and depress them about the condition.

Conclusion

AIDS and HIV infection can present in a multitude of clinical guises. Its diagnosis and management presents many challenges both to the hospital clinician and general practitioner. Advances in drug treatment are proceeding at a rapid pace and there has been real progress in reducing morbidity and mortality from the disease. With the increasing longevity of survivors, decreasing stigmatization, and normalizing of care, there is likely to be greater involvement of general practitioners in the management of HIV/AIDS patients.

References

Advisory Council on the Misuse of Drugs (1988). *AIDS and drug misuse, Part 1*. HMSO, London.

Brettle, R. P., Bisset, K., Burns, D., and Davidson, J. (1987). HIV and drugs misuse: the Edinburgh experience. *British Medical Journal*, **295**, 421–4.

Bury, G. and O'Kelly, F. D. (1989). HIV infection in a Dublin general practice. *Journal of the Royal College of General Practitioners*, **39**, 101–3.

Center for Disease Control and Prevention (1992). 1993 revised classification system for HIV infection and expanded surveillance case definition for AIDS among adolescents and adults. *Morbidity and Mortality Weekly Report*, **41**, 1–19.

Concorde Coordinating Committee (1994). Concorde: MRC/ARNS randomised, double-blind, controlled trial of immediate and deferred zidovudine in symptom-free HIV infection. *Lancet*, **343**, 871–88.

Connor, E. M., Sperling, R. S., Gelber, R., *et al.* (1994). Reduction of maternal – infant transmission of HIV-1 with zidovudine treatment. *New England Journal of Medicine*, **331**, 1173–80.

Cravell, A. M. and Hart, G. J. (1990). Help-seeking and referrals in a needle exchange: a comprehensive service to injecting drug users. *British Journal of Addiction*, **85**, 235–40.

Delta Coordinating Committee (1996). Delta: a randomised, double-blind, controlled trial comparing combinations of zidovudine plus didanosine or zalcitabine with zidovudine alone in HIV-infected individuals. *Lancet*, **348**, 283–91.

Department of Health (1993). *HIV & AIDS: issues in primary care* (vols **1–3**). DoH, London.

Gillies, P., Slack, R., Sfoddart, N., and Conway, S. (1992). HIV-related risk behaviour in UK holiday-makers. *AIDS*, **6**, 339–40.

Guthrie, B. and Barton, S. (1995). HIV at the hospital/general practice interface: bridging the communication divide. *International Journal of STD & AIDS*, **6**, 84–8.

Hendriks, J. C. M., Medley, G. F., van Griensven, G. J. P., *et al.* (1993). The treatment-free incubation period of AIDS in a cohort of homosexual men. *AIDS*, **7**, 231–9.

Mansfield, S. and Singh, S. (1993). Who should fill the care gap in HIV disease? *Lancet*, **342**, 726–8.

Miller, E., Waight, P. A., Tedder, R. S., Sutherland, S., *et al.* (1995). Incidence of HIV infection in homosexual men in London, 1988–1994. *British Medical Journal*, **311**, 545.

Morcroft, A. J., Johnson, M. A., Sabin, C. A., Lipman, M., *et al.* (1995). Staging system for clinical AIDS patients. *Lancet*, **346**, 12–17.

Phillips, A., *et al.* (1994). Use of CD4 lymphocyte count to predict long-term survival free of AIDS after HIV infection. *British Medical Journal*, **309**, 309–13.

Poznansky, M. C., Coker, R., Skinner, C., Hill, A., *et al.* (1995). HIV-positive patients presenting with an AIDS defining illness: characteristics and survival. *British Medical Journal*, **311**, 156–8.

Quagliarello, V. Q., Viscoli, C., and Horwitz, R. I. (1995). Primary prevention of cryptococcal meningitis in HIV-infected patients. *Lancet*, **345**, 548–52.

Robertson, J. R. (1994). *Drug services, changing priorities (1994)*. In *Heroin addiction and drug policy: the British system* (ed. J. Strang and M. Glossop). Oxford University Press, Oxford.

Ronald, P. J. M., Robertson, J. R., Wyld, R., and Wrightman, R. (1993). Heterosexual transmission of HIV in injecting drug users. *British Medical Journal*, **307**, 1184–5.

Shilts, R. (1987). *And the band played on: politics, people and the AIDS epidemic*. St. Martins Press, New York.

Smith, S., Parker, C., Shaunak, S., Ash, S., and Bhatt, R. (1993). GPs should be more involved. *British Medical Journal*, **307**, 801–2.

Smith, S., Robinson, J., Hollyer, J., Bhatt, R., Ash, S., and Shaunak, S. (1996). Combining specialist and primary health care teams for HIV-positive patients: retrospective and prospective studies. *British Medical Journal*, **312**, 416–20.

Tolley, K., Maynard, A., and Robinson, D. (1991). *HIV-AIDS and Social Care*. Centre for Health Economics, University of York, Discussion Paper No 81.

Appendix

The National AIDS Manual is a compendium of topics of information and a directory of all UK services which is regularly updated by the National Aids Trust. There is usually a copy obtained by subscription in each Health District, major libraries and health information centres.

Members of the public may obtain information and advice by telephoning the National AIDS Helpline 0800 567123 or the general Health Information Line 0800 665544. More detailed advice and counselling may be obtained locally from the GU Medicine clinic, District HIV/AIDS Co-ordinator or support groups who may be listed in local directories. If there are problems finding our about local groups the following national charitable organisations provide assistance:

Body Positive Helpline 0171 373 9124
Terence Higgins Trust Helpline 0171 242 1010
Terence Higgins Trust Office 0171 831 0330

Outside the UK many countries have similar networks of national and local groups dealing with HIV/AIDS.

CHAPTER TWELVE

Urological problems

David Gillatt and Brian Cox

It is in the area of urology that doctors deal with problems that are unique to men. Yet even in this specialty there is a striking absence of information concerning the effects of urological problems and their management on men as people. Men's lack of knowledge about their genito-urinary system has been uncovered by opinion pollsters rather than the medical profession. We still know little about men's health beliefs, fears and coping strategies in this area. Urologists are not solely responsible for this state of affairs as it merely reflects a wider blindness to a men's agenda in health and illness. This chapter deals with the epidemiology and management of common diseases that affect the male genito-urinary tract. It deals with management issues that general practitioners are likely to come across in sharing care with their specialist colleagues.

Urinary tract infections

It is accepted wisdom in urology that urinary tract infections in men are always potentially complicated and an underlying predisposing factor should be sought. The term 'urinary tract infection' (UTI) encompasses a range of conditions, from pyelonephritis to cystitis, with a variety of aetiologies. In addition to this, men may suffer from inflammation or infection of the prostate. In young adults, bacteriuria is 30 times more prevalent in women than in men, but by the age of 70 years it is only twice as common in women (Schaeffer 1992). A review of patients presenting at Southmead Hospital showed that 25% of men below the age of 50, presenting with UTI, had a predisposing cause. This group often had other symptoms, such as loin pain from a ureteric stone. While bacteriuria is commoner in men with advancing age, other predisposing causes, such as bladder out-flow obstruction secondary to benign prostatic hyperplasia, also become more prevalent.

The majority of urinary tract infections are caused by faecal organisms such as *Escherichia coli* or *Proteus*. Many recurrent infections are, in fact, reinfections by these organisms. A lower UTI should ideally be investigated with urine culture, urine for cytology, and plain X-ray of the abdomen to exclude a bladder stone, with upper-tract imaging (ultrasound or intravenous urogram) if there is loin pain or haematuria. Cystoscopy should be reserved for those patients with persisting symptoms or in whom there may be a clinical suspicion of bladder cancer, as in men over 40 years with haematuria.

Tuberculosis still presents occasionally, with signs of either upper or lower UTI, or occasionally in a patient with asymptomatic sterile pyuria. If there is any history of TB exposure, or a patient has sterile pyuria or unexplained, chronic urinary tract symptoms, TB should be considered.

Stone disease

Urinary tract stones count for a large percentage of urological workload and are responsible for approximately 15% of all acute surgical admissions in England and Wales. Until the twentieth century, urinary tract stones were predominantly bladder calculi. In the 1960s and 70s, a trend away from bladder calculi towards upper urinary tract calculi was noted, wherever countries become more industrialized and diet becomes more nutritious. In Europe and the United States, upper urinary tract calculi are far more common than bladder calculi. Upper urinary tract calculi occur in between 5% and 10% of the population. Urinary tract stones are three times as common in men as in women. The peak age incidence for urinary calculi is in the fourth to sixth decades. The largest number of patients report the onset of urinary stone disease in their second decade of life, with a peak incidence in the fifth decade suggesting that urinary calculus disease has a tendency to persist over a long period of an individual's life. Long-term studies of individuals in military service have shown that the chance of having one or more recurrence of a urinary calculus disease over a period of several years is more than 60% for a male with idiopathic urinary lithiasis (Blacklock 1969). The peak risks of recurrence are either early, at about 18 months, or later, at about eight years. Interestingly, autopsy studies have shown equal incidence of upper urinary tract calcification in males and females.

Anderson (1973) believes that at least two separate epidemiological factors are involved in the genesis of urinary calculi. The first are intrinsic factors related to inherited biochemical or anatomical aspects of the individual. For instance, African Bantu and North American blacks have very low rates of urinary calculi. Superimposed on these factors are other extrinsic or environmental factors which include climate, drinking water, dietary patterns, and occupation. Britain has a relatively high incidence of urinary tract stones. It is difficult to link climate directly to the occurrence of urinary stones, although in most countries there does appear to be a seasonal difference in the clinical presentation of calculi, with the peak incidence occurring in July, August, and September. It is probable that elevated environmental temperature, resulting in a degree of dehydration and therefore a high concentration of urine, may contribute to stone formation. Patients with a tendency towards formation of uric acid or cysteine calculi always have an additional risk as acid urine holds much less of either of these substances in solution. Apart from the volume drunk, it has also been suggested that the mineral content of water may play a part. There is no hard evidence that trace elements in water increase the risk of urinary stones although it has been suggested that zinc is an inhibitor of calcium crystallization and therefore low urinary levels could encourage a tendency towards stone formation. There is no definite proof that water hardness or softness or trace-element content is critical to stone formation. There is little doubt that diet may influence the formation of urinary stones. Ingestion of excessive amounts of purines (uric acid, oxylates, and calcium phosphate) may result in excessive excretion of these components in urine.

Acute stone disease

Urinary calculus usually presents with an acute episode of renal or ureteric colic. The level of the pain associated with the episode often indicates the site of the stone, with the pain moving from the kidney to the flank into the iliac fossa and the groin as the stone moves lower. In general, it is said that a stone less than 4 mm in diameter will pass down the ureter spontaneously in more than 90% of cases, without the need for intervention. Larger stones may of course pass, and stones of over a centimetre in diameter have passed spontaneously. The majority of small stones will cause an acute episode of pain, and if they do not pass spontaneously they will often become asymptomatic. A small percentage will cause some degree of obstruction, although total obstruction is unlikely with a stone less than 4 mm in diameter. However, full investigation is necessary in order to ascertain the degree of obstruction and the function of the contralateral kidney. Investigation of a patient presenting with acute renal or ureteric colic should include urinalysis. It should be recognized that 10% of patients with ureteric stones do not have haematuria, either microscopic or macroscopic. This is especially true of calculus causing complete obstruction. Moderate pyuria may occur. A plain abdominal film will reveal a calculus in 90% of cases. An intravenous urogram is necessary to identify translucent or non radio–opaque calculi, to identify obstruction and to assess function on the contralateral side.

The initial step in management of a patient with acute ureteric colic is pain relief. Pethidine is gradually being superseded by the use of a non-steroidal inflammatory drug, particularly diclofenac, given either orally, intramuscularly, or per rectum. Antibiotics should be considered if there is any sign of fever. In general, a small stone causing minimal obstruction to the ureter, with symptoms controllable by non-steroidal anti-inflammatories, can safely be left, the patient discharged, and subsequently reviewed after four to six weeks with a plain X-ray. For a larger stone, or one causing significant obstruction or persisting symptoms, intervention will be indicated. Depending upon the position of the stone this may be endoscopic to relieve obstruction, or ureteroscopic destruction of the stone, or by utilizing extra corporeal shockwave lithotripsy (ESWL).

Until recently, the standard management of a large renal stone was by surgical removal. However, larger renal stones can be dealt with percutaneously with a track made directly into the kidney and the stone destroyed *in situ*, using ultrasonic or electrohydraulic lithotriptors passed down the percutaneous track and the pieces washed out. The advent of ESWL will now allow any remaining fragments to be cleared, and it is quite effective for non-obstructing ureteric stones with clearance rates of almost 90% in some series. Both ureteroscopy and ESWL require specialist urological intervention although the advent of the mobile lithotriptors has made the full range of stone treatment techniques available to urologists in all district hospitals.

Diseases of the prostate

The prostate is a gland sitting at the base of the bladder and encircling the prostatic urethra and lying between the bladder neck and the distal urethral sphincter. It contributes
approximately 30% of the secretions that make up the ejaculate. This gland is something
of an enigma in that it provides an enormous clinical workload due to inflammation,
benign enlargement, and malignant change while its function is not fully understood.
Our ignorance was summarized by Franks (1983): 'The gland is inaccessible during life,
its secretions are difficult to collect, and it shows no known easily measurable function. It
is not essential for life and is associated in some way with reproduction, but even for this
it is not essential.' In view of all this, perhaps it is small wonder that in a recent survey of
men, MORI found that only 13% of men could correctly identify the prostate gland,
although 16% of women could (MORI 1995). Nonetheless, the prostate is an enormous
source of morbidity and workload in both general and urological practice.

Benign prostatic hyperplasia (BPH)

BPH is a common change associated with increasing age, found in autopsy studies to be
absent below the age of 30 years, but present in 85% of subjects over the age of 80 years in
the UK (Franks 1954). Garraway (1991) has demonstrated in a Scottish community-
based study involving questionnaires, urine flow measurement, and transrectal ultrasound prostatic volume measurements that the prevalence of symptomatic BPH is more
than 25% in men aged 40–79 years. Arrighi (1990) showed that at the age of 55, approximately 25% of men note a decrease in the force of their urinary stream and by the age of
75 this has increased to nearly 50%. In the US, the cumulative prevalence of BPH for a
40-year-old man surviving to the age 80 is 78% and the chance of prostatectomy is 29%
(Glynn 1985), while in the United Kingdom the lifetime risk for requiring a prostatectomy in a man from the age of 50 is approximately 10%. At present, prostatectomy is considered the most effective long-term treatment for BPH. Almost 50000 transurethral
resections of the prostate are performed in the United Kingdom each year. It is one of the
most commonly performed surgical procedures in Western countries, transurethral
prostatectomy (TURP) having become more popular than the retropubic technique during the 1970s. However, a retrospective study involving 54000 patients in Denmark, England, and Canada demonstrated a reoperation rate of at least 12% after TURP compared
with less than 4.4% after the open procedure within eight years of the initial surgery (Roos
1989). In addition, this study suggested a higher long-term mortality associated with
TURP compared to that associated with open prostatectomy. An interview-based study
of 434 postprostatectomy patients in the USA reported the occurrence of short-term
complications of varying severity in 24% of patients; 5% complained of postoperative
erectile dysfunction and 4% of persistent incontinence at 12 months (Fowler 1988). The
authors concluded that a significant improvement in indices of quality of life following
surgery occurred only among patients with severe symptoms or acute retention of urine.
A recent prostatectomy audit from Stirling (McKelvie *et al.* 1992) recorded short-term
post-TURP complications, varying in severity from postoperative urinary retention to
septicaemia, in 40% of 142 patients. The commonest late complication is retrograde
ejaculation.

'Watch and wait' in managing BPH

Men, in a study from Bristol (Ball 1981), were studied for up to five years without treatment. Approximately one-third improved; the majority were symptomatically stable and as few as 20% required surgery. In other words, a 'watch and wait' policy is entirely reasonable in men with mild or moderate symptoms of bladder outflow obstruction and minimal disruption to their lives. Such men are unlikely to develop any serious complications. It is recognized that primary symptoms of bladder outflow obstruction secondary to BPH are reduced urinary stream, hesitancy, and a feeling of incomplete emptying. Secondary or irritative symptoms, because the bladder is working harder against an obstruction, may include frequency of micturition, nocturia, and urgency with occasional urge incontinence. Arrighi (1990) showed that in men with the primary symptoms of bladder outflow obstruction, 38% required prostatectomy. In those with secondary or irritative symptoms, only 8% required an operation. Secondary symptoms can also be caused by other conditions such as bladder stone, detrusor instability, and bladder tumours. It is the practice in most urology units to obtain free urinary flow rates and measurement of residual urine as objective measures of bladder outflow obstruction. A normal peak flow rate will usually exceed 15 ml/sec, and in a younger man 25 ml/sec, with the whole flow being complete within a few seconds. When the flow is obstructed the peak flow is less than 15 ml/sec, and the whole flow is prolonged with some residual urine remaining in the bladder.

Transurethral incision of the prostate and lasers

Increasing awareness of the drawbacks of prostatectomy among urologists and the general public has prompted growing interest in various alternatives to standard operations. These alternatives, some of which are currently undergoing clinical trials, include transurethral incision of the prostate (TUIP), transurethral laser prostatectomy, drug treatment, balloons, stents, and hyperthermia. Transurethral incision of the prostatic urethra and bladder neck under direct vision has gained popularity since its introduction in 1973 for treatment of the small (less than 40 cm^3) obstructing prostate without median lobe enlargement. The advantages of this procedure over TURP include shorter operating time, reduced complications such as haemorrhage and the TUR syndrome, and reduced hospital stay. In the majority of series, the outcome of TUIP is equivalent to that of TURP. The technique is applicable to smaller prostates.

There have been several favourable reports of neodymium YAG laser vaporization of BPH tissue. This is carried out either using conventional endoscopic instrumentation or purpose-built, ultrasound-guided equipment. Very large glands are considered unsuitable for this modality, but the procedure is fast and blood loss and hospital stay are minimized. Since tissue is not obtained for histological examination, prior systematic needle biopsies may be taken if there is clinical suspicion of malignancy. Randomized studies comparing TURP with laser prostatectomy are beginning to suggest that the latter may be as good a method of symptom relief.

Drugs

Drugs which modify smooth muscle activity can provide symptomatic relief to some patients, although these benefits are not always maintained. Alpha-adrenergic blocking agents inhibit myocontractility at the bladder neck and prostatic capsule, thereby reducing the 'dynamic' component of bladder outflow obstruction. Prompt improvement of urinary symptoms and flow rates are seen in over half the patients, at the expense of side-effects which include ataxia, tiredness, headache, and ejaculatory failure. Such effects occur in about one-third of patients taking the non-selective blockers (e.g. indoramin), but are less common in the case of the selective alpha-1 blockers, such as alfluozin or tamsulosin.

The second group comprises drugs which can potentially reverse, or at least arrest, the growth of prostatic 'adenoma' – both the epithelial and stromal (fibromuscular) components. The prostate is responsive to hormonal manipulation; males castrated before puberty apparently do not develop BPH and patients with symptomatic BPH who undergo orchidectomy or treatment with LHRH analogues experience symptomatic improvements and prostatic regression. Androgen receptors (AR) and oestrogen receptors (ER) are present on both epithelial and stromal prostatic cells, although epithelium exhibits predominant AR, while the majority of ER are found in the stroma. Two lines of hormonal manipulation have developed, one concerned with androgens and the other with oestrogens. Neither evoke a state of systemic androgen deprivation, unacceptable in the treatment of benign disease, since there is no interference with the hypothalamo–pituitary–testicular axis of testosterone production. 5-alpha reductase (5-AR) converts serum androgens, predominantly testosterone, into dihydrotestosterone (DHT) in target tissues which include the prostate. DHT is five times more active, in terms of its androgen receptor binding affinity, than testosterone. In the prostate, the DHT concentration is 10–20 times that of testosterone, while this relationship is reversed in the serum. However, in tissues devoid of 5-AR, such as muscle, testosterone is the active androgen. The inhibition of 5-AR induces a reduction of serum DHT concentration without affecting serum testosterone. DHT is considered an important mediator in the pre- and post-natal development of the prostate, forming complexes with androgen receptors which regulate gene expression. In BPH tissue, DHT concentrations tend to be higher than normal prostatic tissue. Moreover, males with congenital 5-AR deficiency do not develop BPH. Finasteride, a recently introduced competitive 5-AR inhibitor, reduces urinary symptom scores and prostatic volume, and increases maximum urine flow rates (by a mean value of only 1.6 ml/sec or 22%) compared to placebo over 12 months, while maintaining normal serum testosterone concentrations (Gormley *et al.* 1992). Curiously, the most common side-effect of finasteride is sexual dysfunction, seen in 5% patients. The results of long-term and combination (alpha-blockade + 5AR inhibition) studies are awaited.

A considerable proportion of men taking finasteride fail to show a response, possibly because their BPH is predominately stromal. Morphometric data indicate that the development of symptomatic BPH is associated with an increase in the proportion of stroma relative to epithelium. The enzyme aromatase metabolizes testosterone into oestradiol; it is found in certain tissues, including the prostate. The predominance of ER in prostatic stroma implicates oestrogens in the pathogenesis of BPH. The clinical efficacy of selective oestrogen withdrawal has, in the past, been impossible to evaluate because antihormones without intrinsic oestrogenic activity were not available; tamoxifen, for example, is unsuitable since it has oestrogenic properties. A specific competitive aromatase inhibitor is currently undergoing safety and efficacy trials in symptomatic BPH patients. Urine flow measurements are especially open to interpretation. It may not be necessary, however, for all patients to be seen by urologists prior to starting drug 'treatment'. Various shared care programmes are being developed in the United Kingdom to allow general practitioners access to investigations. In some cases, general practitioners will interpret the results and decide whether to refer on to a urologist; in others, the urologist will provide a reporting service with advice as to whether the patient needs further hospital evaluation.

Stents

Stents have been utilized to relieve bladder outflow obstruction. They consist of either expandable metal mesh stent, coil, or a plastic intra-urethral catheter. Whichever type is employed, their position in the prostatic urethra is designed to relieve the obstruction at this level. They are expensive, especially the metal stents, and are only of limited use in patients with outflow obstruction. They may have a role in patients with acute urinary retention who are otherwise poor candidates for surgery.

Prostatic carcinoma

Prostatic adenocarcinoma has been traditionally seen as a benign condition affecting elderly men and rarely causing death. The disease is found in as many as 50% of men over the age of 70 years at post-mortem (Breslow 1977), while only a small proportion will have had clinical problems associated with their tumours. In the majority of men with prostatic cancer, the tumour grows at a slow rate and other disease processes often intervene to cause death. Up to 80% five-year survival rate is found if local disease is left untreated (George 1988). Prostatic cancer does, however, occur in an appreciable and increasing number of men between the ages of 45 and 65 years. Increasing incidence and longevity means the death rate from prostate cancer is likely to rise over the next two decades. In England and Wales, the present incidence of the disease is 0.72 new cases per 1000 men between the ages of 55 and 70 years. In 1991, 8500 men died from this disease with about one-third of them being below the age of 65. In the European Union as a whole, it was estimated that there were 85 000 new cases of prostate cancer in 1980, and 35 084 men die annually from the disease. It is believed that it takes from 10 to 20 years to progress from the development of the tumour to the point where it may result in death or disability.

The challenges for the clinician in approaching prostate cancer are threefold. The first is to identify the disease and to do so at an early and potentially curable stage. The second is to stage the tumour, after diagnosis, accurately so that the most appropriate treatment may be offered to each individual patient. The third is that the various therapeutic modalities, both new and traditional measures, must be evaluated in order to identify the benefits and risks that may accrue.

Diagnosis

The simplest and cheapest test available to detect prostatic cancer is digital rectal examination. However, this is a particularly insensitive test, and when performed by non-urologists, the number of cancers detected is very low. Even when performed by a urologist, a nodule will be incorrectly diagnosed as being malignant in as many as 40% of cases, and staging errors will be made in as many as 50% of cases with cancer.

Transrectal ultrasonography is now gaining wide acceptance as a method of imaging the prostate. The majority of modern machines employ hand-held probes, with the patient in the lateral position. The true value of prostatic ultrasonography in routine clinical practice is as yet unclear. The skilled prostatic ultrasonographer can detect prostatic cancers as small as 0.5 cm in diameter (Lee *et al.* 1987). Other series, however, reported that ultrasonography may miss up to 40% of cancers, subsequently detected by random biopsy of the prostate.

Prostate specific antigen: tumour markers for prostate cancer

Prostatic acid phosphatase, the first tumour marker described in the 1930s, unfortunately had a low sensitivity. As few as 25% of patients with prostate cancer have raised serum levels of acid phosphatase. Another marker, prostate specific antigen (PSA), was introduced in the 1980s. PSA is a glycoprotein produced by the epithelial cells lining prostatic acini. It is present in normal, benign, and malignant prostatic tissue and is therefore prostate specific and not prostate cancer specific. Its function is that of a protease, responsible for cleaving fibronectin and aids in the liquefaction of semen. PSA was initially used as a tissue marker by histopathologists to identify the prostatic origin of adenocarcinomas. Several series have shown PSA to be a sensitive serum marker for the presence of prostatic carcinoma. A variety of different kits are now available for measuring the marker. The majority state similar normal ranges but individual laboratory variations should be taken into account.

In general, more than 97.5% of normal asymptomatic men with prostates that feel normal will have a PSA below 4 ng/ml. In this population, 25% of men with a PSA between 4 and 10 ng/ml, and 65% or more of those with a PSA above 10 ng/ml, will have prostate cancer. Unfortunately, symptomatic benign disease can also cause raised levels of PSA. In men presenting to urology clinics with symptomatic BPH, between 30 and 40% will have levels above 10 ng/ml, without evidence of prostate cancer. It has therefore been suggested that in symptomatic urology populations, a higher cut-off point than 4 ng/ml should be taken – up to 10 or even 20 ng/ml – in order to reduce the false positives. In other words, the upper level of normality for PSA will vary according to the patient population being studied. In a normal population it may be reasonable to take 4 ng/ml as the upper limit of normal. In a urology clinic, older patients with symptomatic BPH, in order to reduce the number of false positives without significant loss of sensitivity, it may be more reasonable to investigate those with a level of over 10 ng/ml. The level of concern about the presence of prostate cancer should also be taken into account. In other words, in a young man aged 55 with minimal urinary symptoms and a PSA of 6 ng/ml, investigation is probably mandatory. In these cases, active treatment for a localized prostate cancer may well be considered. However, in a man of 75 with a PSA of 6 ng/ml, clinically benign prostatic hyperplasia, and some urinary symptoms, the PSA level may safely be ignored as he is unlikely to have prostate cancer and, even if a localized tumour was present, active treatment would not be immediately indicated. Serum PSA is also a useful staging tool. In increasing tumour stage an increasing level of PSA will be found. A level of more than 30 ng/ml will usually be associated with tumour spread outside the prostate. A level of 60 ng/ml or above will be associated with advanced disease, and certainly a level of 100 ng/ml will usually indicate metastatic disease.

Screening

The effectiveness of screening to reduce prostate cancer mortality is not known (Schroder 1995). There is little evidence that digital rectal examination is a useful screening procedure (Denis *et al.* 1995) but research into the value of the PSA test in asymptomatic men, with or without digital rectal examination, is in progress.

There is no doubt that localized tumours of the prostate can be detected. The level of PSA plus digital rectal examination identified prostate cancer in about 1.7% of asymptomatic men screened, aged 55–70 years (Chadwick *et al.* 1991). Two major problems are the relatively low specificity of the test and concern that treatment of many men with small and perhaps innocuous tumours might result in considerable iatrogenic morbidity. As the PSA level increases with age and gland size, various refinements have been proposed. These include age-specific normal values (Oesterling *et al.* 1993), the change in PSA with repeated measurements (the PSA velocity) (Carter *et al.* 1992), the ratio of PSA level to gland volume (the PSA density) (Benson *et al.* 1992), and the ratio of free to complexed PSA in the serum (Stenman *et al.* 1991). Also, it has been reported that there is some physiological variation in PSA levels (Stamey *et al.* 1995). Nonetheless, PSA levels are extremely useful in monitoring the progress of prostate cancer among those with urinary symptoms and in assessing the effectiveness of treatment.

Staging

The accurate staging of prostatic cancer involves assessment of the local extent of the tumour, the lymph node status, and the presence or absence of distant metastases. It is important to obtain such data in order to be able to offer appropriate treatment, estimate likely prognosis, and to assess the outcome of treatment. The histological grade of the cancer also is related to the extent of the tumour. If the histological grade of the tumour is high, there is a strong likelihood of advanced disease being present. Unfortunately, even when digital staging and histological assessment are combined, staging errors of between 7% and 56% have been reported. Despite the introduction of high-tech imaging, including transrectal ultrasonography and MRI, it is still difficult to detect early spread outside the prostate. One of the main problems when staging prostatic cancer is that, in a large proportion of patients with apparently localized tumours, spread to regional lymph nodes has already occurred; and once regional lymph-node spread has occurred, prognosis is significantly worsened.

Effect of stage and grade on prognosis

At any age, a patient with a high-grade or aggressive tumour has a median survival of approximately two years (from diagnosis and after commencing hormonal therapy). With lower-stage disease, prognosis depends upon the patient's age and the aggressiveness of the tumour. A well-differentiated, early lesion confined to one lobe of the prostate is associated with a progression rate of less than 20% at five years and a mortality of 10%. This increases linearly, but obviously in a man over the age of 70, a slowly progressive tumour such as this will not affect his overall life expectancy. A moderately differentiated nodule within one lobe of the prostate and confined to the gland is associated with a five-year survival of 80%, although 50% of tumours will have shown signs of progression, a ten-year survival of 60%, and a fifteen-year survival of 35%. In these cases there may have been symptomatic progression either locally or with distant metastases. Moderately differentiated localized disease is still slow growing but an appreciable number of patients will progress to metastases and die during a ten-year period, especially if the disease affects both lobes of the gland. Therefore, in younger patients with a ten-year life expectancy there may be an argument for considering curative treatments for localized prostate cancers.

Treatment

Localized disease

When curative treatment is being considered, two treatment options are available; radical surgery and radiation therapy. Radical prostatectomy is now performed via the retropubic approach and involves removal of the whole prostate and seminal vesicles. It is usually combined with pelvic lymphadenectomy. The morbidity of this approach is less than with a perineal approach and the nerve-sparing approach has further reduced complications such as impotence. The results of radical surgery depend on the stage and grade of the cancer. Patients with focal early tumours confined to one lobe of the prostate have 10-year survival rates comparable with men of the same age without cancer (Nichols 1977). However, older patients with such tumours can usually have a normal life span with conservative therapy (Hanash *et al.* 1972). More widespread disease within the gland or a definite T2 nodule is likely to progress if untreated, and recurrence rates of only 24% within 15 years following surgery have been achieved (Jewett 1975). The results of surgery for more advanced disease are less promising with Schroeder and Belt (1975) reporting a 10-year survival rate of 36% for T3 tumours treated by radical prostatectomy and oestrogens. However, tumour-associated morbidity is less in patients treated surgically.

The second method of treating localized prostatic cancer is with radiation therapy. The most optimistic advocates of radiotherapy claim a 15-year survival of 50–60% for T2 tumours and 18% for T3 disease. The morbidity of radiation therapy includes radiation cystitis, portcullis, and fistula formation.

Advanced disease

Once the disease has spread beyond the confines of the prostate, cure is impossible at the present time. Hormonal manipulation is the standard treatment for advanced prostatic cancer and is aimed primarily at palliation. Androgen withdrawal has become the mainstay of treatment for patients with metastatic and locally advanced prostatic cancer. The androgen dependence of prostatic adenocarcinoma was first established more than 50 years ago by Huggins and Hodges (1940). Oral oestrogens and bilateral orchidectomy subsequently became the standard primary treatments for advanced prostatic cancer. However, in recent years it has become evident that the use of oestrogens may be associated with an increase in cardiovascular morbidity and mortality. As a result, bilateral orchidectomy has become the 'gold standard' against which all other therapies must be judged. At the present time, many new theories concerning hormonal treatment exist and newly developed pharmaceutical preparations are being evaluated in many centres.

Physiology

The basis for hormone treatment for prostatic cancer is the androgen dependence of prostatic tumour cells. The available treatments produce a response by depriving the cells of androgens. This can be achieved by interfering at one of several points along the hypothalamic–pituitary–gonadal axis or by blocking androgen receptors at the level of the prostate. Despite the apparent hormone dependence of prostatic cancer, ultimately, almost all these cancers, even after hormonal treatment, will progress. Prostatic cancers consist of varying proportions of androgen-dependent and androgen-independent cells. Once androgens are withdrawn, the dependent clones will regress. However, the independent clones will continue to progress until the tumour again reaches clinically significant proportions. It is evident that, if this theory is correct, the response of the tumour will depend upon the proportion of androgen-dependent cells present.

Conventional methods of androgen withdrawal

1. *Bilateral orchidectomy.* Bilateral orchidectomy has become the standard form of hormonal manipulation, producing a rapid reduction in circulating testosterone to 'castration' levels (< 2 nmol/L) within 12 hours. The procedure is simple and safe and may be performed in unfit patients using a spinal or local anaesthetic. Complications are hot flushes and impotence, occurring in 58–85% of men so treated. This must be tempered by the finding in the same study that 70% of men with advanced prostatic cancer were no longer sexually active prior to castration. The psychological effects of castration have often been quoted as a reason for not performing orchidectomy, although little data exists to support this contention. In an attempt to help prevent psychological problems, a subcapsular orchidectomy is often used in order to leave a palpable intrascrotal remnant.

2. *Antiandrogens.* Antiandrogens are compounds which block the effect of androgens. They achieve this by inhibiting the metabolism of androgens at the cellular level. These compounds produce their effect by a variety of mechanisms and often act in other ways apart from simple androgen blockade. Several such agents have been produced; however, only one, cyproterone acetate, is widely used. One pure antiandrogen, flutamide, is also available.

3. *Luteinizing hormone releasing hormone agonists.* Luteinizing hormone releasing hormone (LHRH) is produced by the neuroendocrine cells of the hypothalamus in a pulsatile fashion. Various synthetic analogues have been produced, most of them are more potent than the natural compound. LHRH normally causes the anterior pituitary to release luteinizing hormone (LH) and follicle stimulating hormone (FSH), which in turn acts upon the testes. LH acts upon the Leydig cells of the testes which produce testosterone. Administration of an LHRH analogue will cause an initial rise in testosterone production (Siddall *et al.* 1986). However, chronic administration of a LHRH analogue will result in pituitary depletion of LH and a down regulation of LHRH receptors within the pituitary. This insensitivity of the pituitary to LHRH results in a reduction in LH and therefore in testosterone production. This is the basis of the use of LHRH analogues for androgen reduction in prostatic cancer. The initial surge in testosterone levels is termed the flare reaction and usually will be complete within 12–14 days. Initially, daily doses of LHRH analogues were required either by subcutaneous injection or frequent intranasal

application in order to achieve androgen suppression. Depot preparations are now available, reducing the frequency of treatment to one injection every 28 days, and the future holds the promise of depot injections lasting up to three months. The complications of LHRH analogues are the same as those of bilateral orchidectomy – hot flushes and erectile impotence. It would seem that LHRH analogues provide an alternative to surgical castration.

4. *Combination therapy: total androgen suppression.* It has been suggested that in addition to medical or surgical castration, blocking adrenal androgens with an anti-androgen can improve response rates. A combination of an LHRH analogue and flutamide has been shown in some trials to bring about marginal improvement in survival in men with low volume metastatic disease.

The most useful palliation for patients with painful relapse is radiotherapy and high-dose intravenous oestrogens. External beam radiotherapy is useful for relieving localized pain from metastatic disease. Whole or half-body radiotherapy is valuable in patients with more diffuse widespread pain secondary to their disease. Oral steroids, such as hydrocortisone or dexamethasone, are valuable in the terminal stages of the disease.

Conclusion

We are in the fortunate position of being able to offer effective treatment, and when that fails, to be able to provide reasonable palliation. Apart from preventing serious complications, pain will be reduced and, although difficult to quantify, patients report a general improvement in well-being once hormonal therapy is instituted. The only way of improving survival at this time is by identifying tumours whilst still at a curable stage.

Bladder cancer

Bladder cancer is one of the commoner malignancies and, in general, the majority of tumours of the urinary bladder are transitional cell carcinomas (TCC). A small proportion will be adenocarcinomas, either primary tumours associated with urachal remnants or secondary lesions usually involving the bladder by direct spread from a sigmoid or rectal carcinoma. Squamous cell carcinoma also occurs and is often associated with chronic irritation with schistosomiasis being the commonest cause worldwide.

Transitional cell carcinoma is one of the few malignancies with a well-documented environmental aetiology. In as many as one-third of cases environmental agents such as smoking or occupational exposure can be identified. Occupational risks include dye, chemical and rubber workers, and those exposed to paints.

Haematuria is a presenting symptom of bladder malignancy in up to 90% of cases. In addition, some patients will present with dysuria, frequency, and apparent urinary infection. It is important to diagnose bladder carcinoma early as there is some evidence that early diagnosis will improve prognosis. A patient over the age of 40 presenting with painless haematuria should undergo full investigation, including urine cytology which will be positive in 70% of bladder tumours, imaging the urinary tract with ultrasound scan or intravenous urography, the latter still being preferred by many, and cystoscopy. Approximately 20% of men over the age of 40 presenting with macroscopic haematuria will have bladder cancer. Another 25–30% will have other pathology but in about 50% no cause for the haematuria will be identified.

The treatment of bladder cancer depends upon its stage. At diagnosis approximately 25% of transitional cell carcinomas will have shown signs of invasion into the bladder muscle or spread beyond the bladder. A muscle invasive tumour, if still confined to the bladder, will usually be treated radically either with radical radiotherapy or cystectomy. A tumour which has spread beyond the bladder involving local structures with lymph node metastases or distant metastases has gone beyond cure and palliative treatment will be offered, either radiotherapy or chemotherapy. Occasionally, palliative urinary diversion will be necessary.

Seventy per cent of TCC at diagnosis, however, will still be superficial and confined to the superficial layers of the bladder wall. The majority of these cases can be kept under control by endoscopic resection and regular cystoscopic review. A small proportion will show signs of progression and will ultimately require more radical treatment. A proportion will also have poor prognostic signs at diagnosis, including poor differentiation, early signs of lamina propria invasion, multifocality, or association with a carcinoma *in situ*. These may also come to early radical treatment. In those showing signs of problematic features or progression, intravesical chemotherapy or intravesical immunotherapy with BCG may be used in an attempt to halt progression.

Testicular cancer

The detection of a testicular mass by the patient or physician is the usual presentation. Testicular tumours can be divided into two main categories: seminomas and non-seminomatous tumours. Non-Hodgkin's lymphomas are the commonest other type of testicular cancer and occur more commonly in older men.

The concept of carcinoma *in situ* of the testis acquired at an early age, probably during fetal development, has been proposed (Skakkebaek 1972). It appears to be a precursor of both seminoma (except spermatocytic seminoma) and non-seminomatous tumours of the testis (Muller *et al.* 1984; Muller *et al.* 1987; Skakkebaek *et al.* 1987). Regression of carcinoma *in situ* of the testis has not been reported (Giwercman 1992). Carcinoma *in situ* of the contralateral testis is present in about 5 per cent of men with a diagnosis of testicular cancer and the presence of carcinoma *in situ* appears to significantly increase the risk of the development of a second testicular tumour. Research into the possible development of a screening test of semen to detect carcinoma *in situ* of the testis is being undertaken (Giwercman 1992).

A reduced sperm count is common among men presenting with testicular cancer and this may be associated with atrophy of the contralateral testicle. As a result, some men are infertile at the time of diagnosis. Shielding of the contralateral testicle is undertaken when localized disease is treated by radiotherapy alone without loss of fertility. Fertility is usually affected by chemotherapy but some men recover from iatrogenic azoospermia and quite a few father children (Fossa *et al.* 1985; Roth *et al.* 1988). Bilateral, radical, retroperitoneal, lymph-node dissection usually results in infertility by producing retrograde ejaculation or ejaculatory failure. Where facilities exist, the banking of sperm should be offered to patients prior to treatment.

Epidemiology

Survival after diagnosis is good (Adami *et al.* 1992, Stiller and Bunch 1990). The incidence of testicular cancer has been doubling every 25 years in several populations: the United Kingdom, Denmark, and among United States whites (Forman *et al.* 1990). In Denmark, the risk of testicular cancer has been found to be lower for men born during the Second World War and this may have been, among other things, due to altered maternal diet, average maternal age, or average parity of mothers during wartime (Moller 1989).

Differences exist between the epidemiology of seminoma and teratoma of the testis. The age at which the incidence of teratoma is maximal is at about 30 years of age while the incidence rate of seminoma is a maximum at about 40 years of age (Nethersell *et al.* 1984). In general, few aetiological studies have examined these two predominant types of testicular cancer separately, but when this has been possible few notable differences have been found (Pike *et al.* 1997). Because of the large variation in the incidence rates of testicular cancer around the world, a predominant cause of this cancer is thought to be environmentally determined. However, migrants from low-risk to high-risk countries appear not to increase their risk in their new country (Forman *et al.* 1990).

The main risk factors for germ cell tumours of the testis are undescended testes, white race, and previous testicular cancer (Forman *et al.* 1990). Maldescent of one testis increases the risk of testicular cancer for both testes and orchidopexy does not appear to eliminate the increased risk (Vogelzang and Lange 1991). Undescended testes are associated with between a fourfold and 10-fold increase in the risk of testicular cancer (Forman *et al.* 1990). Urogenital developmental abnormalities associated with gonadal dysgenesis, generalized testicular atrophy, and orchitis after mumps are possible aetiological factors for germ cell cancers of the testis. The maternal or pregnancy characteristics associated with an increased risk of testicular cancer are: low birth weight; high maternal weight relative to height; high maternal age; being a first born son; and nausea, hyperemesis, or uterine bleeding during pregnancy (Forman *et al.* 1990). Also, inguinal hernia in the absence of cryptorchidism, high socio-economic status, and non-racial genetic factors appear to be associated with an increased risk of testicular cancer. These risk factors suggest an influence of the hormonal environment *in utero* in the later development of testicular cancer.

Numerous other factors have been inconsistently linked to the development of testicular cancer. These include: being single, living in a rural environment, being a farmer, an early onset of puberty, obesity, exogenous oestrogen use of the mother during pregnancy, the wearing of tight jeans or tight underwear or increased scrotal temperature, acne, the season of birth, testicular trauma, certain infectious agents, and industrial exposure to dimethylformamide (Forman *et al.* 1990). Insufficient evidence currently exists to consider these exposures to be causal. Also, it has been suggested that some patients with a genetically determined predisposition to ichthyosis may be at increased risk of testicular cancer (Lykkesfeldt *et al.* 1991). Neither cigarette smoking, alcohol consumption, radiation exposure, not vasectomy (Brown *et al.* 1987; Nienhuis *et al.* 1992) appear to be associated with an increased risk of testicular cancer.

Prevention and control

There is evidence that diagnosis occurs earlier now than in the past (Kennedy *et al.* 1987). Testicular self-examination has occasionally been advocated in the hope that early detection of testicular cancer could lead to reduced mortality from this disease. Earlier diagnosis will inevitably be associated with increased survival from diagnosis compared to disease detected later through lead-time bias. No randomized controlled trial of the effect of this method of detection on mortality has been undertaken and any recommendation for self-examination does not have a strong scientific basis (Hayward *et al.* 1991).

Disparities in trends in mortality rates of testicular cancer between countries have been attributed to variations in the use of proven therapy, particularly the use or availability of cisplatinum (Boyle *et al.* 1990). In Ireland, a national programme to reduce mortality from testicular cancer has been established through a tumour registry which involves ensuring that appropriate therapy is used for all patients with testicular cancer (Thornhill and Walsh 1991).

Screening of the general population by testicular examination is not recommended by most well-known authorities in North America and several authors recommend against such screening (Hayward *et al.* 1991).

Urinary incontinence

The urinary tract should be anatomically complete and functioning at birth. Whilst the urinary tract is functioning as a conduit for urine it is uncontrolled. In the infant, the bladder fills and micturition occurs spontaneously as a spinal cord reflex. Distension of the bladder stimulates the afferent rim of the reflex arc, resulting in contraction of the bladder detrusor muscle. Even in infants, the voluntary external urinary sphincter contracts to prevent incontinence. However, relaxation occurs during micturition to allow bladder emptying. By the age of four years most children should have developed an adult pattern of urinary control and will be continent day and night. Normal continence in the adult depends upon an adequate reservoir that is the urinary bladder in which the detrusor muscle relaxes during filling, allowing adequate capacity for storage. Continence is maintained by the distal-urethral sphincter, located within the wall of the urethra, just distal to the apex of the prostate. The bladder neck sphincter, contiguous with the prostatic urethra, is mainly responsible for preventing retrograde ejaculation but may have some role in continence in men.

Incontinence in men can be divided into the following:

1. *Urge incontinence which may be secondary to detrusor instability or hypersensitivity of the bladder.* If due to the former, it is secondary to unstable waves of contraction occurring in the detrusor muscle at inappropriate times, producing high pressure within the bladder and urine leakage as the resistance due to the distal urethral sphincter is overcome. This may be secondary to bladder outflow obstruction, or a primary idiopathic condition. It can be identified on a frequency volume chart, the patient often voiding small volumes frequently, both day and night time, with associated incontinence. It should be confirmed urodynamically (see above). Detrusor instability in the absence of obstruction should be corrected initially by bladder

retraining. In this technique the patient is told to try to hold on to his urine when he has the urge to void for a set amount of time beyond the initial point. By doing this regularly, the bladder can be retrained in a proportion of patients. The second-line treatment is medical therapy with anticholinergic agents such as oxybutinin. These agents may have side-effects due to the anticholinergic effect. If used in patients with symptoms secondary to bladder outflow obstruction it may exacerbate the condition.

2. *Stress incontinence or incontinence secondary to distal urethral sphincter weakness.* In men, the most frequent cause of this is damage, either surgically after transurethral resection of prostate, or radical prostatectomy. It may also occur if prostate cancer has invaded the distal sphincter. It is analogous to stress incontinence seen in parous women. Stress incontinence can be diagnosed clinically if a man leaks urine when he coughs or laughs or stands up quickly. It should be confirmed using urodynamic studies which will reveal a weak distal sphincter and leakage of contrast medium per urethra on coughing or straining. Stress incontinence can be improved by pelvic floor exercises. If severe, an artificial urinary sphincter placed around the bulba urethra may be indicated.

3. *Post-micturition dribbling.* Many men complain of dribbling urine after completion of micturition. This is, in fact, quite a common complaint with up to 25% of normal men having some degree of post-micturition dribbling due to trapping of urine in the urethra. It is rarely associated with any serious bladder pathology. Urethral massage from the perineum forwards can help clear the trapped urine.

4. *Incontinence may occur secondary to chronic urinary retention.* This is a form of over-flow incontinence and clinical examination, combined with ultrasonic measure-ment of residual urine, should help identification of this condition.

References

Adami, H.-O., Glimelius, B., Sparen, P., Holmberg, L., Krusemo, U. B., and Ponten, J. (1992). Trends in childhood and adolescent cancer survival in Sweden 1960 through 1984. *Acta Oncologica,* **31**, 1–10.

Anderson, D. A. (1973). Environmental factors in the etiology of urolithiasis and urinary calculi. In urinary calculi. International symposium on renal stone research (Eds L. Cifuentes, A. Rapado, A. Hodgkinson). S. Karger, New York.

Arrighi, H. M., Guess, H. A., Metter, E. J., *et al.* (1990). Symptoms and signs of prostatism as risk factors for prostatectomy. *Prostate,* **16**, 253–61.

Bagshaw, M. A. (1985). Potential for radiotherapy alone in prostatic cancer. *Cancer,* **55**, 2079.

Ball, A. J., Feneley, R. C., and Abrams, P. H. (1981). The natural history of untreated prostatism, *British Journal of Urology,* **53**, 613–6.

Benson, M. C., Whang, I. S., Panturk, A., Ring, K., Kaplan, S. A., Olsson, C. A., *et al.* (1992). Prostate specific antigen density: a means of distinguishing benign prostatic hypertrophy and prostate cancer. *Journal of Urology,* **147**, 815–16.

Blacklock, N. J. (1969). The pattern of urolithiasis in the Royal Navy. In: Renal Stone Research Symposium (ed A. Hodgkinson, B. E. C. Nordin) J. A. Churchill, London.

Boyle, P., Maisonneuve, P. and Kaye, S. (1990). Therapy for testicular cancer in Central and Eastern Europe. *Lancet*, **335**, 1033. (Letter).

Breslow, N., Chan, C. W., Dhom, G. (1977). Latent carcinoma of prostate at autopsy in seven areas. *International Journal of Cancer*, **20**, 680–8.

Brown, L. M., Pottern, L. M., and Hoover, R. N. (1987). Testicular cancer in young men: the search for causes of the epidemic increase in the United States. *Journal of Epidemiology and Community Health*, **41**, 349–54.

Carter, H. B., Pearson, J. D., Metter, E. J., Brant, L. J., Chan, D. W., Andres, R., *et al.* (1992). Longitudinal evaluation of prostate-specific antigen levels in men with and without prostate disease. *Journal of the American Medical Association*, **267**, 2215–20.

Chadwick, D. J., Kemple, T., Astley, J. P., MacIvor, A. G., Gillat, D. A., Abrams, P., *et al.* (1991). Pilot study of screening for prostate cancer in general practice. *Lancet*, **338**, 613–16.

Del Regato, J. A. (1967). Radiotherapy in the conservative treatment of operable and locally inoperable carcinoma of the prostate. *Radiology*, **88**, 761.

Denis, L., Murphy, G. P., and Schroder, F. H. (1995). Report of the consensus workshop on screening and global strategy for prostate cancer. *Cancer*, **75**, 1187–207.

Flocks, R. H. (1973). The treatment of stage C prostatic cancer with special reference to combined surgical and radiation therapy. *Journal of Urology*, **109**, 461.

Forman, D., Gallagher, R., Moller, H., and Swerdlow, T. J. (1990). Aetiology and epidemiology of testicular cancer: report of consensus group. *EORTC Genito-urinary Group Monograph*, **7**, 245–53.

Fossa, S., Ous, S., Abyholm, T., Norman, N., and Loeb, M. (1985). Post-treatment fertility in patients with testicular cancer. II. Influence of cisplatin-based combination chemotherapy and of retroperitoneal surgery on hormone and sperm cell production. *British Journal of Urology*, **57**, 210–14.

Fowler, F. J., Wennberg, J. E., Timothy, R. P., *et al.* (1988). Symptom status and quality of life following prostatectomy. *Journal of the American Medical Association*, **259**, 3018.

Franks, L. M. (1954). Benign nodular hyperplasia of the prostate: a review. *Annals of the Royal College of Surgeons of England*, **14**, 92–106.

Franks, L. M. (1983). Origins of benign prostatic hypertrophy. In *Benign prostatic* hypertrophy (ed. F. Hinman), p. 141. Springer, New York.

Garraway, W. M., Collins, G. N., and Lee, R. J. (1991). High prevalence of benign prostatic hyperthrophy in the community. *Lancet*, **338**, 469–71.

George, N. J. R. (1988). Natural history of localised prostatic cancer managed by conservative therapy above. *Lancet*, **1**, 494.

Giwercman, A. (1992). Carcinoma *in situ* of the testis: screening and management. *Scandinavian Journal of Urology and Nephrology*, Suppl. **148**, 1–47.

Glynn, R. J., Campion, E. W., Bouchard, G. R., et al. (1985). The development of benign prostatic hyperplasia among volunteers in the normative ageing study. *American Journal of Epidemiology*, **121**, 78–90.

Gormley, G. J., Stoner, E., Bruskewitz, R. C., Imperato-McGinley, J., Walsh, P. C., McConnell, J. D., et al. (1992). The effect of finasteride in men with benign prostatic hyperplasia. The Finasteride Study Group. *New England Journal of Medicine*, **327**, 1185–91.

Hanash, K. A., Utz, D. C., Cook, E. N., et al. (1972). Carcinoma of the prostate: a 15-year follow-up. *Journal of Urology*, **107**, 450–3.

Hayward, R. S. A., Steinburg, E. P., Ford, D. E., Roizen, M. F., and Roach, K. W. (1991). Preventive care guidelines: 1991. *Annals of Internal Medicine*, **114**, 758–83.

Huggins, C. and Hodges, C. V. (1941). Studies on prostatic career. *Cancer Research*, **1**, 293–7.

Jewett, H. J. (1975). The present status of radical prostatecting for stages A and B prostatectomy. Urology clinics of North America, 2. *Radiology*, **163**(2), 515–20.

Kennedy, B. J., Schmidt, J. D., Winchester, D. P., Peace, B. L., Natarajan, N., and Mettlin, C. (1987). National survey of patterns of care for testis cancer. *Cancer*, **60**, 1921–30.

Lee, F., Littrup, P. J., Torp-Pedersen, S. T., Mettlin, C., McHugh, T. A., Gray, J. M. et al. (1988). Prostate cancer: comparison of transrectal US and digital rectal examination for screening. *Radiology*, **168**, 389–94.

Lykkesfeldt, G., Bennett, P., Lykkesfeldt, A. E., Micic, S., Rorth, M., Skakkebaek, N. E., et al. (1991). Testis cancer. Ichthyosis constitutes a significant risk factor. *Cancer*, **67**, 730–4.

McKelvie, G. B., Morison, M., Hehir, M., Rogers, A. C. (1992). A prostatectomy audit: phase I-insights and questions. *British Journal of Urology*, **69**, 163–8.

Moller, H. (1989). Decreased testicular cancer risk in men born in wartime. *Journal of the National Cancer Institute*, **81**, 1668–9. (Letter).

MORI (1995). *Men's Health. Research study conducted for the Reader's Digest*. MORI, London.

Muller, J., Skakkebaek, N. E., Nielsen, O. H., and Graem, N. (1984), Cryptorchidism and testis cancer. Atypical infantile germ cells followed by carcinoma in situ and invasive carcinoma in adulthood, *Cancer*, **54**, 629–34.

Muller, J., Skakkebaek, N. E., and Parkinson, M. C. (1987). The spermatocytic seminoma: views on pathogenesis. *International Journal of Andrology*, **10**, 147–56.

Nethersell, A. B. W., Drake, L. K., and Sikora, K. (1984). The increasing incidence of testicular cancer in East Anglia. *British Journal of Cancer*, **50**, 377–80.

Nichols, R. T., Barry, J. M., and Hodge, C. V. (1977). The morbidity of radical prostatectomy for multifocal stage 1 prostatic adenocarcinoma. *Journal of Urology*, **117**, 83.

Nienhuis, II., Goldacrc, M., Scagroatt, V., Gill, L., and Vessey, M. (1992). Incidence of disease after vasectomy: a record linkage retrospective cohort study. *British Medical Journal*, **304**, 743–6.

Oesterling, J. E., Jacobson, S. J., Chute, C. G., Guess, H. A., Girman, C. J., Panser, L. A., et al. (1993). Serum prostate specific antigen in a community-based population of healthy men: establishment of age-specific reference ranges. *Journal of the American Medical Association*, **270**, 860–4.

Pike, M. C., Chilvers, C. E. D., and Bobrow, L. G. (1987). Classification of testicular cancer in incidence and mortality statistics. *British Journal of Cancer*, **56**, 83–5.

Roos, N. P., Wennberg, J. E., Malenka, D. J., *et al.* (1989). Mortality and reoperation after open and transurethral resection of the prostate for benign prostatic hyperplasia. *New England Journal of Medicine*, **320**, 1120–4.

Roth, B. J., Griest, A., Kubilis, P. S., Williams, S. D., and Einhorn, L. H. (1988). Cisplatin-based combination chemotherapy for disseminated germ cell tumours: long-term follow-up, *Journal of Clinical Oncology*, **6**, 1239–47.

Schaeffer, A. (1992). Infections of the urinary tract. In Campbells Urology vol 1, 6th edition (ed.P. C. Walsh, A. B. Renk, T. A. Stacey, E. D. Vaughan). pp. 731–806. WB Saunders, Philadelphia.

Schally, A. V., Arimura, A., Babay, *et al.* (1971). Isolation and properties of the FSH and LH releasing hormone. *Biochemistry and Biophysics Research Communications*, **43**, 393.

Schroder, F. H. (1995). Detection of prostate cancer. *British Medical Journal*, **310**, 140–1.

Shroeder, F. H. and Belt, E. (1975). Carcinoma of the prostate. A study of 213 patients with stage C tumours treated by total perineal prostatectomy. *Journal of Urology*, **114**, 257–60.

Siddall, J. K., Hetherington, J. W., Cooper, H., *et al.* (1986). Biochemical monitoring of carcinoma of prostate treated with an LHRH analogue. *British Journal of Urology*, **58**, 676–82.

Skakkebaek, N. E. (1972). Possible carcinoma *in situ* of the testis. *Lancet*, **2**, 516–17.

Skakkebaek, N. E., Berthelsen J. G., Giwercman A., and Muller, J. (1987). Carcinoma *in situ* of the testis: possible origin from gonocytes and precursor of all types of germ cell tumours except spermatocytoma. *International Journal of Andrology*, **10**, 19–28.

Stamey, T. A., Presigiacomo, A., and Komatsu, K. (1995). Physiological variation of serum prostate-specific antigen (PSA) from a screening population in the range 4–10 ng/ml using the Hypritech Tandem-R PSA assay. *Journal of Urology*, **153**, 420A. (Abstract).

Stenman, U. H., Leinonen, J., Alfthan, H., Ranniko, S., Tuhkanen, K., and Alfthan, O. (1991). A complex between prostate-specific antigen and alpha 1-antichromotrypsin is the major form of prostate-specific antigen in serum of patients with prostate cancer: assay of the complex improves clinical sensitivity for cancer. *Cancer Research*, **51**, 222–6.

Stiller, C. A. and Bunch, K. J. (1990). Trends in survival for childhood cancer in Britain diagnosed 1971–85. *British Journal of Cancer*, **62**, 806–15.

Thornhill, J. A. and Walsh, A. (1991). A national programme for testis cancer, the Irish Testis Tumor Registry (ITTR). *Archivio Italiano di Urologia, Nefrologia, Andrologia*, **63**, 37–42.

Vogelzang, N. J. and Lange, P. H. (1991). Tumours of the testes. In *Comprehensive textbook of oncology; volume two* (2nd edn) (ed. A. R. Moosa, S. C. Schimpff, and M. C. Robson). Williams and Wilkins, Baltimore.

CHAPTER THIRTEEN

Cardiovascular disease

Hugh Bethell

Cardiovascular disease is not just the major cause of death in the developed world; it is also responsible, more than any other group, for the excess of death among men. Some recent studies have suggested that cardiovascular disease is seen as a male preserve to the extent that women are under-represented both in research and in treatment. It also presents a paradox of its own as it affects men's health; while we know so much about the causes of cardiovascular disease in general, the reasons for the male excess are still unclear. Obviously, it would be impossible to deal with every aspect of cardiovascular disease in a few pages. This chapter therefore concentrates on those aspects that relate more clearly to men and those that shed any light on more general implications for men's health.

Cardiovascular disease is the largest cause of death in the United Kingdom, and is commoner among men than in women, particularly before the age of 75. The same pattern is true throughout the developed world, with rates for coronary heart disease (CHD) deaths among men in 1985 about three to four times higher than women's for 30–69 year olds (Waldron 1995). This differential is of great importance to both sexes – one sex it disables or kills prematurely while of the other it creates widows with years of solitary life ahead. In England and Wales, diseases of the circulatory system were responsible for 116800 deaths in men in 1995, with malignant neoplasms the next largest group at 73600. The comparable figures for women were 126500 and 67600 (ONS 1997). The excess of death among women from circulatory disease is surprising until it is remembered that it is a heterogeneous group comprising all causes and all ages. Looking only at deaths from ischaemic heart disease, the figures are 73100 for men compared with 60700 for women. Breaking down the whole group of circulatory disease by age, the figures are, for those aged 45–74, 52600 for men compared with 27900 for women, and for those aged 75 and over, 62300 for men and 97700 for women. The pattern varies in the countries of the European Union, with circulatory diseases causing between 9% (in Portugal) and 31% (in Eire) of deaths in men under the age of 65 (Department of Health 1993). However,

Khaw (1993) has pointed out that for women overall, CHD remains the leading cause of death and an important cause of disability. The tendency to see CHD as a 'male disease' has, she suggests, led to the majority of research into the causes, prevention, diagnosis, and treatment being carried out in men. Some recent evidence has examined the extent to which this has influenced doctors' attitudes to the management of patients with CHD and will be discussed below.

Hypertension

Blood pressure changes with the time of day, the day of the week, alterations in mood, variations in posture, the time of the last meal (and what it contained), the ambient temperature, and with myriad daily influences on the external and internal milieu. Moreover, these changes can be quite extreme and an individual may show a range of levels from the low to the very high in a short space of time. A particular influence on blood pressure may be doctors themselves, causing 'white coat' hypertension, when the blood pressure is high when measured by the physician and normal at other times (Mancia *et al.* 1983). This can be identified by asking patients to take their own pressures, but self-recording is not always reliable. A recent innovation has been ambulatory blood pressure monitoring. The patient wears a cuff attached to a machine which automatically inflates the cuff and records the blood pressure at intervals through the day and night. This usually reveals much lower pressures than are found in the surgery or hospital clinic. However, since all the results of controlled trials of treatment have been based on surgery or clinic measurements, it is impossible to tell at this stage what role ambulatory readings will play in the future. It is possible that ambulatory monitoring will lead to a revision of the diagnostic criteria for hypertension (Chatellier *et al.* 1993).

As blood pressure rises there is an increased risk of heart failure, renal failure, heart attack, and strokes. Unfortunately, there is no clear cut-off point at which this happens. The risks increase progressively with increased pressure, with an exponential shape to the risk curve which gets steeper as the pressure rises. Before deciding what level of blood pressure warrants reduction, there are two practical points:

1. A close approximation to intra-arterial pressure requires that the correct-sized cuff be used for its measurement. The 'standard' size cuff, 10 cm × 22 cm, is too small for accuracy in most adults, the 'large' size, 13 cm × 35 cm, being more appropriate. Obese patients need an 'outsize' cuff. Other problems with maintenance of sphygmomanometers can also lead to inaccurate readings.
2. Because of the great variability of blood pressure, it is important to record it on several occasions. By convention, it is generally agreed that three readings are required and even then it is usually best to delay drug treatment until non-pharmacological approaches have been given an adequate trial.

There is also a general agreement that patients with blood pressures above 160/95 benefit from treatment – that is not to say that everyone who has a pressure above this level *must* be treated, but certainly it is a level below which drug therapy is seldom indicated, except perhaps in those with diabetes mellitus. The British Hypertension Society has produced guidelines for the management of hypertension which place emphasis on the importance of considering coexisting risk factors and damage to target organs (Sever *et al.* 1993). However, Fahey has shown that the guidelines produced in different countries have widely different effects in terms of the level at which treatment is judged to have 'controlled' hypertension (Fahey and Peters 1996). Of the guidelines examined by Fahey, only those from New Zealand are explicit in terms of the absolute risk to individuals. They make it apparent that while men and women have similar distribution of blood pressure, the risk to individual men of CHD at each level of blood pressure, and therefore the benefit of treatment, is greater. Elderly males have the highest absolute risk and therefore benefit most from treatment; young females have very low absolute risk and therefore have least to gain in absolute terms (Jackson *et al.* 1993).

Management of hypertension

No drug therapy should be contemplated until non-pharmacological treatment has been applied. The height of the pressure and the presence of complications will decide how long this preliminary phase should last. Patients should be encouraged to make changes which are likely to reduce their own pressure without resorting to pills; and the greater the changes possible, the longer delayed should medication be. Patients may be able to help themselves by losing weight, aiming for a body mass index of 25 or less; giving up salt, which is an acquired taste (this should be done in a progressive way; firstly by giving up salty foods such as ham, bacon, and cheese, secondly, not adding salt on the plate, and finally, removing it from the cooking); reducing alcohol intake if this is excessive; taking up exercise; and reducing stress. Regular aerobic exercise, three or four times per week for half an hour or so, to a level which produces mild breathlessness, can result in significant falls in blood pressure (World Hypertension League 1991). Exercise also aids weight control, reduces blood cholesterol, and helps to dissipate stress. Anger, irritation, and frustration all seem to increase blood pressure, probably through noradrenaline secretion (Glass 1982). Overwork, long hours, and fatigue, particularly for those in subordinate roles, aggravate these emotional reactions. Patients should be advised to learn relaxation, the art of delegation, avoidance of unnecessary conflict, and long hours at work, and encouraged to enjoy more leisure and take up non-competitive sporting activities, all of which should help blood pressure control (Johnston 1991).

There is no doubt that patients find such advice hard to follow. Most hypertensive men are middle-aged or older, and the discovery of a raised blood pressure is unlikely to have such an impact that they readily change a well-accustomed way of life which has evolved over several decades. For instance, in one study both subjects and researchers found it very difficult to reduce their salt intake. At the end of the trial only two subjects said that they preferred the low-sodium diet, and they were found on urine testing not to be complying with the diet (Hart 1984). Most doctors find it extremely difficult to persuade their patients to lose weight. For men, there is the additional problem that it is often someone else who does the cooking in the household. This means that they may not be in control of what they eat and may have low levels of knowledge about nutrition when choosing their own meals. Most fat people grow inexorably fatter as they get older, however emphatically they are advised to lose weight. The Allied Dunbar National Fitness Survey (1992) has taught us just how unfit British men are, and this has triggered moves to encourage more exercise in the population. Following the example of the 'Oasis' project in Sussex, a large number of community sports centres have gone into partnership with local GPs to create exercise 'prescription' schemes. The GP prescribes the course, the patient is assessed by the sports centre staff and set a programme of, say, eight weeks' exercise, either free or at reduced rate, and the patient is then reassessed by the GP. The benefit to the sports centre is that people who would not usually take exercise start to do so, perhaps bringing in their family and friends, and continue to take part, at full cost, when the prescription has been fulfilled. It is important that the exercise is tempered to the individual's inclinations and capabilities or it will not be continued for long. Finally, it is my experience that men of working age find it impossible to reduce the stress levels under which they live because of economic necessity. Those who have retired usually have no need of this advice.

With such reservations in mind, general practitioners must consider carefully the balance of risks and benefits of counselling patients in this way during a period of observation before starting drug treatment. Some patients' pressures will fall without complying with any of these points; some will take the health message to heart with improvement in their health and prognosis; others may be either alienated by being given the advice or made to feel guilty by their inability to follow it.

Follow-up

It is essential to have an efficient follow-up system for patients with raised blood pressure, whether or not they are deemed to need treatment. Middle-aged men are usually infrequent consulters and tend to be at work during surgery hours. Some long-standing hypertensives can be relieved of their medication without recurrence (Aylett and Ketchin 1991). It is worth trying to tail well-controlled hypertensives off treatment from time to time, and this is particularly worthwhile after a change in lifestyle, i.e. at retirement.

Coronary artery disease

Coronary disease kills about 180 000 people annually in the UK, three-quarters of them men. The UK is near the top of the international league for coronary disease and parts of the country, notably Scotland, have the highest heart attack rate in the world. Men develop the disease on average 10 years earlier than women, and it accounts for about 50% of the deaths of men of working age. One man in 12 dies of a heart attack before retiring age.

Epidemiology

There is no single cause of coronary atheroma and its clinical consequences. Rather, there is a large number of 'risk factors' which are associated with the disease: some well-known, some becoming apparent, and some as yet undiscovered. Broadly, these risk factors can be divided into the fixed and the modifiable.

Fixed risk factors

1. *Age.* The prevalence of coronary disease and the incidence of new coronary events rise with age. The older you are the more likely you are to have angina and to suffer

a heart attack. Although heart attacks cause an absolutely greater number of deaths in the elderly, they are responsible for a smaller proportion of the death rate than in middle-aged men in whom other causes of death are less common. Myocardial infarction causes about 50% of the death rate in middle-aged men and about 25% in the elderly.

2. *Family history.* A family history of coronary disease confers a greater risk through a variety of mechanisms. The most clear-cut is familial hypercholesterolaemia, but there are less well-defined, probably polygenic, inherited elevations of blood lipids. Tendencies towards glucose intolerance, hypertension, and obesity may be inherited, as may raised fibrinogen levels and large platelets. Some familial trends have an environmental basis, i.e. diet, obesity, and cigarette smoking.

3. *Ethnicity.* Most of the differences between races in coronary disease prevalence are environmental. The risk of heart attack in Japan is extremely low, but the risk to Japanese who move to the USA and adopt the American lifestyle rapidly rises to native American levels (Nichaman *et al.* 1975). In the UK, however, Asians from the Indian subcontinent have a substantially greater risk of heart disease than the rest of the population, and this risk is associated with higher rates of diabetes and of 'central' obesity (Knight *et al.* 1992).

4. *Nutrition in fetal and early life.* Over the past few years, much debate has been generated by the idea that the uterine environment and patterns of growth in childhood influence the later development of coronary disease. In the UK, a strong geographic relationship has been shown between infant mortality in 1921–25 and coronary mortality in 1968–78 (Barker and Osmond 1986). Follow-up studies show an inverse relationship between weight at age one year and risk of dying of a heart attack in later life (Barker *et al.* 1989). Evidence of poor nutrition in fetal life and early childhood is associated with impaired glucose tolerance and raised blood pressure in middle age, and has led to the concept of 'programming' of the individual for coronary disease (Barker 1993).

Modifiable risk factors

1. *Cigarette smoking.* Of all self-inflicted causes of ill health, cigarette smoking is second to none. It is a major risk factor for coronary disease and the one which can be changed with more effect than any other. About 35% of men smoke, but as many as 70% of men who have a heart attack are smokers. A myocardial infarction is a most effective anti-smoking event, and most smokers can give up the habit after the attack. The mechanisms by which cigarette smoking causes or aggravates atheroma are not clear, but probably include the toxic effects of carbon monoxide, the vasospastic properties of nicotine, and the shortened clotting time produced by smoking.

2. *Raised blood lipids.* There is a direct relationship between total cholesterol and coronary risk, with an exponential shape to the curve. The best indicators of risk are a

high level of low-density lipoprotein cholesterol and a low ratio of high-density lipoprotein cholesterol to total cholesterol. The risk of heart disease increases with cholesterol level throughout its range, but overall mortality is lowest where the level is below 5.2 mmol/L, and this is the level below which the British Hyperlipidaemia Association recommends we aim (Betteridge 1993). However, the mean level in the population is nearer 6.0. The main determinants of blood cholesterol are heredity, diet and metabolic disorders such as diabetes. Type A behaviour is thought to raise blood cholesterol, and those who take regular aerobic exercise have higher HDL cholesterol than sedentary people.

3. *Hypertension.* There is a direct relationship between blood pressure and coronary risk and this holds good for both systolic and diastolic pressures. The effect is exponential, being small at levels within the normal range and rising rapidly above this; it is presumably mediated by mechanical effects upon the arterial wall. Treating hypertension reduces coronary risk by less than would be expected, and this may be because the most commonly used drugs, diuretics and beta-blockers, have adverse effects on blood lipids.

4. *Raised fibrinogen.* The relationship between plasma fibrinogen level and coronary risk is as strong as the cholesterol link (Yarnell *et al.* 1991). Fibrinogen is raised by heavy drinking and by smoking and accounts for at least 50% of the atherogenic effect of cigarettes (Meade *et al.* 1986). It is also an important risk factor in non-smokers. Raised fibrinogen increases blood viscosity, stimulates platelet aggregation, and promotes the laying down of fibrin on atheroma plaques.

5. *Obesity.* Obesity contributes to increased coronary risk by raising blood cholesterol and blood pressure, but is also a weak risk factor in its own right. 'Central' obesity is a better predictor of risk than the body mass index.

6. *Diabetes mellitus.* This is included among the modifiable risk factors because behaviour influences both the development of diabetes and the quality of its control. Diabetics have a risk of coronary disease three times that of the general population. In patients without overt diabetes, the links between insulin resistance, hypertension, and atheroma may be fundamental to the development of coronary disease (Reaven 1988). Insulin resistance is characterized by central obesity, resistance to insulin-stimulated glucose uptake with relative glucose intolerance, hyperinsulinaemia, increased triglycerides, decreased HDL cholesterol, and hypertension. The syndrome, which is sometimes called 'syndrome X', has both genetic and acquired contributions, as seen in Asians living in the UK who have a particularly high prevalence of the condition (Knight *et al.* 1992). Coincidentally, it has also been linked to the other 'syndrome X' which is the symptom of angina pectoris with angiographically normal coronary arteries (Swan *et al.* 1994).

7. *Lack of exercise.* Regular vigorous exercise counteracts raised blood pressure (World Hypertension League 1991), lowers blood cholesterol and triglycerides (Haskell

1986), aids weight control (Findlay *et al.* 1987), modifies high fibrinogen (Ferguson *et al.* 1987), and reduces insulin resistance (Schneider *et al.* 1984). Numerous epidemiological surveys have shown that those who exercise regularly have a low risk of developing coronary disease (Kannel and Sorlie 1979; Morris *et al.* 1990; Paffenbarger *et al.* 1993).

8. *Stress.* The evidence that stress contributes to heart disease was provided by the Western Collaborative Group Study (Rosenman *et al.* 1975). The trialists followed up for seven years nearly 4000 men who had been divided into those showing the type A behaviour pattern and those with type B behaviour. The type As had three times more coronary events that the type Bs. Type A behaviour includes aggression, competitiveness, goal-seeking, and time consciousness – it creates stress for the individual (and those around him) and is associated with anger, irritability, and frustration, emotions which increase noradrenaline secretion.

9. *Social class.* It is a popular misconception that heart attacks, being related to stress, are commoner among managers than workers. The opposite is true. Coronary disease is far more prevalent in social classes IV and V than in I and II (Pocock *et al.* 1987). This differential is mediated by poorer diet, more smoking, less recreational exercise, and greater frustration in daily living in the lower socio-economic groups (Shewry *et al.* 1992).

Reasons for the male excess of coronary heart disease

Waldron (1995) has reviewed the various explanations for the male excess in CHD. Among biological factors, sex hormones and body fat distribution are thought to be most important. The protective effect of oestrogens is inferred from the increased risk that comes after menopause or oophorectomy, and is thought to operate by increasing the level of high-density lipoprotein (HDL) cholesterol, which is generally 25% higher in women, and which may explain up to half of the difference in CHD mortality between men and women. The effect of male sex hormones is less certain, but it is also thought that higher levels of testosterone in men may cause lower levels of HDL cholesterol. Whereas obesity is felt to be a risk factor of itself, Waldron (1995) points out that there is a marked difference between men and women in body fat distribution, with men tending to accumulate fat in the upper body and women more in the buttocks and thighs. The waist-to-hip ratio may be associated with the ratio between HDL and LDL cholesterol and a predictor for coronary heart disease. Another biological factor which may be important is differential reaction between the sexes to stress; factors that appear not to explain the sex difference include blood pressure and blood-clotting mechanisms, where the pattern of distribution is similar between the sexes. Behavioural factors considered by Waldron include smoking, commoner among men and thought to be responsible for between a quarter and a half of the sex differences in CHD mortality. Diet may be important (beyond any effect on body fat) as women tend to eat more vegetables and fruit and may therefore have a higher intake of antioxidants. Any effect of exercise, on the other hand, should work to the advantage of men, who tend to take more exercise than women.

Finally, men have higher scores than women on measures of hostility and distrust of others and this may contribute to their greater risk of ischaemic heart disease. It is clear that this is nowhere near a complete answer: in a longitudinal survey of men and women in Scotland, after correction for cholesterol levels, smoking, diastolic blood pressure, body mass index, and social class, men in the age group 60–64 still had twice the ischaemic heart disease mortality as women of the same age (Isles *et al.* 1992).

Angina

At rest, the heart pumps about five litres of blood per minute – at peak exercise this may increase to 25 litres. Heart muscle is extremely efficient at removing oxygen from its blood supply, where the oxygen saturation is reduced to about 30% during its passage from aorta to coronary sinus, compared with central venous oxygen saturation of 70%. During vigorous exercise, myocardial workload increases by up to five times and nearly all of the extra oxygen required must be supplied by an equivalent increase in coronary blood flow. Fortunately, the capacity of the normal coronary arteries greatly exceeds the demands made of them, so that problems are not met until there is severe coronary narrowing. Most patients with angina have significant disease of two or three arteries – when they exercise the increased demand of the myocardium cannot be met and angina results.

Angina brought on by predictable amounts of exercise over many months, without changing in severity or frequency, is referred to as chronic stable angina. Unstable or crescendo angina is the name given to the condition when it is progressing in terms of severity or the effort required to induce pain, and which threatens to progress to myocardial infarction.

At the onset of angina there is a characteristic change in the ECG, which is flat or a downward-sloping depression of the ST segment of 1 mm or more. Holter monitoring has shown that most patients with angina have episodes of painless ST segment depression in everyday life. These are known as 'silent ischaemia' (Cohn 1986). It is not known why some patients with ischaemic episodes have no pain; some always have pain while most sometimes do and sometimes do not. It is also not known whether silent ischaemia is dangerous.

Those caring for patients with angina have to consider whether they will benefit from angioplasty or coronary artery bypass grafting (CABG). Controlled trials have shown that the prognosis of coronary patients is improved after bypass grafting if there is triple-vessel disease or disease of the main stem of the left coronary artery (Veterans Administration Coronary Artery Bypass Surgery Cooperative Study Group 1984). There have, however, been no studies of patients with triple-vessel disease which compare CABG with treatment regimes that include the most recent lipid-lowering drugs. The results of controlled trials of angioplasty are awaited. One or two-vessel disease is only an indication for surgical intervention if the symptoms cannot be controlled by medication. In practice, the decision on whether to use angioplasty (percutaneous transluminal coronary angioplasty or PTCA) or CABG is usually made on feasibility grounds. PTCA should be used for the same indications as CABG because occasionally it results in coronary artery dissection or acute closure, necessitating rescue CABG. There is a 30% restenosis rate after PTCA and comparison between the two procedures shows that PTCA produces less immediate mortality and morbidity but CABG produces better long-term symptom relief (Bonner et al. 1993).

Recent studies have explored how far the view of coronary heart disease as a male disease has influenced doctors' decision-making. A survey of hospitals in 11 European countries revealed that women were less likely than men to receive thrombolytic therapy following myocardial infarction (European Secondary Prevention Study Group 1996). Men in Northern Ireland were more than five times as likely as women to have coronary catheterization; after adjusting for admissions to hospital for ischaemic heart disease, the ratio was greater than two (Kee et al. 1993). Similarly, data from two of the regions around London showed that in all age groups and diagnostic groups, men were more likely than women to undergo angioplasty or CABG (Petticrew et al. 1993). A large study in Canada reported that women had a slightly longer time waiting for CABG following registration on a waiting list (Naylor et al. 1995), although there was no difference in waiting time between men and women in Northern Ireland (Kee and Gaffney 1995).

Myocardial infarction

Myocardial infarction is caused by sudden blockage of a coronary artery by a clot – a coronary thrombosis. It is the commonest presentation of coronary disease. About 25% of heart attack patients have pre-existent angina, about 25% have suffered atypical chest pain over the previous days or weeks, and about 50% have no recognized preceding symptoms, though a period of fatigue and declining abilities is extremely common (Nixon and Bethell 1974). Between 30% and 40% of infarcts discovered at post-mortem or by community surveys have not been diagnosed previously. Some may have been truly silent, but probably a large proportion produced symptoms which were not recognized by the patient or his doctor. The commonest misdiagnosis is indigestion, and many patients delay calling the GP because of this assumption. It is all too easy for the GP to make the same mistake (Finlayson and McEwen 1977).

Heart attack patients need urgent attention to prevent arrhythmic deaths and start thrombolysis. Roughly 50% of heart attack victims die and 50% of these die before medical help arrives, the cause being ventricular fibrillation very soon after the onset. These deaths are tragic since the prognosis of those resuscitated from ventricular fibrillation is as good as it is for those who have not suffered this complication. The occurrence of ventricular fibrillation is an electrical accident which is totally unrelated to the size of the infarct. Some general practitioners give thrombolytic drugs before admission and this has been tested and found feasible by a trial in Grampian Region (GREAT Group 1992). It is necessary to take an ECG to confirm the diagnosis, to have a defibrillator, and to adhere to strict guidelines on contraindications before giving the drug. We are some distance from this becoming a routine in British general practice, as was shown by the finding of the Royal College of General Practitioners' trial of thrombolysis which had to be abandoned because there were so few patients in the treatment group.

After thrombolysis and treatment of complications in hospital, most patients will be mobilized early and ready to come home after about a week. They should be discharged with clearly written advice about activities soon after discharge, and such problems as sexual intercourse, driving, and flying. It is helpful if they are told about some of the common and benign post-infarct symptoms such as fatigue, missed beats, and niggling, left-sided chest pains. These can be ignored. It may be wise to warn of the more serious symptoms such as anginal pain at rest or with small exertions, undue breathlessness, and rapid palpitations accompanied by lightheadedness.

The anxiety generated by the acute attack settles while in hospital, but may return with a vengeance when patients come home (Dellipiani *et al.* 1976). Their wives are usually even more anxious. It is often accompanied by depression. A visit by the GP and/or a trained health visitor or cardiac nurse can be invaluable in the first few days at home to allay anxiety and encourage gentle mobilization. The rate at which he gets back to normal depends upon his age and the severity of the attack, and it is helpful if the advice can be tailored to the individual.

In most areas there will be opportunities for patients to join a cardiac rehabilitation programme (Horgan *et al.* 1992). Exercise is the centrepiece of most cardiac rehabilitation programmes. It helps the patient regain full activity and it contributes to long-term prevention. This is one area where there is an advantage in being male: men are both more likely to enroll in and less likely to withdraw from cardiac rehabilitation programmes than women (McGee and Horgan 1992).

Benefits of exercise

The benefits of exercise are:

(1) increased physical fitness (Bethell and Mullee 1990). The fitter the individual, the less the cardiac workload for any given activity. The increased fitness produced by exercising coronary patients is mediated mainly by peripheral training effects. Only if the exercise is vigorous and maintained for a year or more is a cardiac effect found;

(2) decreased angina (Todd and Ballantyne 1990). Because increased physical fitness reduces the work performed by the heart for any particular external workload, it takes a greater effort to bring on angina. This effect has been shown to be as great as beta-blockade;

(3) enhanced coronary blood flow. Physical training can allow patients with angina to exercise to a greater myocardial workload before developing ST segment depression (Raffo *et al.* 1980). Although increased collaterals have not been demonstrated, thallium scanning has shown better myocardial perfusion (Doba *et al.* 1990);

(4) reduced ventricular arrhythmias and increased heart rate variability (Herzeanu *et al.* 1993);

(5) improved lipid profiles. To achieve this aim requires prolonged vigorous training and weight loss (Haskell 1986);

(6) lower blood pressure for hypertensive patients (World Hypertension League 1991);

(7) improved fibrinolysis. This has been shown for patients following both myocardial infarction (Estelles *et al.* 1989) and coronary bypass grafting (Wosornu *et al.* 1992);

(8) weight loss. This effect does not come easily, particularly for those who have given up smoking (Hartnung and Rangel 1981);

(9) psychological benefit. Those who run cardiac rehabilitation programmes often cite this as the main benefit of their treatment. However, controlled trials have found this very difficult to demonstrate (Langosch 1988);

(10) improved chance of return to work. Although increased fitness would be expected to facilitate the return to employment of men in manual jobs, few trials have shown such a benefit. This is probably because most manual jobs require low levels of physical fitness. Undoubtedly, some men do find it easier to go back to work if they have undertaken an exercise course, but they are in a minority (Bertie *et al.* 1992). One group who really do need to be fit to return to work after a heart attack are the holders of Large Goods Vehicle and Passenger Carrying Vehicle driving licences. They must complete nine minutes of the Bruce protocol treadmill test if they are to regain their licences, which are automatically taken away after a heart attack or CABG;

(11) improved survival. The meta-analyses of exercise-based cardiac rehabilitation have shown a reduced mortality of between 20% and 25% for the treated groups (O'Connor *et al.* 1989, Oldridge *et al.* 1988). This effect is greater for 'multifactorial' rehabilitation.

It is likely that most of the cardiac rehabilitation programmes in this country are too brief and too gentle to produce most of these benefits.

Prevention of coronary heart disease

The prevalence of coronary disease in middle-aged men, and its place as the chief cause of death at all ages over 40, make primary prevention extremely attractive. In the USA and Australia, public health measures have been accompanied by a drop of 25% in coronary mortality in the past 20 years, and an association for the two phenomena is widely claimed. However, there has also been a slight fall in mortality in the United Kingdom in the last few years, where much less effort at prevention has been made.

The Department of Health has, in its document *The health of the nation,* laid the responsibility for reducing the burden of coronary disease firmly on the shoulders of general practice (Secretary of State for Health 1991). However, all the research into action on multiple risk factors has failed to demonstrate substantial benefit. Most recently, the OXCHECK (Imperial Cancer Research Fund OXCHECK Study 1994) and Family Heart Study (1994) groups have both reported modest changes from intensive intervention. Despite the enthusiasm of some doctors, there does not seem to be a rational, well-founded basis for primary coronary prevention to be carried out in general practice, where the approach is the indiscriminate application of public health conclusions to individual patients.

Secondary prevention of coronary disease has been largely ignored until recently. The appeal of primary prevention is great, but it is more difficult to achieve and to apply than secondary prevention, and it has not been shown to be effective. Secondary prevention is effective (O'Connor *et al.* 1989; Oldridge *et al.* 1988) and represents a much more efficient use of resources for several reasons: the messages are more readily accepted by the patients and have more impact; also the target population is much smaller and at much higher risk than the general population. It is more realistic to tailor intervention to the needs of individual patients. Apart from meticulous attention to other risk factors and review of cardiovascular status to identify signs of heart failure, a number of drugs have been clearly demonstrated to confer long-term benefit:

(1) aspirin reduces mortality of patients with coronary disease by about 20% (Antiplatelet Trialists' Collaboration 1994);

(2) beta-blockers improve the prognosis after myocardial infarction (Beta-blocker Heart Attack Trial Research Group 1982) but there is a dilemma. Those with small infarcts and no evidence of residual ischaemia have such a good prognosis that beta-blockers are unlikely to improve it. Those with moderate-sized infarcts definitely benefit while those with large infarcts, who should gain most from beta-blockade, are least likely to tolerate it due to aggravation of cardiac failure;

(3) lipid-lowering drugs. The 4S study was a randomized controlled trial of simvastatin in 4444 men with coronary disease whose blood cholesterol remained above 5.5 despite their best dietary effects, but who had a normal triglyceride level (Scandinavian Simvastatin Survival Study Group 1994). The trial showed a 42% fall in coronary mortality and a 30% fall in total mortality in the treated group compared to the controls. The more recently completed CARE study tested the effect of treating much lower levels of blood cholesterol (The Cholesterol and Recurrent Events Trial Investigators 1996). More than 4000 men and women recovering from acute myocardial infarction with a total cholesterol of 6.2 mmol/L or less (mean 5.4) were randomized to receive either pravastatin or placebo. The treated group showed a 24% reduction in acute coronary events, a 24% reduction in revascularization, but no significant difference in overall mortality;

(4) angiotensin-converting enzyme (ACE) inhibitors. These reduce mortality in patients with heart failure (The CONSENSUS trial study group 1987) and in patients with severe left ventricular damage from acute myocardial infarction (The Acute Infarction Ramipril Efficacy (AIRE) Investigators 1993; Yusuf et al. 1992).

Peripheral vascular disease

Peripheral vascular disease (PVD) is very much a problem for men in whom it is 10 times more common than in premenopausal women and about five times more common overall. It also has high prevalence: 5% of men under the age of 50 are affected and 20% of those over the age of 65. Risk factors are similar to those for coronary artery disease, with particular weight carried by smoking and diabetes mellitus.

PVD is usually a manifestation of more generalized arterial disease and those who present with symptoms often have evidence of atheroma in other sites. Patients with intermittent claudication have a 20% five-year probability of dying from myocardial infarction or stroke (Ruckley 1986).

The presenting symptom is usually intermittent claudication which builds up over several months, gradually restricting the walking distance until it becomes a nuisance to the patient. The severity of the condition at presentation therefore depends upon the activity level of the patient. Middle-aged, vigorous men appear at an early stage while elderly, sedentary men tend to present when the disease is far advanced. They are more likely to have compromised circulation to the feet with cold or painful toes or ulceration of vulnerable points such as the skin over the malleoli or tips of the toes. Impotence is commonly associated and may be the presenting symptom together with buttock pain in the LeRiche syndrome which is caused by occlusion of the aortic bifurcation. A planned walking programme often increases walking distances appreciably (Clifford et al. 1980). The resulting development of collateral vessels is promoted by muscle ischaemia and the patient should be told to walk until the pain becomes unbearable, then to stop until it subsides before setting off again. If the symptoms are sufficiently bad to interfere substantially with daily life or if the limb is severely ischaemic, the patient should be offered angiography to delineate the extent of the disease, with a view to angioplasty or bypass surgery. Relatively short segments of narrowing in large vessels can be opened up by balloon angioplasty with a one-year patency of 80% (Lamberton 1986). Bypass grafting has a five-year success rate of between 50 and 80% (Sonnenfelt 1982). There are some patients with severe PVD who cannot be treated by revascularization because there are no vessels beyond the occlusion sufficiently large to accept a graft. For them, amputation may become necessary.

Aortic aneurysm

Aneurysm of the abdominal aorta is five times more common in men than in women and it affects 2% of men over the age of 60 (Taylor and Wolfe 1991). It is usually asymptomatic until it ruptures, with a very high mortality – nearly 100% if untreated and about 50% with emergency surgery. Symptoms, if present, may include abdominal or back pain, intermittent claudication, or the feeling of a throbbing lump in the abdomen. The aneurysm is easily felt in thin patients but may very difficult to detect in the obese.

Investigation is by ultrasound scanning to measure the diameter of the swelling. Aneurysms under 4 cm across are unlikely to rupture and should be followed up by regular scanning. Those over 5 cm are very likely to do so and should be repaired, and in this case the operation carries a mortality of between 2% and 5%. Those in between should be followed carefully and operated on if the aneurysm causes symptoms or enlarges. The possibility of screening men over 60 for aortic aneurysms has been raised.

Conclusions

After so many years of human endeavour expended on research, we understand a great deal about cardiovascular disease. It is, above all others, the male disease, responsible for the premature deaths of large numbers of young and middle-aged men. Much can be done in terms of treatment, but while we understand so little of the behavioural aspects there are still major limitations. Efforts at primary prevention have failed to deliver the health gains that had been hoped for; in contrast, the gains for secondary prevention look promising. Finally, the evidence presented here suggests that exercise may be a very rewarding method for helping affected men.

References

Allied Dunbar National Fitness Survey (1992). The Sports Council and Health Education Authority.

Antiplatelet Trialists' Collaboration (1994). Collaborative overview of randomised trials of antiplatelet therapy: prevention of death, myocardial infarction and stroke by prolonged antiplatelet therapy in various categories of patients. British Medical Journal, 308, 81–106.

Aylett, M. and Ketchin, S. (1991). Stopping treatment in patients with hypertension. *British Medical Journal*, **303**, 345.

Barker, D. J. P. (1993). Fetal origins of coronary heart disease. *British Heart Journal*, **69**, 195–6.

Barker, D. J. P. and Osmond, C. (1986). Infant mortality, childhood nutrition and ischaemic heart disease in England and Wales. *Lancet*, **i**, 1077–81.

Barker, D. J. P., Winter, P. D., Osmond, C., *et al.* (1989). Weight in infancy and death from ischaemic heart disease. *Lancet*, **ii**, 577–80.

Bertie, J., King, A., Reed, N., *et al.* (1992). Benefits and weaknesses of a cardiac rehabilitation programme. *Journal of the Royal College of Physicians*, **26**, 147–51.

Beta-blocker Heart Attack Trial Research Group (1982). A randomised trial of propranolol in patients with acute myocardial infarction. *Journal of the American Medical Association*, **247**, 1707.

Bethell, H. and Mullee, M. (1990). A controlled trial of community based coronary rehabilitation. *British Heart Journal*, **64**, 370–4.

Betteridge, D. J., Dodson, P. M., Durrington, P. N., *et al.* (1993). Management of hyperlipidaemia: guidelines of the British Hyperlipidaemia Association. *Postgraduate Medical Journal*, **69**, 359–69.

Bonner, H., de Vries, C., Michels, R., and El Gamal, M. (1993). Initial and long-term results of coronary angioplasty and coronary bypass surgery in patients of 75 or older. *British Heart Journal*, **70**, 122–5.

Chatellier, G., Battaglia, C., Pagny, J. Y., *et al.* (1993). Decision to treat mild hypertension after assessment by ambulatory monitoring and World Health Organization recommendations. *British Medical Journal*, **305**, 1062–6.

Clifford, P. C., Davies, P. W., Hayne, J. A., and Baird, R. N. (1980). Intermittent claudication. Is a supervised exercise class worthwhile? *British Medical Journal*, **280**, 150–3.

Cohn, P. F. (1986). Total ischemic burden: definition, mechanisms and therapeutic implications. *American Journal of Medicine*, **81** (suppl. 4A), 2–6.

Dellipiani, A. W., Cay, E. L., Philip, A. E., *et al.* (1976). Anxiety after a heart attack. *British Heart Journal*, **38**, 752–7.

Department of Health (1993). *On the State of the Public Health 1992*. HMSO, London.

Doba, N., Shukuya, M., Yoshida, H., *et al.* (1990). Physical training of the patients with coronary heart disease: non-invasive strategies for the evaluation of its effects on the oxygen transport system and myocardial ischaemia. *Japanese Circulation Journal*, **50**, 1409–18.

Estelles, A., Aznar, J., Tormo, G., *et al.* (1989). Influence of a rehabilitation sports programme on the fibrinolytic activity of patients after myocardial infarction. *Thrombosis Research*, **55**, 203–12.

European Secondary Prevention Study Group (1996). Translation of clinical trials into practice: a European population-based study of the use of thrombolysis for acute myocardial infarction. *Lancet*, **347**, 1203–7.

Fahey, T. P. and Peters, T. P. (1996). What constitutes controlled hypertension? Patient-based comparison of hypertension guidelines. *British Medical Journal*, **313**, 93–6.

Family Heart Study Group (1994). Randomised controlled trial evaluating cardiovascular screening and intervention in general practice: principal results of the British Family Heart Study. *British Medical Journal*, **308**, 313–20.

Ferguson, E., Bernier, L., Banta, G., *et al.* (1987). Effects of exercise and conditioning on clotting and fibrinolytic activity in man. *Journal of Applied Physiology*, **62**, 1416–21.

Findlay, I., Taylor, R., Dargie, H., *et al.* (1987). Cardiovascular effects of training for a marathon run in unfit, middle-aged men. *British Medical Journal*, **295**, 521–4.

Finlayson, A. and McEwen, J. (1977). *Coronary heart disease and patterns of living.* Croom Helm, London.

Glass, D. C. (1982). Psychological and physiological responses of individuals displaying type A behaviour. *Acta Medica Scandinavica*, **660** (suppl.), 193–202.

GREAT Group (1992). Feasibility, Safety and efficacy of domiciliary thrombolysis by general practitioners: Grampian region early anistreptase trial. *British Medical Journal*, **305**, 548–53.

Hart, J. T. (1984). Salt restriction for borderline hypertension. *Journal of the Royal College of General Practitioners*, **34**, 140–5.

Hartnung, G., Rangel, R. (1981). Exercise training in post-myocardial infarction patients: comparison of results with high risk coronary and post-bypass patients. *Arch. Phys. Med. Rehabil.*, **62**, 147–56.

Haskell, W. (1986). The influence of exercise training on plasma lipids and lipo proteins in health and disease. *Acta Medica Scandinavica*, **suppl. 711**, 25–37.

Herzeanu, H. L., Shemish, J., Aron, L. A., *et al.* (1993). Ventricular arrhythmias in rehabilitated and non-rehabilitated post-myocardial infarction patients with left ventricular dysfunction. *American Journal of Cardiology*, **71**, 24–7.

Horgan, J., Bethell, H. J. N., Carson, P., *et al.* (1992). British Cardiac Society. Working party report on cardiac rehabilitation. *British Heart Journal*, **67**, 412–18.

Imperial Cancer Research Fund OXCHECK Study Group (1994). Effectiveness of health checks conducted by nurses in primary care: results of the OXCHECK study after one year. *British Medical Journal*, **308**, 308–12.

Isles, C. G., Hole, D. J., Hawthorne, V. M., and Lever, A. F. (1992). Relation between coronary risk and coronary mortality in women of the Renfrew and Paisley survey: comparison with men. *Lancet*, **339**, 702–6.

Jackson, R., Barham, P., Bills, J., Birch, T., McLennan, L., MacMahon, S., *et al.* (1993). Management of raised blood pressure in New Zealand: a discussion document. *British Medical Journal*, **307**, 107–10.

Johnston, D. W. (1991). Stress management in the treatment of mild primary hypertension. *Hypertension*, **17** (suppl. III), 63–8.

Kannel, W. B. and Sorlie, P. (1979). Some health benefits of physical activity: the Framingham Study. *Archives of Internal Medicine*, **139**, 857–61.

Kee, F. and Gaffney, B. (1995). Priority for coronary artery surgery: who gets by-passed when demand outstrips capacity? *Quarterly Journal of Medicine*, **88**, 15–22.

Kee, F., Gaffney, B., and O'Reilly, D. (1993). Access to coronary catheterisation: fair shares for all? *British Medical Journal*, **307**, 1305–7.

Khaw, K. T. (1993). Where are the women in studies of coronary heart disease? *British Medical Journal*, **306**, 1145–6.

Knight, T. M., Smith, Z., Whittles, A., *et al.* (1992). Insulin resistance, diabetes and risk markers for ischaemic heart disease in Asian men and non-Asian men in Bradford. *British Heart Journal*, **67**, 343–50.

Lamberton, A. (1986). Percutaneous luminal angioplasty. *British Journal of Surgery*, **73**, 91–7.

Langosch, W. (1988). Psychological effects of training in coronary patients: a critical review of the literature. *European Heart Journal*, **8** (suppl. m), 37–42.

Mancia, G., Bertinien, G., Grassi, G., *et al.* (1983). Effects of blood pressure measurement by the doctor on patient's blood pressure and heart rate. *Lancet*, **ii**, 695–8.

McGee, H. M. and Horgan, J. H. (1992). Cardiac rehabilitation programmes: are women less likely to attend? *British Medical Journal*, **305**, 283–4.

Meade, T., Mellows, S., Brozovic, M., *et al.* (1986). Haemostatic function and ischaemic heart disease: principal results of the Northwick Park Heart Study. *Lancet*, **ii**, 533–7.

Morris, J. N., Clayton, D. G., Everitt, M. G., *et al.* (1990). Exercise in leisure time: coronary attack and death rates. *British Heart Journal*, **63**, 325–34.

Naylor, C. D., Sykora, K., Jaglal, S. B., Jefferson, S., and the Steering Committee of the Adult Cardiac Care Network of Ontario (1995). Waiting for coronary artery bypass surgery: population-based study of 8517 consecutive patients in Ontario, Canada. *Lancet*, **346**, 1605–9.

Nichaman, M. Z., Hamilton, H. B., Kagan, A., *et al.* (1975). Epidemiologic studies of coronary heart disease and stroke in Japanese men living in Japan, Hawaii and California. *American Journal of Epidemiology*, **102**, 491–501.

Nixon, P. G. F. and Bethell, H. J. N. (1974). Preinfarction ill health. *American Journal of Cardiology*, **33**, 446–9.

O'Connor, G., Buring, J. E., Goldhaber, S. Z., *et al.* (1989). An overview of randomised trials of rehabilitation with exercise after myocardial infarction. *Circulation*, **80**, 234–44.

Oldridge, N. B., Guyatt, G. H., Fischer, M. E., and Rimm, A. A. (1988). Cardiac rehabilitation after myocardial infarction. Combined experience of randomised clinical trials. *Journal of the American Medical Association*, **260**, 945–50.

Office for National Statistics. *Mortality statistics, cause. Review of the Registrar General on deaths by cause, sex and age, in England and Wales, 1995.* Stationery Office, London.

Paffenbarger, R. S., Hyde, R. T., Wing, A. L., *et al.* (1993). The association of changes in physical activity level and other lifestyle characteristics with mortality among men. *New England Journal of Medicine*, **328**, 538–45.

Petticrew, M., McKee, M., and Jones, J. (1993). Coronary artery surgery: are women discriminated against? *British Medical Journal*, **306**, 1164–6.

Pocock, S. J., Cook, D. G., Shaper, A. G., *et al.* (1987). Social class differences in ischaemic heart disease in British men. *Lancet*, **ii**, 197–201.

Raffo, J., Luksic, I., Kappagoda, C., *et al.* (1980). Effects of physical training on myocardial ischaemia in patients with coronary artery disease. *British Heart Journal*, **43**, 262–9.

Reaven, G. M. (1988). Banting Lecture 1988. Role of insulin resistance in human disease. *Diabetes*, **37**, 1595–607.

Rosenman, R. H., Brand, R. J., Jenkins, D., *et al.* (1975). Coronary heart disease in the Western Collaborative Group Study. Final follow-up experience of 8.5 years. *Journal of the American Medical Association*, **233**, 872–7.

Ruckley, C. V. (1986). Claudication. *British Medical Journal*, **292**, 970–1.

Scandinavian Simvastatin Survival Study Group (1994). Randomised trial of cholesterol lowering in 4444 patients with coronary artery disease. *Lancet*, **344**, 1383–9.

Schneider, S., Amorosa, L., Khachadurian, A., *et al.* (1984). Studies on the mechanism of improved glucose control during regular exercise in type 2 diabetes. *Diabetalogia*, **26**, 355–60.

Secretary of State for Health (1991). *The health of the nation.* HMSO, London.

Sever, P., Beevers, G., Bulpitt, C., *et al.* (1993). Management guidelines in essential hypertension: report of the second working party of the British Hypertension Society. *British Medical Journal*, **306**, 983–7.

Shewry, M. C., Smith, W. C. S., Woodward, M., and Tunstall-Pedoe, H. (1992). Variation in coronary risk factors by social status: results from the Scottish heart health study. *British Journal of General Practice*, **42**, 406–10.

Sonnenfelt, T. (1982). Reconstructive vascular surgery for intermittent claudication. *Acta Medica Scandinavica*, **212**, 145–9.

Swan, J. W., Walton, C., Godsland, I. F., *et al.* (1994). Insulin resistance syndrome as a feature of cardiological syndrome in non-obese men. *British Heart Journal*, **71**, 41–4.

Taylor, P. R. and Wolfe, J. H. N. (1991). ABC of vascular diseases. Treating aortic aneurysms. *British Medical Journal*, **303**, 1127–9.

The Acute Infarction Ramipril Efficacy (AIRE) Investigators (1993). Effect of ramipril on mortality and morbidity of survivors of acute myocardial infarction with clinical evidence of heart failure. *Lancet*, **342**, 821–8.

The Cholesterol and Recurrent Events Trial Investigators (1996). The effect of pravastatin on coronary events after myocardial infarction in patients with average cholesterol levels. *New England Journal of Medicine*, **335**, 1001–9.

The CONSENSUS Trial Study Group (1987). Effects of enalapril on mortality in severe congestive cardiac failure: results of the cooperative North Scandinavian Enapril Survival Study Group. *New England Journal of Medicine*, **316**, 1429–35.

Todd, I. and Ballantyne, D. (1990). Anti-anginal efficacy of exercise training: a comparison with beta-blockade. *British Heart Journal*, **64**, 14–19.

Veterans Administration Coronary Artery Bypass Surgery Cooperative Study Group (1984). Eleven-year survival in the Veterans Administration randomized trial of coronary bypass surgery for stable angina. *New England Journal of Medicine*, **311**, 1333–9.

Waldron, I. (1995). Contributions of biological and behavioural factors to changing sex differences in ischaemic heart disease mortality. In *Adult mortality in developed countries: from description to explanation* (ed. A. D. Lopez, G. Caselli, and T. Valkonen). Clarendon Press, Oxford.

World Hypertension League (1991). Physical exercise in the management of hypertension: a consensus statement. *Journal of Hypertension*, **9**, 283–7.

Wosornu, D., Allardyce, W., Ballantyne, D., and Tansey, P. (1992). Influence of power and aerobic exercise training on haemostatic factors after coronary artery surgery. *British Heart Journal*, **68**, 181–6.

Yarnell, J., Baker, I., Sweetnam, P., *et al.* (1991). Fibrinogen, viscosity and white blood cell count are major risk factors for ischaemic heart disease. The Caerphilly and Speedwell Collaborative Heart Disease Studies. *Circulation*, **83**, 836–44.

Yusuf, S., Pepone, C., Garces, C., *et al.* (1992). Effect of enalapril on myocardial infarction and unstable angina in patients with low ejection fraction. *Lancet*, **340**, 1173–8.

PART IV

PART IV

CHAPTER FOURTEEN

Violence in the home

Fiona Bradley

The doctor never looked at me. He studied parts of me but he never saw all of me. He never looked at my eyes. Drink, he said to himself. I could see his nose moving, taking in the smell, deciding.

The woman who walked into doors by Roddy Doyle

We considered leaving this topic out of a book on men's health because it seemed to be a women's problem. The perpetrator is usually male but the patient is usually female. At the core is the need of one gender to control the other. Doctors (and perhaps authors) turn a blind eye to it, fearing the opening of a can of worms or perhaps offending women by mentioning it. It is more difficult in general practice where the perpetrator is likely to be a patient also. This is a disturbing chapter which challenges our attitudes while providing guidance. Asking makes a difference and, indeed, may set in train a series of solutions that are not easy. The GP author explains the strategy of censure by the criminal justice system working together with a therapeutic response. It is a bleak, dark side of men's health and we are glad we have included it in this book.

Over the past 30 years, societies throughout the world have increasingly acknowledged that violence in the home is commonplace. This violence may take many forms (including physical, sexual, and emotional) and may affect young and old alike, although the focus of this chapter is on violence in adult relationships. Violence in the home is a complex issue which can obviously never be solved by health care professionals alone, but needs to be considered in a societal context. However, because of its far-reaching implications for health and the utilization of health care resources, violence in the home is now recognized as an important (if often hidden) health problem, particularly relevant to general practice.

Discussion of violence in the home (even among doctors) tends to be characterized by confusing and rather sensationalist terminology ('battered this and battered that'), predictable but unhelpful questions ('Why doesn't she just leave?' or 'What about battered men?'), and stereotypical views of victims and perpetrators ('alcoholic, psychopathic husband and neurotic, inadequate wife'). The aims of this chapter are to consider what we actually mean by violence in the home and how often it occurs; to address some of the predictable questions; to challenge the stereotypes; and to move on to consider our own attitudes as GPs and the contributions we can make in addressing this challenging problem.

Violence in the home – naming the issue

Since the early 1970s, when violence in the home first became the subject of social science and medical research, a number of different names have been used to describe and thus define the issue (for example, family violence, domestic violence, marital violence, violence against women, battered women, and spouse abuse). The first difficulty with some of these descriptions (for example, family violence, domestic violence, marital violence) is that they imply that both women and men are equally likely to be violent to their intimate partners. The evidence is that in marital or cohabiting relationships, women are the usual victims of violence and men its usual perpetrators (Dobash and Dobash 1979), and therefore such gender-blind terms are misleading and euphemistic. Secondly, the word 'violence' is often taken to mean solely physical force, whereas 'abuse' can include physical, sexual, *and* emotional interactions. This chapter will therefore use 'domestic violence against women', a phrase chosen by the authors of a recent *British Medical Journal* editorial (Richardson and Feder 1995), to describe a phenomenon which encompasses not only physical injury, but threats, sexual abuse, emotional torment and controlling behaviour. Since it is also the case that men may be on the receiving end of violence – at the hands of either female partners, or from other men in the context of gay relationships – the issue of men who are victims of violence will also be considered. The term 'elder abuse' will be used when referring to violent or emotional abuse of older people within the home. The problem of violence to children is outside the scope of this chapter.

What about battered men?

Although it is my contention that the evidence is that women are the usual victims of domestic violence, this view is not universally held. Almost always, in every public forum where the topic of domestic violence against women is discussed, the question 'What about battered men?' is raised.

The idea that men and women suffer equally from violence in the home is based mainly on the results of two national surveys undertaken in the United States (Straus and Gelles 1990). In order to estimate the prevalence of violence in the home, both of these surveys used a measure call the 'Conflict Tactic Scales' (CTS), which consists of a series of questions about how respondents might settle a dispute with their partner (Straus 1979) (Box 14.1). The first survey in 1974 found that 11.6% of men were victimized by their wives and 12.1% of women were victimized by their husbands. The corresponding figures in 1985 indicated that men had become slightly more likely (12.1%) than women (11.3%) to be victims. The researchers also concluded that men were more likely to suffer 'severe

---

Box 14.1 *Introduction to, and items on, the Conflict Tactic Scales*

No matter how well a couple get on, there are times when they disagree, get annoyed with the other person, or just have spats or fights because they are in a bad mood or tired or for some other reason. They also use many different ways of trying to settle their differences. The following is a list of things that partners might have done during an argument or other relationship stress:
- discussed an issue calmly
- got information to back up his/her side of things
- brought in or tried to bring in someone to help settle things
- insulted you or swore at you
- sulked or refused to talk about an issue
- stomped out of the room/house/yard
- cried
- did or said something to spite you
- threatened to hit you or throw something at you
- threw, smashed, bit, or kicked something
- threw something at you
- pushed, grabbed, or shoved you
- slapped you
- kicked, bit, or hit you with a fist
- hit or tried to hit you with something
- beat you up
- choked you
- threatened you with a knife or gun.

---

violence' compared to women. The CTS is the focus of much controversy and debate because it examines violent incidents in isolation, without considering the context, intent of the action, outcome in terms of injuries, or meaning of the event (see Nazroo 1995). In fact, men tend to be violent towards their women partners in the context of a pattern of controlling behaviour, and the violence may result in psychological or physical ill health for the woman. In contrast, women are usually violent in self-defence, and violence by women to their male partners is unlikely to have the same meaning or health effects.

Indeed, the counter-intuitive claim that men are as likely as women to be the victims of domestic violence is challenged by a large body of work by those who view the problem predominatly in terms of 'violence against women' and abused women. This work actually predates the recognition of battered wives in the 1970s. It includes criminal justice statistics and national surveys in Britain and North America, and qualitative work involving case-history analysis, ethnography, and in-depth interviewing. For example, an analysis of Scottish police and court records found that 99% of reported assaults between spouses involved men assaulting their partner (Dobash and Dobash 1977–8), and the British Crime Surveys of 1982 and 1984 indicated that all victims of domestic violence reported in this context were women (Worral and Pease 1986). In a review of surveys of crime and criminal justice statistics, Dobash and Dobash (1992) report similar findings from Canada and throughout the United States.

Prevalence of domestic violence against women

Assessing the prevalence of domestic violence against women is obviously difficult because of the sensitive nature of the issue. There is no universally recognized definition of what constitutes domestic violence, and estimates of prevalence vary according to the definition used in a study, the study's focus (for example, crime surveys compared to community surveys), and also the study methodology (face-to-face interviews, self-completed questionnaires).

In the community

As already mentioned, a 1985 probability sample national survey in the United States suggested that 11.3% of women had been subject to violence by their husbands during the previous year (although some commentators cast doubt on the methodology of this work and the validity of its findings). Starke and Flitcraft (1991) reviewed population studies in the USA and reported that they indicate that as many as 20–25% of adult women have been abused by a male intimate.

The most comprehensive community survey to date was carried out in Canada in 1993 (Johnson and Sacco 1995). A representative sample of 12 300 women aged 18 years or over were interviewed by telephone. The survey, which focused specifically on violence in the home, reported a 64% response rate overall, and in households where a woman could actually be contacted, 91% agreed to be interviewed. According to the survey, 29% of Canadian ever-married or cohabiting women have been assaulted by a spouse or live-in partner. Interestingly, rates of violence in previous relationships were significantly higher (48%) than in relationships that were current at the time of the interview (15%). This challenges the stereotype that battered women choose violent partners and are stuck in a cycle of violent relationships. However, the survey also showed that there is a continued risk of violence to women by ex-partners despite a divorce or separation, and that when men assault their spouse this is not usually an isolated incident – violence is usually repeated.

To date, no such extensive community surveys have been carried out in Britain or Ireland, although a study in London found that 27% of women responding to a questionnaire said they had suffered physical injury from their partners at some stage (Mooney 1993), and an Irish national random survey of 679 women indicated that 18% of respondents in intimate relationships had been subject to male violence (Kelleher et al. 1995). Thus, existing research indicates that about a quarter of women in the community have at some time suffered violence at the hands of an intimate partner.

In medical settings: turning a blind eye

Doctors working in accident and emergency settings were among the first to identify domestic violence against women as a health problem. In Stark and Flitcraft's (1979) seminal study carried out in an American emergency room, retrospective analysis of the case notes of 520 women who sought aid for injuries indicated that up to a quarter of the women were definitely or probably experiencing domestic violence. Doctors had identified only 14 battered women in this group (2.8%), demonstrating a startling ability, or perhaps determination, to turn a blind eye to the problem of 'women who walk into doors'.

In recent years, a number of studies carried out in primary care settings have examined the prevalence of domestic violence among women attenders. Hamberger and colleagues (1992) surveyed 394 women attending a community clinic in midwestern USA. They found that 22.7% reported having been physically assaulted by their partners within the past year and 38.8% at some time in their lives. Many of the reported assaults were severe (for example, 5% were choked, 3% had received multiple blows, and 3% had been threatened with a knife or gun). Despite this, only 23 women (6.5%) had been asked by their doctor about problems in relationships and only six women (1.5%) had been directly asked about abuse.

Also in the USA, a self-administered survey of almost 2000 women attenders (carried out in four community-based primary care practices with academic links) found that 5.5% of women had experienced domestic violence in the previous year and 21.4% at some time in their adult life (McCauley et al. 1995). The authors suggest that the relatively low prevalence identified by their survey could be explained by the relatively older age and higher socio-economic status of the patients in the study, as 14% of both women between 18 and 35 and women with annual family incomes less than $10000 reported current abuse. However, the suggestion that violence is commoner in poorer families is controversial, and in the extensive Canadian study cited already, there was no association between male unemployment and increased violence.

Most recently, Mazza and colleagues carried out a questionnaire-based prevalence survey of 2181 women in 15 general practices in Melbourne (1996). She found that 28% of women in a current relationship had experienced either physical and/or emotional violence from their partner in the previous year and that nearly three-quarters of victimized women had never discussed the abuse with their doctor. Contrary to popular belief, the main reason why women did not discuss the issues was not because they were afraid, embarrassed, or untrusting, but because they were never asked.

To date, no studies of the prevalence of domestic violence among women presenting to general practice have been reported from Britain or Ireland, although it is safe to assume that in the last year at least 5% and probably nearer a quarter of our women patients have experienced violence from their husband or partner. Because of the paucity of our information, we do not know whether prevalence varies between practices, either because of differences between groups of patients or because of different doctors attracting different patients, and this is an area for future research.

Understanding domestic violence against women

Theories about why men are violent

Although there is now a substantial body of research examining women's experiences of domestic violence, we know much less about the men who perpetrate such violence.

At present, we do not have a comprehensive understanding of the causes of domestic violence against women, although the many social science theories fall into three main groups.

Firstly, intra-individual theories have tried to explain the violence in terms of the psychological characteristics of abusers and abused, seeking to describe both a typical wife batterer and a typical victim. This approach underlies much medical and psychiatric research. Early campaigners, particularly Erin Pizzey of Britain's first refuge at Chiswick, reinforced the tendency to see the men who abuse as alcoholic or psychopathic and the women experiencing domestic violence as inadequate and immature (see Dobash and Dobash 1992). The drunken husband coming home and beating his wife is a common stereotype. Alcohol may be seen as both the cause of, and an excuse for, his violence (by helping agencies and women experiencing violence alike). In contrast, a woman who has a drug or alcohol problem may be blamed for the violence and her behaviour seen as provocative (see Frieze and Browne's review, 1990). In fact, most research has failed to uncover a typical victim personality among women. However, in relation to alcohol, most comparative studies examining the issue have found that abusive men *are* more likely to drink heavily than non-violent men. The recent Canadian national survey indicated that half of the men who were being violent to their wives were usually drinking (Rodgers 1994). Abusive men with drug or alcohol problems may be violent to their partners both when drunk *and* sober. There is debate about whether women experiencing domestic violence are more likely to misuse alcohol or drugs. In Frieze and Browne's review, they found that most comparative studies failed to show an association, whereas other authors have concluded that women experiencing domestic violence are at increased risk of misusing drug or alcohol themselves (Richardson and Feder 1996).

Although focusing on personality types of violent men or battered women does not explain domestic violence, it *is* true that the highest rate of assault of wives or partners is by young men, affecting younger women, and that rates decline with age (McCauley *et al.* 1995; Rodgers 1994). The Canadian study did not identify any significant relationship between male unemployment and rates of offending. Thus, focusing on the individual characteristics of either men who batter or women who experience violence as an approach to explaining domestic violence has proved mainly unhelpful, which is not surprising considering the pervasive nature of the phenomenon in our community. Despite this, as Stark and Flitcraft (1979) have noted, all too often the medical reaction to abused women is to focus on the women's individual characteristics and responses, labelling them as either psychiatrically ill or neurotic.

The psychosocial approach to understanding domestic violence has focused on the interaction between individuals and their environment. In particular, learnt behaviour has been suggested as a reason for violence in families. It is certainly true that violent men are more likely to have experienced violent behaviour in their own family of origin, but learning theory fails to explain why more men than women learn violence or why many victims of child abuse do not become abusers themselves, and indeed, this explanation is rejected by many victims themselves.

Finally, sociocultural theories propose that social phenomena (such as cultural norms and values, inequality between the sexes, and institutional structures) are important determinants of individual violence. Consideration of a societal dimension goes some way to explaining the universal and pervasive nature of domestic violence against women. Activist researchers such as the Dobashes have pointed to the importance of considering domestic violence within the numerous contexts (historical, individual, institutional, cultural) in which it occurs, otherwise we are in danger of seeing the problem in terms of 'an unfortunate personal pathology' rather than that of a social problem requiring change. This is particularly true for general practitioners, who are so attuned to dealing with individuals.

While there is continuing debate in both the academic literature and among activists about the exact aetiology of battering, there is agreement that at a given point in time, perpetrators choose to be violent (Letellier 1996). Victims of violence, the police, and health care providers alike may see a violent man as losing control. Violent behaviour is a deliberate and systematic strategy used to control one's partner. Attributing the violence to outside causes (most typically alcohol, but often some behaviour of his spouse, such as being late in preparing a meal) removes the concept of responsibility for his actions from the perpetrator, and it is important for GPs not to collude with this sort of explanation. GPs need to have a clear understanding of the dynamics of violent behaviour as it will affect both their attitude to women experiencing violence and their ability to respond appropriately.

Why don't battered women leave?

Although commonly asked, for those of us who believe that men are the usual perpetrators of domestic violence this is an uncomfortable question as it focuses attention on the woman and her behaviour, rather than the man and his behaviour. However, addressing it does allow us to recognize the process which occurs in domestic violence and is an important prerequisite for effective care (Alpert 1995). Most studies indicate that the majority of battered women (73–85%) do not experience violence until they are married or have made a major commitment to their partner. In fact, early in the relationship the man's behaviour may be seen as attentive and involved, but as time goes by it becomes more controlling and isolating. Also, violence by men towards their wives or partners is often seen initially as an isolated incident, but then escalates in severity and frequency (Frieze and Browne 1990). In Alpert's excellent review she points to a number of factors which make it difficult for women to leave violent or abusive relationships.

Firstly, women are rightly afraid for the safety of themselves and their children. It is not unusual for violent men to threaten to harm or even kill their partner if she attempts to leave home. The most dangerous time for a woman experiencing domestic violence is when she does attempt to leave.

Secondly, many abusive men behave in a strongly controlling fashion towards their partners. This may have the dual effect of causing financial dependence and social isolation, both of which contribute to women's difficulties in leaving home.

Thirdly, abused women commonly experience feelings of failure, low self-esteem, self-blame, and guilt about their situation and their perceived inability to change it. As GPs we must be wary of unrealistically expecting women to leave home straightaway once they have disclosed domestic violence. Also, we need to avoid suggesting (either overtly or implicitly) that it is the woman's responsibility to stay in the relationship or even to try to make it better.

Finally, although it is often disheartening and frustrating for members of the primary health care team to witness women living in a situation of ongoing violence, it is not true that many women stay in violent relationships. The Canadian national survey found that repeated or ongoing abuse was more often reported in relationships that had ended, suggesting that many women leave relationships where there is more frequent or serious violence (Rodgers 1994).

Men who experience violence in the home

Heterosexual men who experience violence from their partners

In the vast majority of relationships where there is violence, women are the usual victims of violence and it is predominatly perpetrated by men. However, this is not universally true, so GPs must not be blind to the possibility that men can and do experience violence. However, it is always important to consider the context of violence. For example, in some states in the USA where arrest is mandatory when the police are called to violence in the home, women who are defending themselves from ongoing abuse have been arrested (Hamberger and Potente 1994).

There is little in the medical literature on men who *do* suffer significant abuse from their female partners, and how they might present to GPs or other health services. This may reflect a hidden issue or it may imply a non-issue. Further work will be needed to illuminate the situation.

Violence in gay men's domestic partnerships

If domestic violence against heterosexual women is a mainly hidden problem for general practice, then violence in gay relationships has until recently been completely invisible. Many GPs make the assumption that patients are heterosexual. Consequently, gay men often feel uncomfortable about revealing their sexual orientation or discussing relationships with their GP (Harrison 1996), let alone disclosing that they are being battered. To date, studies estimating the rates of gay partner assault are mainly from North America and based on small sample sizes (see Hamberger 1996 for a review of current knowledge). Some authors suggest that violence is as prevalent in same-sex relationships as in heterosexual relationships, and that about one in five men in an intimate relationship with another man will be battered, but further research is needed to confirm this estimate. At present, there are no studies of the characteristics of the perpetrators of gay male violence, but it seems likely that they are a similarly heterogeneous group to violent heterosexual men.

Elder abuse

Although those most likely to experience domestic violence from their partners are younger women, elderly patients, both men and women, are also at risk. Case reports of 'granny battering' first appeared about 20 years ago (Burston 1975) and since then there has been a limited amount of research, mostly in North America, but also in Britain (see Lachs and Pillemer 1995 for a review of current knowledge).

Elder abuse can include physical violence (such as slapping and hitting), psychological or emotional abuse, material exploitation (such as the misappropriation of money or property), and finally, intentional neglect (such as the withholding of food or medication). In community surveys it has been estimated that 3–4% of the population over the age of 65 years have experienced some form of maltreatment, most commonly physical abuse. About two-thirds of abusers are spouses, and often, elder abuse is a form of domestic violence against women. The remainder of elder abuse is perpetrated by adult children living with the older person.

As with other forms of violence in the home, relatives with alcohol or substance misuse problems are more likely to become abusive. Family members who are dependent on an elderly person for either finance or housing also have a higher risk of becoming abusive, but again, as with other forms of violence in the home, there is no typical picture of either the abused or abuser. Consequently, the American Medical Association suggests that all older adults should be asked about family violence. In the United States, mandatory reporting laws in many states require health care workers to report suspected abuse of elderly persons to an official state agency, but a recent government report there has questionned the effectiveness of this strategy.

In many ways, the approach to intervening with an elderly person who is being abused will be the same as that for other women who experience domestic violence (see later). However, it is also important that GPs consider whether the patient retains decision-making capacity. Even if the person is competent it may be useful to involve care-of-the-elderly specialists and other community support services.

General practice responses to domestic violence

Barriers to involvement

Several qualitative studies have used interviews or focus groups to explore general practitioner attitudes to domestic violence (for example, Brown *et al.* 1993; Sugg and Inui 1992). These have concentrated on physicians' responses to the women involved. GP attitudes to the perpetrators of such violence and whether or how to intervene with them has not been examined. Study findings do indicate that there are a number of issues which militate against GPs intervening effectively with women experiencing violence.

A powerful barrier to involvement by GPs is the fear that if we attempt to explore the issues of domestic violence with a woman patient, we will be confronting more than we can handle, what Sugg and Inui describe as 'opening Pandora's box to release a myriad of evils'. This feeling of the potential for being overwhelmed is added to many doctors' worries about offending patients by asking them about abuse and also by the time constraints of general practice. Doctors also feel powerless in the face of domestic violence, and frustrated at their inability to 'fix it', both of which may contribute to reluctance to make efforts to identify or engage with the issue during a consultation. The reality is that women who have experienced domestic violence may be difficult patients, frequent attenders with ongoing physical and psychological problems, and thus challenging to work with in general practice (Alpert 1995).

A barrier to even considering the possibility of domestic violence in a differential diagnosis is the close identification that many doctors have with their patients, particularly those with similar backgrounds to themselves. It may be that we are more willing to ask patients of lower socio-economic status about abuse, but fail to consider the possibility with patients who are 'like us'. Also, unusually among the caring professions dealing with domestic violence, GPs frequently find themselves looking after both the victim and the perpetrator of the violence. This dual responsibility adds further to the pressures to turn a blind eye, and exacerbates GPs' unease about their role when actually faced with a woman who is experiencing violence from her partner.

All these difficulties are compounded by many doctors' lack of knowledge or specific training in detecting or dealing with domestic violence against women.

Overcoming the barriers

GPs asking about violence – bringing it out in the open

Several authors have tried to identify specific markers of domestic violence against women which could be used as indicators for enquiry during primary care consultations (for example, McCauley *et al.* 1995). Although a number of features are certainly associated with domestic violence (for example, depression, anxiety, and somatization), they are so common in general practice that they lack any predictive value.

As an alternative to trying to identify high-risk groups, many individuals and organizations have advocated that GPs should routinely ask all patients (most importantly women, but also men) about whether they are experiencing domestic violence (for example, Alpert 1995; American Medical Association 1992; Heath 1992; Richardson and Feder 1996; Sassetti 1993) – in effect, a form of screening. Although doctors are sometimes reluctant to ask about violence and fear offending their patients, in fact, in one American primary care survey of women, three-quarters of respondents favoured being asked routinely about physical abuse; and in a study from Northern Ireland, two-thirds of women thought doctors should ask about violence (McWilliams and McKiernan 1993). Burge has pointed out that women who have experienced violence suggest that from their perspective, the single most important intervention a GP can make is to ask about the abuse.

Until very recently, the vast majority of published work and debate about GP identification of domestic violence focused exclusively on raising the issue with women and ignored the issue of whether we should be confronting the (mostly) men who perpetrate the violence. Given that GPs will often be in the position of being responsible for the care of both the woman experiencing violence and the man perpetrating it, this is something which we need to consider and address. Richardson and Feder (1996) suggest that as health care providers we should be aiming to challenge perpetrators' attitudes and behaviour as well as improving services for victims.

Guidance for intervening with violent men – censure and therapy

Research on intervening with men who are violent at home is both controversial and in its relative infancy. As yet there is no work which specifically considers intervention with perpetrators in the context of general practice, so hard and fast guidelines are difficult. In an era of limited resources, the provision of treatment programmes for violent men may be seen as a threat to the resourcing of services for women who experience violence, but we must address this side of the equation if we are to have any impact on what is currently an epidemic. General practitioners and members of the primary health care team need to be aware of treatment programmes which currently exist and consider working with other professionals to develop new approaches for the future.

The vast majority of existing work on intervening with violent men has been carried out in the context of criminal justice systems, mostly in North America and more recently in Britain (see Dobash *et al.* 1995 for a comprehensive review). Three main approaches have been evaluated.

Firstly, a number of American studies have examined the effectiveness of automatic arrest of the perpetrator when the police are called to an incident of domestic violence (compared with offering advice or asking either the man or the woman to leave the household). On balance, it appears that in most cases this is an appropriate action and does result in a modest reduction in the subsequent incidence of violent episodes. This approach also reinforces to society the message that domestic violence is a criminal offence, not to be tolerated. However, any effect is short-lived, and without community support for women to protect themselves, arrest and prosecution may result in more severe violence upon the perpetrator's release (Morley 1995).

In Britain and Ireland, the use of a civil injunction ('barring order') is a commoner response than arrest, and the number of injunctions is increasing annually. Unfortunately, the use and enforcement of such injunctions are not always consistent and women report that many men do not take them seriously. However, evidence from the United States indicates that injunctions can be useful if they are properly enforced.

The third and most innovative approach to intervening with violent men combines the censure of arrest or injunction with a therapeutic element in the form of an organized programme. Most existing programmes are based on the pioneering work first started in Duluth, Minnesota in the early 1980s. Cognitive-behavioural methods and re-education in a group setting are used to focus on the offending behaviour and on how to change it. In their carefully designed evaluation of two Scottish programmes, Dobash *et al.* (1995) have shown that women whose partners have been on one of the innovative programmes report a reduction in violence and controlling behaviour by their partners compared to women whose partners have not been on a programme.

Although general practice has not yet become involved in either the direct provision of, or even the referral to, services for perpetrators of violence, this is an area that we need to consider further so that we can contribute to the development of coherent responses in the future. As Ferguson and Synott (1995) have said, the crucial point is that it is the violent man who *is* the problem and who *has* the problem and who needs to become a focal point of intervention. Some community mental health services and psychotherapists *have* begun to develop services which deal with perpetrators on an individual level as well as in group programmes. Also, the self-help group MOVE (Men Overcoming Violent Emotions) aims to acknowledge, confront, and address domestic violence, and is a resource that can be suggested to the minority of violent men who present themselves to us in general practice.

At this early stage in the evolution of general practice and community-based responses to violent men, a number of guiding concepts and principles can be outlined (adapted from Alpert 1995; Dobash *et al.* 1995; Ferguson and Synott 1995; Hamberger 1996; Jordan and Walker 1994; and Murphy 1994):

1. Many violent men do not recognize that a problem exists and often do not report violent behaviour accurately.
2. Domestic violence against women should be clearly defined as criminal behaviour.
3. Legal sanctions should be applied if violent behaviour does not stop.
4. In treatment, cessation of violence takes priority over family reunification.
5. Couples counselling or family therapy in a primary-care setting should usually be avoided. Both these approaches risk failing to shift the burden of the problem away from the woman, failing to address the core problem of the man's violence, and may even increase the immediate danger to the woman.
6. Groupwork, particularly in any initial intervention with batterers, is the preferred approach.
7. In any therapy, cognitive and behavioural approaches which focus on stopping the offending behaviour should be used, while psychodynamic approaches are inappropriate.
8. Any therapy for domestic violence perpetrators should be part of a coordinated community response that includes criminal justice interventions *and* comprehensive services for victims.

Caring for women who experience violence – the GP can make a difference

As already stated, many GPs are uncertain how to approach women who are experiencing domestic violence, feel powerless to intervene, and often even avoid asking about such violence. However, one striking finding of Sugg and Inui's (1992) study of GP attitudes to domestic violence was that a few doctors stood out from the rest because of their level of ease in dealing with the issue. They differed from their colleagues in that they identified domestic violence often in their practices and they had a comfortable and business-as-usual approach to asking about violence. They saw their role as validating a patient's feelings, discussing safety issues, and referring patients to other helping agencies. They were not expecting a quick fix, but expected that if change occurred it would take time.

So, domestic violence against women is usually a hidden problem in general practice, overlooked by most of us. But GPs *can* make a difference. Several authors have given guidance for general practice intervention (Alpert 1995; Asher 1993; American Medical Association 1992; Burge 1989; Heath 1992; Hendricks-Mathews 1991; Knowlden and Frith 1993; Sassetti 1993). The following is a brief distillation of the main features of effective GP care for women experiencing domestic violence:

Ask about domestic violence

It is clear that women experiencing violence want GPs to ask them directly about this, and most other women do not mind being asked about their relationships. When women present with vague chronic complaints, unexplained injuries, depression, or anxiety, think of abuse and *ask*. Consider asking all patients (male and female) during a routine consultation. Although it may feel awkward at first, you will soon develop a style of questionning that suits you. For example:

(1) 'Many patients tell me they have been hurt by someone close to them. Could this be happening to you?' *or*

(2) 'I notice you have some bruises. Could you tell me how they happened? Did someone hit you?'

Provide the right environment – ensure confidentiality

Women may be ashamed to admit that they are being hit. They are also often worried that their partner will find out that they have disclosed the situation, particularly if the GP is the partner's doctor. It is therefore important to remain non-judgemental and relaxed, and to reassure explicitly about confidentiality. This can be a particular issue for first-generation immigrant women, who may be unfamiliar with the concept of confidentiality, and may also have the added difficulty of consulting through an interpreter.

Validate the experience and act as an advocate

A woman who discloses an experience of domestic violence will feel vulnerable and fear judgement. Support her with a statement such as 'You did not deserve to be hit' or 'Violence like that is wrong'. In this situation, GPs will sometimes find that they know and like the perpetrator of domestic violence, so it is important not to fall into the trap of minimizing the situation (for example, 'I'm sure he didn't mean it') as this will reinforce the woman's sense of shame, blame, and powerlessness. Instead, we must clearly acknowledge the abuser's behaviour to be wrong and illegal.

Document the history and physical findings

This is important for both women who disclose and for those in whom you suspect domestic violence as it may provide vital evidence in any future legal proceedings. Document both the history and examination findings in as much detail as possible. Record the woman's story of events and, if she denies being assaulted, any inconsistencies in your physical findings. Drawing a body map is a helpful way of recording injuries.

Facilitate referral while leaving the door open

Discuss the woman's options with her and provide information about the community resources and legal alternatives available to help. If you are uncertain about what is available, Women's Aid provide 24-hour helplines throughout Britain and Ireland (see p. 256). Remember that women are often unable or do not want to leave their violent partner, so avoid unrealistic expectations and make it explicit that the door is open to discuss the issue again in the future. Although care for a woman experiencing domestic violence is likely to be long term, do check about present danger. The most dangerous time for a battered woman is when she decides to leave her abuser, so make sure that women who are seriously considering leaving home have considered their own and their children's immediate safety. Advocates from Women's Aid will have more time to explore the practical and legal issues in detail.

In summary, GPs do not need to know all and do all, but to screen, document, validate, and refer. Alpert (1995) has suggested an acronym, 'RADAR', as an aide-memoire for busy physicians, and using this tool will provide a simple, straightforward approach for busy GPs:

Remember to ask about violence and victimization in the course of the routine patient encounter;

Ask directly 'Have you been hit, hurt, or frightened by someone with whom you are in a relationship?';
Document findings in the medical record;
Assess immediate safety;
Review options and refer as appropriate.

References

Alpert, E. (1995). Violence in intimate relationships and the practicing internist: new 'disease' or new agenda? *Annals of Internal Medicine*, **123**, 774–81.

American Medical Association, Council on Scientific Affairs (1992). Violence against women – relevance for medical practitioners. *Journal of the American Medical Association*, **267**(23), 3184–9.

Asher, M. L. (1993). About domestic violence: SAFE questions. *Journal of the American Medical Association*, **269**(18), 2367. (Letter).

Brown, J., Lent, B., and Sas, G. (1993). Identifying and treating wife abuse. *The Journal of Family Practice*, **36**(2), 185–91.

Burge, S. (1989). Violence against women as a health care issue. *Family Medicine*, **21**(5), 368–73.

Burston, G. R. (1975). Granny-battering. *British Medical Journal*, **19**, 970–7.

Dobash, R. E. and Dobash, R. P. (1977–8). Wives: The 'appropriate' victims of marital violence. *Victimology*, **2**, 426–42.

Dobash, R. E. and Dobash, R. P. (1979). *Violence against wives*. The Free Press, New York, and MacMillan Distributing, Basingstoke.

Dobash, R. E. and Dobash, R. P. (1992). *Women, violence and social change*. Routledge, New York and London.

Dobash, R. E., Dobash, R. P., Cavanagh, K., and Lewis, R. (1995). Evaluating criminal justice programmes for violent men. In *Gender and crime*. (ed. R. E. Dobash, R. P. Dobash, and L. Noaks) University of Wales Press, Cardiff.

Ferguson, H. and Synott, P. (1995). Intervention into domestic violence in Ireland: developing policy and practice with men who batter. *Administration*, **43**(3), 57–81.

Frieze, I. H. and Browne, A. (1990). Violence in marriage. In *Crime and justice: a review of research*, (ed. L. Ohlin and M. Tonry) Vol. II, pp. 163–218. University of Chicago Press, Chicago.

Hamberger, L. K. (1996). Intervention in gay male intimate violence requires coordinated efforts on multiple levels. In *Violence in gay and lesbian domestic partnerships*. Harrington Park Press, New York. (An imprint of the Haworth Press.)

Hamberger, L. K. and Potente, T. (1994). Counselling heterosexual women arrested for domestic violence: implications for theory and practice. *Violence and Victims*, **9**(2), 125–37.

Hamberger, L. K., Sauders, D., and Hovery, M. (1992). Prevalence of domestic violence in community practice and rate of physician inquiry. *Family Medicine*, **24**(4), 283–7.

Harrison, A. E. (1996). Care of lesbian and gay patients: educating ourselves and our students. *Family Medicine*, **28**(1), 57–8.

Heath, I. (1992). *Domestic violence: the general practitioner's role.* Royal College of General Practitioners members' reference book, London.

Hendricks-Mathews, M. (1991). Battered women: you can make a difference. *American Family Physician,* **44**, 1894–6.

Johnson, H. and Sacco, V. (1995). Researching violence against women: statistics from Canada's national survey. *Canadian Journal of Criminology,* **37**(3), 281–304.

Jordan, C. E. and Walker, R. (1994). Guidelines for handling domestic violence cases in community mental health centers. *Hospital and Community Psychiatry,* **45**(2), 147–51.

Kelleher, P., Kelleher, C., and O'Connor, M. (1995). *Making the links – towards an integrated strategy for the elimination of violence against women in intimate relationships with men.* Women's Aid, Ireland.

Knowlden, S. and Frith, J. (1993). Domestic violence and the general practitioner. *Medical Journal of Australia,* **158**, 402–6.

Lachs, M. and Pillemer, K. (1995). Abuse and neglect of elderly persons. *New England Journal of Medicine,* **332**(7), 437–43.

Letellier, P. (1996). Twin epidemics: domestic violence and HIV infection among gay and bisexual men. In *Violence in gay and lesbian domestic partnerships.* Harrington Park Press, New York. (An imprint of the Haworth Press.)

Mazza, D., Dennerstein, L., and Ryan, V. (1996). Physical, sexual and emotional violence against women: a general practice-based prevalence study. *Medical Journal of Australia,* **161**, 14–17.

McCauley, J., Kern, D., Kolodner, D., Dill, L., Shroeder, A., DeChant, H., *et al.* (1995). The 'battering syndrome': prevalence and clinical characteristics of domestic violence in primary care internal medicine practices. *Annals of Internal Medicine,* **123**(10), 737–46.

McWilliams, M. and McKiernan, J. (1993). *Bringing it out in the open: domestic violence in Northern Ireland.* HMSO, Belfast.

Morley, R. (1995). The sociologist's view – more convictions won't help victims of domestic violence. *British Medical Journal,* **311**, 1618–19.

Murphy, C. M. (1994). Treating perpetrators of adult domestic violence. *Maryland Medical Journal,* **43**(10), 877–83.

Mooney, J. (1993). *The hidden figure: domestic violence in North London.* Islington Council, London.

Nazroo, J. (1995). Uncovering gender differences in the use of marital violence: the effect of methodology. *Sociology,* **29**(3), 475–94.

Richardson, J. and Feder, G. (1995). Domestic violence against women. *British Medical Journal,* **311**, 964.

Richardson, J. and Feder, G. (1996). Domestic violence: a hidden problem for general practice. *British Journal of General Practice,* **46**, 239–42.

Rodgers, K. (1994). Wife assault: the findings of a national survey. *Statistics Canada Catalogue,* 85–002, **14**(9).

Sassetti, M. (1993). Domestic violence. *Primary Care,* **20**(2), 289–305.

Starke, E. and Flitcraft, A. H. (1979). Medicine and patriarchal violence: the social construction of a 'private' event. *International Journal of Health Services*, **9**(3), 461–93.

Starke, E. and Flitcraft, A. H. (1991). Spouse abuse. In *Violence in America: a public health approach* (ed. M. Rosenberg and J. Mercy). Oxford University Press, Oxford.

Straus, M. A. (1979). Measuring intrafamily conflict and violence: the conflict tactics scales. *Journal of Marriage and the Family*, **41**, 75–88.

Straus, M. A. and Gelles, R. J. (1990). Societal change and change in family violence from 1975 to 1985 as revealed in two national surveys, In *Physical violence in American families*. Transaction, New Bruswick, NJ.

Sugg, K. and Inui, T. (1992). Primary care physicians' response to domestic violence – opening Pandora's box. *Journal of the American Medical Association*, 267(23), 3157–60.

Worral, A. and Pease, K. (1986). Personal crime against women: evidence from the British Crime Survey. *The Howard Journal*, **25**, 118–24.

Women's Aid in Britain and Ireland – 24-hour helplines

Welsh Women's Aid	01222	390874
Women's Aid Federation England	0117	963 3542
Women's Aid Scotland	0131	221 0401
Women's Aid Northern Ireland	01232	331818
Women's Aid Ireland (freephone)	1800	341900

PART V

PART V

CHAPTER FIFTEEN

Getting help

Andrew Wilson

In a recent MORI poll, 13% of men could correctly identify the location of their prostate gland while 16% of women knew where it was (MORI 1995). Men use their GPs less than women and are also more willing to make do with locums and unfamiliar partners. GP impact on men's lifestyles is limited. They are absent from preventive and counselling settings and even when things are bad, need strong pressure from partners to seek medical help. Men engage in riskier health practices than females but feel more in control of their health. It all sounds hopeless but this chapter describes some innovative developments in the care of men's health. General practice has been flexible and effective in its response to women's health – so why not men's health next?

Introduction

Previous chapters have attributed some of the differences between men's and women's health to men's reluctance to acknowledge their own symptoms and to seek advice. This chapter examines how men seek help when ill and how they try to preserve their health. The present contribution of general practice and other agencies to men's health is reviewed, and suggestions made for a more effective service.

Seeking help

From birth until the age of five, boys attend their general practice more frequently than girls. Between the ages of five and 14 there is little difference in attendance rates, and from then on throughout the age groups, men are less frequent consulters (Table 15.1). Their consultations may also be shorter (Westcott 1977). Lack of contact with GPs is particularly striking in middle age. Cook *et al.* (1990) found that, in all social classes, 10% of men aged 46–65 did not consult their GP over a three-year period, and a further 44% consulted on average twice a year or less.

Table 15.1 *Consultation rates with the general practitioner or practice nurse by age and sex (4th National Morbidity Survey)*

		ALL	0–4	5–15	16–24	25–44	45–64	65–74	75–84	85+
% consulting at least once per annum	*Male*	70.0	100	70.3	61.9	60.7	69.2	81.3	90.0	90.1
	Female	85.7	100	74.5	89.4	86.5	83.1	83.9	90.8	92.3
Average number of consultations per annum	*Male*	2.7	5.1	2.0	1.7	1.9	3.1	4.3	5.1	5.8
	Female	4.2	4.8	2.2	4.3	4.3	4.3	4.7	5.4	5.5

Men's relationships with their general practitioner appear more remote than women's – they are more prepared to see a locum or partner rather than wait for their individual doctor, and are more likely to use casualty services as an alternative to general practice (Cartwright and Anderson 1981). Men's gender preferences mirror women's – in the above study, 25% of men reported occasions when they would like to consult a male doctor compared to 21% of women expressing occasional preference for a female doctor.

Males are less likely to use other sources of help or advice about health. At school, girls seek more help from the nurse (Lewis *et al.* 1977). Men are also less likely to seek help from practitioners of alternative medicine. In one survey, two-thirds of the users of a range of these therapies were female (Thomas *et al.* 1991). The 'absent man' has been noted in a variety of clinical settings, such as child health clinics, family planning centres, and antenatal classes. Men are also unlikely to be the first to seek help when there are marital, child care, or other relationship problems (Lewis and O'Brien 1987).

Why is it that men seem reluctant to use services and seek help? From an early age, boys perceive themselves to be less vulnerable or susceptible to illness than girls (Lewis *et al.* 1977). One explanation for the continuing difference is the influence of adult role models showing that men 'ride things out' and the feeling that to admit to being unwell is 'cissy'. Boys have been shown to develop wider circles of friends than girls, but fewer close relationships or confidants (Skelton 1988). This learned stoicism may be why men seem less perceptive to symptoms and less able to accept that they may be unwell. Men and women differ in their experience, expression, understanding, and response to pain (Bendelow 1993). Men are less likely to accept an emotional influence on pain, and to acknowledge emotional pain as valid. Stoicism may also explain their reluctance to use preventive services, as discussed in a later section.

It is in areas where help is available for emotional or personal difficulties where men are most notably absent. O'Brien (1990) suggests three reasons for this. Firstly, men seem less likely to perceive such problems, for example they are less likely than women to report marital unhappiness or institute divorce proceedings. Secondly, where such problems are recognized, men may be reluctant to articulate and disclose them. Thirdly, there are institutional barriers. Centres providing health care and counselling services may be perceived by users and even, perhaps unconsciously, by providers as 'women's places', where the hours of availability and style of work inhibit men's participation.

Illness behaviour in men

Although there is a consensus that men fail to perceive symptoms of physical and psychological distress, it is less clear whether gender differences exist when symptoms are acknowledged. Two reviews (Lewis *et al.* 1977; Waldron 1976) report no consistent gender differences in response to symptoms, especially those suggesting serious disease. In their classic longitudinal study of 76 men with heart attacks, Finlayson and McEwan (1977) found a strong tendency for men to normalize their symptoms and delay seeking help. As one subject's wife reported: 'He said the pain was like a horse sitting on his chest, but when it was over didn't see the need for going to the doctor. "If it happens again, I'll go," he said. Men *are* difficult.' When help was summoned, wives were found to be instrumental in two-thirds of cases. However, husbands also encourage wives to seek help, for example prompting earlier attendance with suspicious breast lumps (Elwood and Moorehead 1980). For several conditions, late presentation prevents optimal management. Reducing delay in seeking help for heart attack has become more important with the advent of thrombolytic therapy (British Heart Foundation Working Party 1989). Prognosis of testicular cancer is related to stage at presentation (Bosl *et al.* 1981). Much of the variance in presentation remains unexplained by factors such as age, ethnic group, social class, and social support (Dent *et al.* 1990).

Sickness behaviour in men

Parsons (1951) conceptualized sickness as a form of deviance from normal social functioning. He described the sick role as having two rights (exemption from usual role, and from responsibility for current state) and two obligations (to want to get well and to cooperate with health services). Men's social role outside the home is more likely to involve full-time employment. Real fears about loss of job because of sickness absence and subsequent unemployment may add to the psychological barriers to taking time off work. Men are also less familiar with health services, and are less likely to have considered themselves sick previously. These factors all suggest that adopting the sick role may be more difficult for men. Although the process of becoming sick is highly influenced by several sociocultural factors, little work has been done to explore differences between men and women. One aspect that has been researched is adherence to medical treatment, which has been found not to relate to gender (Becker and Maiman 1975).

Similarly, no consistent gender differences in adaptation to significant chronic diseases have been reported. Again, sociocultural influences are important. In their study of men with heart attacks, Finlayson and McEwan (1977) found the attitude of wives to be critical in the ability of men to accept their diagnosis. Successful adaptation was seen more often in marriages where roles were less traditional and the relationship was more of a partnership. They also found that non-manual workers were much more likely to return to work, make major lifestyle changes, and maintain a sense of optimism following a heart attack. The effect of illness on the family is emphasized by Shanfeld (1990), who found that a man's heart attack was likely to lead to redistribution of tasks within and outside the home, and significant psychological ill health in the wife, with inhibition of aggressive and sexual impulses.

How men try to preserve their health

As well as a different perception of illness, men perceive health differently from women. They are more likely to engage in hazardous activities, including smoking, heavy drinking, and dangerous sports, but paradoxically feel more in control of their health than women, and are more likely to report taking action, such as regular exercise, to improve or maintain it. In a large survey of health and lifestyle, 51% of men but only 38% of women agreed that they were conscious of the effects of their own behaviour on their health (Cox *et al.* 1987).

Waldron (1976) attempted to determine how far these lifestyle factors contributed to the differential mortality between men and women. She concluded that approximately two-thirds of the difference was due to behavioural patterns, including smoking, coronary prone behaviour, alcohol, and occupational risks, and that some of the remaining difference was due to underuse of health care provision, particularly preventive services.

A major contributor to women's health has been the women's movement, including self-help and support groups. Men are less likely to take advantage of such approaches. Allen and Whatley (1986) noted the unlikelihood of 'a group of men taking turns doing testicular self-examination, noting differences among their genitals that show a range of healthy variations', and the lack of awareness in men about prostatic disease compared with women's awareness of breast cancer. In the United States, groups such as 'Men Against Sexism' have addressed how sexism is damaging to men's health. For example, differing parental attitudes to risk in boys and girls may explain the greater chance of accidental death in male children and young men.

Men seem less prepared than women to accept the current provision of health promotion by general practice. The largest trial of well-person checks in general practice found attendance by men was lower than women (79% versus 85%) (Thorogood *et al.* 1993). Published results on specific screening tests, such as testing for faecal occult blood, have shown lower compliance rates in men (Mant *et al.* 1992). Although not all studies have shown such gender differences (for example, Stott and Pill 1988), there are consistent findings about factors associated with men's attendance for a health check. Attenders are more highly educated, less likely to smoke or drink to excess, and more likely to have positive views about their ability to influence their own health. Marital status makes a difference in some but not all studies. The clear conclusion is that those most in need of a health check are the least likely to attend, another example of the inverse care law (Waller *et al.* 1990).

Health promotion for men

Most general practices rely on a combination of opportunistic health promotion and invitation to clinics to provide health promotion. As men consult less often than women, and are less likely to accept invitations to a health check, they have been described as elusive (Jackson 1991). Empirical studies support this description.

The impact of GP-based preventive services on men's health can be assessed in two main ways: firstly, by population surveys, and secondly, by audits of general practice. Surveys have shown that only a minority of the population recall receiving any lifestyle advice from their GP. A recent survey of 5000 people aged 35–64 found that advice about smoking was recalled by 27% of smokers, about diet by 12%, about exercise by 4.5%, and about alcohol by 3% of those who drunk too much (Silagy *et al.* 1992). An earlier survey reported very similar results but also found that a majority of respondents felt their GP should be interested in lifestyle issues (Wallace *et al.* 1987). Both surveys found that amongst heavy drinkers, more males reported advice, and that in the overweight, women were more likely to report advice on diet. Levels of smoking advice were similar, but more men received advice on exercise. Both studies concluded that there was a need for more lifestyle advice in general practice, but perhaps more importantly, it should be efficacious and targeted at those most at risk (Pill *et al.* 1989).

Audits of GPs' records for evidence of health promotional activities in men have shown wide variation. Hart *et al.* (1991) reported levels above 98% for blood pressure screening, following decades of sustained effort in a stable community. More typical are the results from a recent audit of 24 practices in north-east Scotland which examined records of men aged 35–64. The median rate (range) of recording for blood pressure was 67% (35–99), weight 25% (10–100), height 7% (1–99), and smoking 54.5% (11–100) (Maitland *et al.* 1991). Several audits of screening for hypertension have, as predicted, found higher levels of coverage in women than men (Baker 1990; Hall 1985). In Scotland, rates of undetected hypertension were almost twice as high in men (31% versus 17%) and fewer men had achieved adequate control (25% versus 42%) (Smith *et al.* 1990).

In conclusion, the impact of general practice advice on lifestyle is very limited and few practices are running effective screening and treatment programmes for hypertension in men.

Services for men in general practice

Few services in practice are specifically tailored to men's needs. Most practices offer health checks at the time of registration, and there are a range of clinics and services which may attract both men and women. These include family planning services, parentcraft groups, stress management, and elderly health checks as well as disease-specific clinics.

Well-man checks

Well-man checks followed in the wake of well-woman clinics and generally replicated the contents minus the smear and breast self-examination. This detailed content was outlined in the 1989 contract for general practitioners (Department of Health 1989).

The contract required checks to be available to newly registered patients and those not seen in the previous three years. The right to a check-up for the latter group has been enshrined in the Patient's Charter (Department of Health 1992). Those who do not consult their doctor spontaneously tend to be healthier than those who do, and so if the checks are worthwhile, it does not make sense to restrict them to non-attenders (Thompson 1990). The utility of the check is being debated in terms of content, eligible age group, and frequency (Noakes 1991). Certain aspects of the check, such as urinalysis, seem to be based on no scientific evidence (Mant and Fowler 1990).

Two large UK trials of interventions by practice-based nurses to reduce cardiovascular risk have been completed (Family Heart Study Group 1994; ICRF OXCHECK Study Group 1995). Both involved more intensive interventions than is standard practice. The OXCHECK Study offered an initial appointment of 45 minutes to men and women. The Family Heart Study targeted men and their families, offering an adult couple a 90-minute initial appointment. Both studies achieved some success in reducing risk, through cholesterol reduction and, less consistently, blood pressure control and smoking cessation. The individual approach of OXCHECK was less successful with men than women in reducing cardiovascular risk at one year (reductions of 7% and 13% respectively). Equivalent figures for the Family Health Study were 13% and 10%. Although there were other important differences in study design, this comparison may support a family-orientated approach to prevention in men. Whether such approaches can be cost-effective depends on duration of benefit. Because men are more likely to develop heart disease than women, even the OXCHECK Study suggested that cost per life-year gained was less for men than women (Wonderling *et al.* 1996). For the same reason, general practice has been encouraged to prioritize older men, and to target patients with raised blood pressure or a history of coronary heart disease (Field *et al.* 1995).

Screening for hypertension is a procedure for which there is strong evidence of potential gain (Medical Research Council Working Party 1985), but explaining the significance of a blood pressure reading and future management requires time and skill, as does negotiating changes in lifestyle.

Practices differ in the emphasis they give to discussion and counselling, and the mechanistic elements of the check. Simply measuring height, weight, and blood pressure and testing the urine is less time-consuming than discussion of lifestyle and requires less skill. The emphasis in many practices has been on throughput in order to achieve contractual obligations, and so for all these reasons the physical 'MOT' elements may have been predominant. This approach was encouraged by the 1993 arrangements for funding of health promotion, which included targets for coverage of blood pressure screening and recording of other cardiovascular risk factors (General Medical Services Committee 1993). This mechanistic approach may explain why such checks can do psychological damage (Stoate 1989).

In 1996, arrangements for health promotion were again amended, towards a more flexible programme based on *Health of the nation* targets, responsive to local needs.

Innovative developments in men's health in general practice

One way of addressing the failure of men to seek appropriate help about their health is to make the service more suited to their needs. Most general practitioners and policy-makers are male, and the lack of attention given to men's health may reflect the denial responses previously described as attributes of the male client. Several innovative service developments have been described.

Extended surgery hours

One reason for the poor uptake of preventive services by men, and perhaps their reluctance to consult with problems, may be inconvenient surgery hours. This difficulty is likely to be most apparent for those in manual employment who may experience difficulty in getting time off work. A recent development has been the establishment of evening surgeries and clinics. These have proved popular with clients and such developments are likely to be supported by the health authority.

Family interventions

The role of other family members in determining lifestyle and illness behaviour is well-recognized (Richardson 1945). Not surprisingly, couples and their children show a concordance in such habits as diet, exercise, and alcohol consumption (Sackett *et al.* 1975). Less predictably, households show strong similarities in biological variables such as blood pressure, blood sugar, and haemoglobin levels. Both selective marriage and environmental factors are thought to contribute. A study of concordance between married partners for plasma cholesterol, triglycerides, and weight showed this was highest in marriages of shortest and longest duration (Venters 1986). As well as determining health, family members also have an important role in promoting change. For example, Mermelstein *et al.* (1983) found those who nagged about smoking were less likely to have partners who gave up compared with those who gave positive reinforcement. The greater effect on risk reduction in the Family Heart Study compared to the individual approach of OXCHECK has already been mentioned. Family-based approaches have also been suggested in primary prevention programmes for children and may well be helpful in high-risk groups, for example those most at risk of heart disease, or as part of rehabilitation after a myocardial infarction.

Outreach activities

Men may be reluctant to visit practice premises for a variety of psychological and social reasons (Lewis and O'Brien 1987). One obvious response is to bring the service closer to potential users, either to their place of employment or social venues. Jackson (1991) describes a successful innovation where health visitors offered health promotion from a caravan at two industrial sites. Such a confidential service in men's own setting appeared highly acceptable amongst men who were reluctant to use general practice or occupational health services. A specific group whose needs had previously been unmet was contract workers living in bed and breakfast accommodation, not registered with a local general practice. Plans for the next year included siting the caravan in pub car parks. It is important that methods of communicating with GPs are established as part of outreach projects, especially when screening is being undertaken. In one study of blood pressure screening in pharmacies, only a quarter of the notifications of blood pressure readings, which clients were asked to take to their doctor, were later found in the medical record (Hampton *et al.* 1990).

A men's health worker

Allocating responsibility for men's health to one individual within the practice might encourage a coordinated response to provision of services for men. In smaller practices this task may be taken by a health visitor or practice nurse; in larger practices a dedicated worker may be feasible. In the United States, increasing expense and specialization within medicine, and dissatisfaction with 'high-tech' approaches has led to the creation of a range of nurse practitioners, including those for children, the family, and women. Bozett and Forester (1989) suggest a place for a 'men's health nurse practitioner', arguing that 'as once had been the case for women, the total health care needs of men are not being met . . . most physicians are not prepared to meet them'. Amongst these unmet needs, the authors list permission to have health concerns and talk about them, support for lifestyle changes, information about their bodies, and help with fathering and interpersonal relationships.

Identifying key areas of men's lives

Men's health needs and concerns alter over their life span, and it appears that at specific times they may be most in need of advice and most amenable to making changes. Recognizing these times and offering help appropriately is more likely to be beneficial than the ritualistic three-year checks described earlier. The following groups may be identified:

1. *Young single men.* This is an age associated with psychological stress, insecurity, and risk-taking behaviour. Traditionally, contact with general practice is slight. If appropriately delivered, advice about smoking, alcohol, accidents, sexual health, and perhaps psychological approaches such as stress reduction or assertiveness training might be appropriate. Groups led by a men's health visitor would probably be the preferred method.
2. *Men with young families.* This group is likely to be particularly receptive to advice about healthier living (Venters 1986) and issues may involve passive smoking, childhood accident avoidance, and stress reduction. The family is likely to be the best locus for such activities.
3. *Entering middle age: the male climacteric.* Burgoyne (1987) noted the increase in minor symptoms around the age of 50. It has been suggested that this may be because of career disappointment and loss, the death of parents, or children leaving home. This group is likely to consult their general practitioner, who could direct clients towards support groups within the practice.
4. *Retirement/unemployment.* Loss of, or threat to, employment through redundancy is known to have a major impact on health. Planned retirement, although often welcome, is also a major loss and associates with increased morbidity. Preretirement groups may help to mitigate these effects and may be organized either at the workplace or in primary care (Harte 1987).

Other sources of help

The evidence presented clearly shows that compared with women, men are reluctant to seek help from general practitioners, particularly for health promotion and emotional problems. They also make less use of alternative practitioners. In this section, some other potential sources of help for men will be considered.

The men's movement

Men have more social acquaintances than women but fewer confidants (Skelton 1988). The strength of women in sharing problems and supporting each other has been encouraged by the women's movement. O'Dowd (1993) movingly contrasts the 'sisterhood' which supported his wife following the death of their child with the absence of similar support offered to him by other men, except through a 'haze of alcohol'. The male 'pub culture' and its middle class equivalent, 'the golf club', have been identified as two of the few areas in which men may feel able to share feelings and emotions (Smith 1987).

Although there is talk about the 'new man' and the development of a men's movement, the evidence of any significant effect is lacking. Allen and Whatley (1986) suggest that the men's movement cannot directly parallel 'women's liberation' as the aim of the latter was explicitly to liberate women from men. Men are oppressed by class, ethnicity, etc., but not by women. However, they suggest the approach of groups such as 'Men Against Sexism' can contribute to men's health. These groups address ways in which sexism is damaging to men, while exploring how men themselves may reduce its force and impact. Specific health issues may include topics such as the high accident rate in boys compared with girls, risk-taking behaviour by young men, and the needs of isolated widowers. Cultural climates change slowly. A long-term effect of both the men and women's movement may be that men become more able to share problems with each other and with women, and that men and women appreciate more the emotional and psychological needs of men.

Self-help groups

Self-help groups have mushroomed over the last 20 years. These range from groups for specific medical conditions, such as the Psoriasis Association, where the main aim is mutual support and information exchange, to groups whose primary focus is campaigning and political change, for example Gingerbread, a pressure group of single-parent families (Brimelow and Wilson 1982). Most groups are for non-gender-specific problems and open to both sexes, but cultural and practical difficulties may make men's attendance more difficult. There are several self-help groups for gay men, e.g. the Campaign for Homosexual Equality. There are also groups for a variety of men's health problems. Most groups are based locally and in many areas a directory is available.

Conclusion

For men, the process of getting medical help is inhibited by their inattentiveness to body distress signals and to emotional cues. Changes in service provision can, however, encourage participation. Attention is being focused on men's health (Chief Medical Officer's Report 1992) and it is likely and indeed appropriate that general practice will be called upon to respond in an innovative and user-friendly way. General practice has changed in response to women's health issues as well as proving itself flexible in response to the shifting demands of the health service. As the needs of men become more apparent and explicit, further opportunities will present to improve men's health.

References

Allen, D. G. and Whatley, M. (1986). Nursing and men's health. Some critical considerations. In *The nursing clinics of North America*, Vol. 21, no. 1. W. B. Saunders, Philadelphia.

Baker, R. (1990). Problem solving with audit in general practice. *British Medical Journal*, **300**, 378–80.

Becker, M. H. and Maiman, L. A. (1975). Socio-behavioural determinants of compliance with health and medical care recommendations. *Medical Care*, **8**(1), 10–24.

Bendelow, G. (1993). Pain perceptions, emotions and gender. *Sociology of Health and Illness*, **15**(3), 273–94.

Bosl, G. J., Vogelzang, N. J., Goldman, A., Fraley, E. E., *et al.* (1981). Impact of delay in diagnosis on clinical stage of testicular cancer. *Lancet*, **2**, 970–2.

Bozett, F. W., and Forester, D. A. (1989). A Proposal for a men's health nurse practitioner. *IMAGE: Journal of Nursing Scholarship*, **21**, (3), 158–61.

Brimelow, M. and Wilson, J. (1982). A problem shared. *Social Work Today*, **13**(19), 10–11.

British Heart Foundation Working Party (1989). Role of the general practitioner in managing patients with myocardial infarction: impact of thrombolytic treatment. *British Medical Journal*, **299**, 555–7.

Burgoyne, J. (1987). Change, gender and the life course. In *Social change and life course* (ed. G. Cohen), pp. 33–6. Tavistock, London.

Cartwright, A., and Anderson, R. (1981).*General Practice Revisited.* Tavistock, London.

Cook, D. G., Morris, J. K., Walker, M., and Shaper, A. G. (1990). Consultation rates among middle-aged men in general practice over three years. *British Medical Journal*, **301**, 647–50.

Cox, B. D., Blaxter, M., Buckle, A. L. J., *et al.* (1987). *The health and lifestyle survey.* Health Promotion Research Trust, London.

Dent, O. F., Goulston, K. J., Tennet, C. C., Langeluddecke, P., *et al.* (1990). Medical bleeding. Patient delay in presentation. *Diseases of the Colon and Rectum*, **33**(10), 851–7.

Department of Health (1992). *The Patient's Charter and primary health care* (EL(92)88). HMSO, London.

Department of Health (1993). *On the State of the Public Health: the annual report of the Chief Medical Officer of the Department of Health for the year 1992.* HMSO, London.

Department of Health and Welsh Office (1989). *General practice in the National Health Service. A new contract.* DoH, London.

Elwood, J. M. and Moorehead, W. P. (1980). Delay in diagnosis and long-term survival in breast cancer. *British Medical Journal*, **280**, 1291.

Family Heart Study Group (1994). Randomised controlled trial evaluating cardiovascular screening and intervention in general practice: principal results of British family heart study. *British Medical Journal*, **308**, 313–20.

Field, K., Thorogood, M., Silagy, C., *et al.* (1995). Strategies for reducing coronary risk factors in primary care: which is the most cost effective? *British Medical Journal*, **310**, 1109–12.

Finlayson, A. and McEwan, J. (1977). *Coronary heart disease and patterns of living.* Croom Helm, London.

General Medical Services Committee (1993). *The new health promotion package.* GMSC, London.

Hall, J. A. (1985). Audit of screening for hypertension in general practice. *Journal of the Royal College of General Practitioners*, **35**, 243.

Hampton, A., Wilson A., and Hussain, M. (1990). Measuring blood pressure in an inner-city pharmacy: an attempt at coordination with general practice. *Family Practice*, **7**(1), 52–5.

Hart, J. T., Thomas, C., Gibbons, B., Edwards, C., Hart, M., Jones, J., *et al.* (1991). Twenty-five years of case finding and audit in a socially deprived community. *British Medical Journal*, **302**, 1509–13.

Harte, J. (1987). Health and preparation for retirement. *Journal of the Royal College of General Practitioners*, **37**, 483.

ICRF OXCHECK Study Group (1991). Prevalence of risk factors for heart disease in OXCHECK trial: implications for screening in primary care. *British Medical Journal*, **302**, 1057–60.

ICRF OXCHECK Study Group (1995). Effectiveness of health checks conducted by nurses in primary care: final results of the OXCHECK study. *British Medical Journal*, **310**, 1099–104.

Jackson, C. (1991). Men's health: opening the floodgates. *Health Visitor,* **64**(8), 265–6.

Lewis, C. E. and Lewis, M. A. (1977). The potential impact of sexual equality on health. *New England Journal of Medicine,* **297**, 865–9.

Lewis, C. E., Lewis, M. A., and Lorimer, A., Palmer, B. B. (1977). Child-initiated care: the utilization of school nursing services by children in an adult-free system. *Paediatrics,* **60**, 499–507.

Lewis, C., and O'Brien, M. (1987). Constraints on fathers: research, theory and clinical practice. In *Reassessing fatherhood* (ed. C. Lewis and M. O'Brien), pp. 1–19. Sage, London.

Maitland, J. M., Reid, J., and Taylor, R. J. (1990). Two-stage audit of cerebrovascular and coronary heart disease risk-factor recording: the effect of case-finding and screening programmes. *Journal of the Royal College of General Practitioners,* **41**, 144–6.

Mant, D. and Fowler, G. (1990). Urine analysis for glucose and protein: are the requirements of the new contract sensible? *British Medical Journal,* **300**, 1053–5.

Mant, D., Fuller, A., Northover, J., Astrop, P., Chivers, A., Crockett, A., *et al.* (1992). Patient compliance with colorectal cancer screening in general practice. *British Journal of General Practice,* **42**, 18–20.

Medical Research Council Working Party (1985). MRC trial of treatment of mild hypertension: principal results. *British Medical Journal,* **291**, 97–104.

Mermelstein, R., Lichtenstein, F., and McIntyre, K. (1983). Partner support and relapse in smoking cessation programs. *Journal of Consulting Clinical Psychology,* **51**, 465.

MORI (1995). *Men's Health. Research study conducted for the Reader's Digest.* MORI, London.

Noakes, J. (1991). Patients not seen in three years: will invitations for health checks be of benefit? *British Journal of General practice,* **41**, 335–8.

O'Brien, M. (1990). The place of men in a gender-sensitive therapy. In *Gender and power in families* (ed. R. J. Perelberg and A. Miller), pp. 195–208. Tavistock, London.

O'Dowd, T. (1993). The needs of fathers. *British Medical Journal,* **306**, 1484–5.

Parsons, T. (1951). *The Social System.* Free Press, Glense, Il.

Pill, R. M., Jones-Elwyn, G., and Stott, N. C. H. (1989). Opportunistic health promotion: quantity or quality? *Journal of the Royal College of General Practitioners,* **39**, 196–200.

Richardson, H. (1945). *Patients have families.* Commonwealth Fund, New York.

Sackett, D., Anderson, G., Milner, R., Feinleib, M., and Kannel, W. (1975) Concordance for coronary risk factors among spouses. *Circulation* **52**, 589–95.

Shanfeld, S. B. (1990) Myocardial infarction and patients' wives. *Psychosomatics,* **31**(2), 138–45.

Silagy, C., Muir, J., Coulter, A., Thorogood, M., Yudkin, P., and Roe, L. (1992). Lifestyle advice in general practice: rates recalled by patients. *British Medical Journal,* **305**, 871–4.

Skelton, R. (1988). Man's role in society and its effect on health. *Nursing,* **3**(26), 953–6.

Smith, J. (1987). Men and women at play: gender life cycle and leisure. In *Sport, leisure and social relations* (ed. J. Home *et al.*). Routledge and Kegan Paul, London.

Smith, W. C. S., Lee, A. J., Crombie, I. K., and Tunstall Pedoe, H. (1990). Control of blood pressure in Scotland: the rule of halves. *British Medical Journal*, **300**, 981–3.

Stoate, H. G. (1989). Can screening damage your health? *Journal of the Royal College of General Practitioners*, **39**, 193–5.

Stott, N. C. H., and Pill, R. M. (1988). *Health checks in general practice. Why some attend and others do not.* University of Wales College of Medicine, Cardiff.

Thomas, K. J., Carr, J., Westlake, L., Williams, B. T. (1991).Use of non-orthodox and conventional health care in Great Britain. *British Medical Journal*, **302**, 207–10.

Thompson, N. F. (1990). Inviting infrequent attenders to attend for a health check: costs and benefits. *British Journal of General Practice*, **40**, 16–18.

Thorogood, M., Coulter, A., Jones, L., Yudkin, P., Muir, J., and Mant, D. (1993). Factors affecting response to an invitation to attend for a health check. *Journal of Epidemiology and Community Health*, **47**, 224–8.

Venters, M. H. (1986). Family life and cardiovascular risk: implications for the prevention of chronic disease. *Social Science and Medicine*, **22**(10), 1067–74.

Waldron, I. (1976). Why do women live longer than men? *Social Science and Medicine*, **10**, 349–62.

Wallace, P. G., Brennan, P. J., and Haines, A. P. (1987). Are general practitioners doing enough to promote healthy lifestyle? Findings of the Medical Research Committee's general practice framework study on lifestyle and health. *British Medical Journal*, **294**, 940–2.

Waller, D., Agass, M., Mant, D., Coulter, A., Fuller, A., Jones, L. (1990). Health checks in general practice: Another example of the inverse care law? *British Medical Journal*, **300**, 1115–8.

Westcott, R. (1977). The length of consultations in general practice. *Journal of the Royal College of General Practitioners*, **27**, 552–5.

Wonderling, D., Langham, S., Buxton, M., *et al.* (1996). What can be concluded from the OXCHECK and British Family Heart Studies: commentary on cost-effectiveness analysis. *British Medical Journal*, **312**, 1274–8.

Wood, D. A., Davies, G., Kinmouth, A. L., *et al.* (1992). *The family heart study: a national randomised controlled trial of cardiovascular screening and lifestyle intervention in general practice.* Proceedings of the 'working group on epidemiology and prevention, European Society of Cardiology, September 1992.

INDEX